RESTRUCTURING CANADA'S HEALTH SERVICES SYSTEM

HOW DO WE GET THERE FROM HERE?

PROCEEDINGS OF THE FOURTH CANADIAN CONFERENCE ON HEALTH ECONOMICS

RESTRUCTURING CANADA'S HEALTH SERVICES SYSTEM

HOW DO WE GET THERE FROM HERE?

PROCEEDINGS OF THE FOURTH CANADIAN CONFERENCE ON HEALTH ECONOMICS

AUGUST 27-29, 1990

UNIVERSITY OF TORONTO

TORONTO, ONTARIO

CANADA

RAISA B. DEBER

GAIL G. THOMPSON

Editors

Sponsored by the Canadian Health Economics Research Association and The Institute of Health Management, University of Toronto

CANADIAN HEALTH ECONOMICS RESEARCH ASSOCIATION

ASSOCIATION CANADIENNE POUR LA RECHERCHE EN ECONOMIE DE LA SANTÉ

University of Toronto Press

Toronto   Buffalo   London

© University of Toronto Press 1992
Toronto   Buffalo   London
Printed in Canada

ISBN 0-8020-5871-X (cloth)
ISBN 0-8020-6005-6 (paper)

Printed on acid-free paper

Design by IMS Creative Communications

Canadian Cataloguing in Publication Data

Canadian Cataloguing in Publication Data
Canadian Conference on Health Economics (4th : 1990 : University of Toronto)
   Proceedings of the Fourth Canadian Conference on Health Economics : restructuring
Canada's health services system

ISBN 0-8020-5871-X (bound)   ISBN 0-8020-6005-6 (pbk.)

1. Medical economics – Canada – Congresses.
2. Medical care, Cost of – Canada – Congresses.
3. Health planning – Canada – Congresses. I. Deber, Raisa B., 1949-   . II. Thompson,
Gail G. (Gail Gordon). III. Title. IV. Title: Restructuring Canada's health services system.

RA410.55.C3C3 1990   338.4'33621'0971   C91-094891-7

CONTENTS

FOREWORD*
William G. Tholl
President, Canadian Health Economics Research Association (CHERA)

CHERA was formed just seven years ago in Regina through the tireless efforts of a small group of people led by Jack Boan. I am pleased to see that Jack is with us today and will be chairing a session. As a non-profit group, our primary aims are, first and foremost, to facilitate the exchange of health economics research; second, to promote high quality, rigorous health services research; and third, to increase awareness of the positive contribution health research can make to health policy development and to effective management of health systems. It is our hope and certainly my belief that this conference will contribute substantially to all three of these goals.

Planning for this showcase event began well over a year ago with an idea. That idea is captured in the theme for this year's conference, *Restructuring Canada's Health Services System: How Do We Get There From Here?* The theme seemed timely then and is even more relevant today. With various task forces, councils, and commissions all advocating change, it is our hope that disseminating the results of research in progress will help inform the policy debate in Canada and foster consensus building.

Having a good idea is one thing, but I don't need to tell you that bringing it to fruition is quite another matter. The first step is to find a partner. CHERA was very fortunate indeed to find a partner with both a long-standing and an outstanding record in health services and health economics research. That partner, of course, is the University of Toronto. Through the hard work of the conference chair, Raisa Deber, and the conference coordinator, Gail Thompson, I think this partnership has produced a program of which we can all be proud. At the end, I have little doubt you will all leave here better informed and with renewed enthusiasm for your own particular missions.

So on behalf of CHERA, thank you, Raisa and Gail, for a job well-done, and thank you to the University of Toronto Department of Health Administration for its support and encouragement.

All our efforts to bring the "doers" and the users of health economics research together in one forum would have been in vain had our ideas not been embraced by key people on both sides of health research. So I want to take this opportunity, on behalf of CHERA, to thank all the participants in the program, but especially those who have travelled so far to be here today.

A good idea, even with the best of moral encouragement, would simply remain in the "world of ought" without the requisite funding. We have been fortunate indeed to have the Ontario Ministry of Health as a major sponsor for this event, and I thank the Honourable Elinor Caplan and Dr. Martin Barkin for their support, financial and otherwise. Specific sessions or speakers have been sponsored by various organizations – the Canadian Hospital Association, the Canadian Medical Association, and the Co-operative Secretariat, Government of Canada – and I thank them as well.

In summary, thanks to all those who have worked to make this conference a reality. At times, it seemed that we might not get here from there! It is my hope as president of CHERA that we will be able to build on the success of this conference and become an even more effective medium for the sharing of health services research.

* edited transcript of opening remarks

PREFACE*
Raisa B. Deber, Conference Chair

This volume contains the proceedings of the Fourth Canadian Conference in Health Economics, entitled *Restructuring Canada's Health Services System: How Do We Get There From Here?* As the discerning reader will recognize, some contributions have been written for this volume; others are edited transcripts of the speaker's remarks. The discussions have also been "Hansardized" a bit by our speakers, to make them say what the speaker intended to say rather than what the tape recorder picked up. We apologize to those unidentified participants whose voices we could not recognize. We hope that this compendium of what we found to be a valuable conference will be useful to those interested in the flourishing of our health care system. Acknowledgements to the many who assisted in this conference are noted in the Closing Remarks, at the conclusion of this volume.

It is quite clear that the Canadian health care system is becoming a victim of its own success. It has done precisely what it was supposed to do – provided universal access to doctors and hospitals without financial barriers to patients. It's an excellent system, it's a model for others, and people come to study the system to see how well it can provide this type of access. But this success has showed the limits of medical care. It's clear that medical care may be necessary for health, but it is not sufficient, and the research looking at utilization rates has also showed that in some cases it may not even be necessary. So there's been a rethinking about precisely what role sick care – doctors and hospitals – should be playing. There is agreement among most who examine the system that there's too much sick care, too much emphasis on doctors and hospitals, and that it is probably not going to be cost-effective to put a lot more money into the existing system, although there are a lot of efficiencies that could be introduced and ways the existing money could be spent more effectively. The rhetoric is constantly talking about the need to restructure and reorient.

But it is interesting that this insight is not yet shared by the public. There are election campaigns going on, and when health care becomes an issue, people are still talking about the old access issues – about more money to doctors, hospitals, and sick care – and the political mileage still is gained by people who are talking the rhetoric of access. The hope is that this conference may help take this next step and, as is appropriate for Canada, we are going to draw insight from one American writer and one British writer. The British writer is Lewis Carroll, who had a dialogue between Alice and the Cheshire Cat in which Alice asked where she should go. The Cat asked her where she wanted to go. Alice said she didn't much care, and the Cat told her then it didn't much matter which way she went – the message being, "If we want to go somewhere else, where?" This translates into the importance of setting goals in deciding where we want to go. The American insight is from the policy analyst Aaron Wildavsky, who pointed out that we never solve problems; we replace them. And the issue about a successful policy is whether we prefer the new problems to the old ones. So the second question then is, "What are the expected results of the changes we're talking about, and do we prefer the new set of problems to the old ones?" The third question is the title of this conference, "*How* do we get there?" The hope is that this conference will help to start answering these questions, looking at the empirical evidence, and seeing where more empirical evidence is necessary, and will help us to open up and facilitate a more informed dialogue with the public, who in the last analysis are the ones who have to decide upon those goals.

* edited transcript of introductory remarks

WHAT
HAPPENS IF
WE DON'T
RESTRUCTURE
THE
SYSTEM?

ONTARIO'S HEALTH CARE SYSTEM AT THE CROSSROADS

Martin Barkin
Deputy Minister of Health, Ontario

As Ontario's Deputy Minister of Health, I am usually asked to speak about health and health care. Today I would like to depart from that tradition and share with you a glimpse of the future challenges facing both Ontario and Canada as a whole.

These insights have come as a result of my chairmanship of a committee established by the Secretary of Cabinet. We sought views about the challenges of the next decade from a variety of sources, including provincial and federal government central and ministry position papers, futurist papers and publications, various "think tank" opinions, and selected academic publications. Individual members of the committee also interviewed a selected list of business, labour, and financial leaders; policy analysts; politicians and political advisors; and pollsters.

The short-term clouds on the economic horizon do not really reflect the objective reality of Ontario's excellent status in comparison with every other jurisdiction in Canada and around the world. Of more basic and long-term significance are the events that are unfolding and will continue to unfold over the next decade and their probable impact on government's directions:

- The Economy and Competitiveness
- Technology
- Demography
- The Changing Nature of Democracy

THE ECONOMY AND COMPETITIVENESS

Although it is true that the next decade will likely be ushered in by reduced economic growth, the real challenge to Ontario will derive from the fact that there will still be economic winners and losers here and around the world. Winners and losers are the stuff of which economic competitiveness is made.

Arguments of economic competitiveness will be invoked to keep government spending and programs within limits, and defining what those limits are will continue to be a significant source of debate between the right and the left.

The economic imperative of wealth-creating growth will continue to cause a re-examination of education systems and will increase our focus on retraining and adjustment of the work force. It will also demand a greater emphasis on undertaking, diffusing, and disseminating basic and applied research. Although the medical research establishment has demands of its own, there will be less convincing evidence for expenditure by governments on this particular form of research as opposed to process research, engineering, communications, and the development of new consumer products.

Competitiveness will influence the way the federal government will manage the economy – balancing the four interrelated components of inflation, deficits, interest rates, and money supply. The government's course of action is more likely to be responsive to trading competitiveness and less to internal social sequelae. Flexibility in program development and enhancement will be severely constrained by the relatively slower rate of growth of transfer payments between the federal government and the provinces and between the provinces and their transfer payment recipients.

Economic competitiveness in its global dimensions has unleashed a tide of neo-conservatism across the industrialized world. Governments are now expected to influence the private sector without being too intrusive and to maintain social programs, but not to the degree that they interfere with either competitiveness or trade treaties. Increasing tensions will arise in areas of automation, layoffs, employment equity, occupational health and safety, environmental restrictions, and regional and targeted subsidies.

"Small" government has become popular, and a wave to sever government from service delivery has swept many western democracies as they sell off decades of accumulated government operations. Air Canada was a start. The British example spread even to public utilities. Canada contemplates Petrocan, and Saskatchewan its natural resources and utilities.

The eastern bloc has also discovered the neo-industrial age and economic competitiveness. Individual initiative has gained credence in the Communist world and thereby enhanced its status in the non-Communist world. Entrepreneurialism is in, and collectivization and state services are on the decline.

TECHNOLOGY

Much has been written about increasing advances in technology, biotechnology, cybernetics, information handling, and communication. All of these will have profound effects into the next century, but will not produce a cataclysmic change within the next 10 years. They will, however, have some influence on agriculture, products, manufacturing processes, and health care. They will contribute significantly to the globalization of industries and financial markets and services, as well as altering both work patterns and the traditional workplace and its hierarchies.

Many will want to look to these new technologies as the catalysts for economic revitalization. The most significant contributors to the economy and to employment will, however, continue to be mainstream and less glamourous industries – industries like the plastics plant in Peterborough that is bringing in its U.S. operations to make ordinary plastic containers for milk, cream, and antibiotics, or the wire plant with its own transport company in Beaverton. These small and medium-sized companies will continue to power economic growth and seek support for their expansion.

DEMOGRAPHY

No changes will demand as much attention from government as changes in demography. Over the next decade, the number of over 65-year-olds will increase by more than 400,000, while the number of children will stay constant. The importance of children to the future of the country will need to be addressed as their proportion decreases. This issue will be increasingly important as the participation of women in the work force approaches 50%, as conventional family structures undergo changes, and as the proportion of single women supporting children grows.

The increase in the number of elderly – notwithstanding their much improved economic status – will continue to capture a larger share of public expenditure in health care, social services, housing, transport, and recreation. Maintaining these programs – let alone expanding or adding to them – will become increasingly difficult because the relative ratio of taxpayers to those supported by taxes is steadily declining. At the same time, the costs of these kinds of services continue to escalate at twice inflation, making government unable to afford them even with increased taxation.

The patterns of population concentration will also change. The trend to urbanization will continue to result in declining northern and rural populations. Within 20 years, the greater Toronto area will add 2 million more people, making it a metropolis of more than 5 million. Infrastructure demands at the centre will increase tension between massive expenditures in the south and demands for expenditures in the north.

Numbers themselves do not reflect the changing face of Ontario. Its immigrant population will grow faster than that of any other province, taking more than 85% of all new Canadians. These people will come from different countries than was the case a generation ago. The next decade will see marked increases from Asia, the Caribbean, and South America. Ontario's visible minorities will double. The impact of the upheavals of eastern Europe will also affect the make-up of Ontario's immigrants.

Ontario's 200,000-strong native population will be more vigorous in seeking greater autonomy. The government's commitment to this course of action will have to seek many new forms of expression, especially in the light of the final days of the Meech Lake accord and the events in Oka, Quebec.

THE CHANGING NATURE OF DEMOCRACY

While democracy gives us a collective view of society, individualism is very much on the upswing. The "Americanization of Canadian parliamentary democracy", as some have described it, refers to the increasing role of the Charter of Rights, the courts, and lobby groups. The courts, as well as the commissioners of Human Rights, Freedom of Information and Privacy, and the Ombudsman, are more frequently being asked to act as quasi-surrogates for government. They may even at times overrule government-initiated policy.

In addition to procedural checks and balances to the exercise of the powers of representative government, other forces are influencing decision-making in our evolving democracies. The combination of modern communications and the increasing sophistication of advocacy groups, activists, and lobbyists is moving our traditional democratic process from virtual dependence on the exclusive overseeing of our elected representatives to something that is much more participatory and at times more chaotic. Increasing accessibility to the deliberations of government and its bureaucracy, a sophisticated mass media, and skilled constituencies are widening and opening as well as complicating the processes of decision-making. Each pressure group seeking public expenditure for its cause uses its unique position to maximum advantage. This has been particularly evident during the recent provincial election campaigns in Manitoba and Ontario.

In view of these trends, democratic governments of the 1990s will have to exercise their mandates – especially when these include reform – differently from the past. They will need to rely less on the traditional legislative and funding levers of government and more and more on the exercise of leadership; achievement of consensus; delegation to agencies, boards, and commissions; use of important advisory structures such as Premier's Councils; and use and, if necessary, creation of credible third parties.

By their very nature these mechanisms are slow, whereas the pace of change, and the rate at which events break, is fast. There will be a growing disparity between the time that it now takes government policy generation to respond and the rate at which new situations arise and demand responses. Government will have to develop different ways of responding to events and, at the same time, adjust expectations to the realities of its own capabilities and limitations.

Choosing the agenda, and conveying the basis for that choice, is important. Equally important will be the development of partnerships that can meet the demands of society in areas where government cannot act alone, or should not act at all.

Ontarians have views and expectations of their government, especially in terms of the overall framework within which they judge it. Like Canadians everywhere, they normally support a government that reflects value systems that embrace the best values of Canadian society. In general, Ontarians value tolerance, fair play, multiculturalism, national unity, equity, social justice, balancing social and economic priorities, and enhanced access to opportunity.

Across Canada, but especially in Ontario, the pluralism, multiculturalism, multilingualism, and other multi-isms that characterize our society reconcile with each other most easily when the economy is strong and the general sense of well-being is high. When the economy falters and that sense of well-being is disturbed, the tendency to reconciliation is marred by the tendency to extremism, and the tendency to care for the disadvantaged is offset by the state of disquietude and growing insularity of the advantaged. At such times, the need for government to articulate and defend its overarching values is even greater.

Values, however, are most forcefully expressed through the government's allocative process. There is an essentially ethical dimension to the decision to allocate limited resources to one purpose as opposed to another. Shall more be devoted to education or research, or transportation, or health care?

Government strives to choose those allocations that are within its value systems and that serve the larger public good. But more often than not, government finds itself in the position of having to decide on an allocation based on its intrinsic merits at the time that the demand presents itself. Only after many such decisions are made does one question their relative importance. So at the federal level, after the fact, we can question the wisdom of funding for nuclear submarines and not for the environment or transfer payments for health care.

We detect also a sense of frustration that government cannot do more in any one of a number of areas without further increases in taxation. And equally troublesome are the difficulties encountered even when the most generous allocations at the macro level fail to translate themselves into effective service delivery at the micro level.

We are one of the wealthiest provinces, with one of the most generous income support systems, and yet we still have homelessness and food banks. We are one of the youngest nations on earth, spending more per capita on health care than any other nation with a national health system, and yet we have shortfalls and waiting lists.

These contradictions are further compounded by the pluralistic nature of our society where different groups hold ethical concepts rooted in different cultures and which, when applied to the same situation, produce diametrically opposing conclusions. What is seen as the right thing to do by one culture may be seen as absolutely wrong by another.

After value systems, all governments are judged by the overall level of well-being – the "quality of life" that prevails during their term of office. Quality of life is vested in the full array of determinants – the creation and distribution of wealth, a spectrum of public policies designed to foster and/or protect general well-being, and programs that enhance the lives of the disadvantaged while encouraging individual responsibility and autonomy.

When the right value system is upheld and overall well-being is maintained, additional judgments rest on other considerations. Specific tangibles, such as local issues, are important symbols – "our school, our hospital, our highway" – items which tend to be specific and easily identified as bonding the government and the community. Social programs that reaffirm the value systems that were described above also form an important basis on which governments are judged. Care for the poor and disadvantaged, the array of social safety nets, attention to specific groups, health care services, public health and health promotion, education, training, academic excellence, and special attention to the many faces of Ontario are all addressed by social programs which have both wide and specific appeal. Finally, a government is judged by the quality of the services which the government itself provides or delivers. When a government pleads for increased efficiencies in nongovernment sectors, it is viewed cynically if the efficiency and effectiveness of its own services are found wanting.

When viewed by its own citizens through various polls and surveys, Ontario's government appears to be reflecting mainstream values. There is concern, however, that these values are not permeating all sectors of society. Certain public reactions around race relations, multiculturalism, and francophone services are illustrative of this dichotomy.

Externally, the quality of life in Canada is seen as very high. The U.N. rates Canada fifth in the world and the U.S. nineteenth. If that is so, then Southern Ontario must rate among the highest.

Within this overall framework of values and services, what do we expect of the provincial government? In simplest terms, this is understood by Ontarians to focus on economic well-being and social equity both for their own sakes and for the consequences of a mutually reinforcing relationship between them.

These are but a few of the challenges facing Ontario. I have not discussed health care or the environment, although both were very much a part of our deliberations. Nor have I discussed the structure of government and the continuous improvement of the quality of the services provided by government to its citizens.

Our overall impression was that this last decade of the twentieth century seems to be one of emerging regional and focal interests. Interest and pressure groups are flexing their muscles and taking advantage of every opportunity to divert the public agenda to their purposes.

Whereas the first decade was characterized by a striving for unity and communications linkages, the last decade is tilting toward disunity – and a breakdown of communications even in the face of the most sophisticated communications technology we could have imagined at the beginning of the twentieth century. Canadians have always prided themselves on their value system of "Peace, Order, and Good Government." As we enter this last decade, all seem to be in short supply.

Perhaps the greatest philosophic insight of the century came out of the mouth of Pogo – Walt Kelly's cartoon anti-hero – "We has seen the enemy and he is us."

DISCUSSION
Chair: Guy Bujold
Health and Welfare Canada

Guy Bujold

There was one question which came to my mind, and it had to do with the changing nature of democracy, and I wonder whether you might give us some insights into what you believe to be, or indeed whether or not you see it as existing, the nature of any change in what has been referred to by some as the Canadian consensus around social programming?

Martin Barkin (Ontario Ministry of Health)

Well, of course, as Canadians have tried to define themselves in the past, they have always defined themselves according to their social programs. In fact, if you ask Canadians what sets them apart from their neighbours to the south, the first line that usually comes is Canadian social programs, and the first of the Canadian social programs that is mentioned is health care. In fact, this audience will remember, in the last federal election when there was some concern that as a result of free trade the Canadian health care system would get to look more like the American health care system, there was about a 25-point drop in the polls in a very short period of time. That consensus on Canadian social policy and its role is rapidly changing, even in Quebec. M. Castonguay, who is the author of one of, I think, the seminal reports that set the pattern for health care in the province of Quebec, has begun to challenge what was the Canadian consensus on health care around the Canada Health Act. And what we see now is an emerging series of interest groups that have a different view of the Canadian social fibre. And trying to balance the protected Canadian social fibre from international competitiveness will probably be the biggest challenge facing national governments in the next decade. I alluded to that earlier in my comment. Defining what we are as Canadians, separating us from a world that has become the global village that Marshall McLuhan, also of this university, foretold almost 20 years ago, that's the real challenge. And what we find is that groups who are very vocal, and very effective, may capture the national agenda, while groups who are not vocal, not well organized, not sophisticated, will find themselves borne along by this tide that emerges. Can Canada become a true participatory democracy, or will we be in the transition a democracy torn by specific interest groups, is a question I have no good answer for, but it's this warning that one needs to sound early on as we enter this last decade of the twentieth century, I think.

UTILIZATION: THE DOCTORS DILEMMA

THE EFFECTS OF MEDICAL CARE POLICY IN B.C.: UTILIZATION TRENDS IN THE 1980s*

Morris L. Barer
Robert G. Evans
Centre for Health Services and Policy Research
University of British Columbia

Dominic S. Haazen
British Columbia Ministry of Health

I am going to try to describe very briefly what has been a fascinating decade in British Columbia in terms of medical policy initiatives and provide a preliminary sense of trends in costs and utilization. This work is a piece of a larger, and still ongoing, project, the intent of which is to: (a) attempt to document what happened in B.C. over the last decade; (b) develop a reliable means of differentiating between utilization and price changes over that period; (c) assess the effects of the separate policy initiatives on utilization of different categories of medical services; and (d) along the way create a data set that will be of use not only to the researchers involved in this project, but to other researchers interested in analyzing the effects on prices and utilization of a rich variety of medical policy initiatives.

When it comes to medical policy, B.C. seems to have a hard time staying out of the news. What occurred over the last 10 years were really three major types of policy (Table 1). Throughout the period the usual fee negotiations took place. The results were a roller-coaster ride, with very large fee increases early in the decade and virtually no increases during the

---

Table 1
A CONCISE POLICY HISTORY

THREE POLICY STREAMS
Fee Negotiations
    Occurred throughout period
    Spectacular failure (success) in 1981/82 and 1982/83
    Fee freeze 1984/85; very few and small increases since
    Rollbacks 1982/83 and 1987/88

Physician Supply and Distribution
    Billing number controls under administrative arrangements December 1983 - March 1985
    March 1985 – billing number policy suspended for 2 months
    May 1985 – billing number policy reinstated
    Court of Appeal decision ends billing number policy, August 1988
    Supreme Court of Canada denies leave to appeal, Fall 1988

Utilization Caps
    Medical association negotiates no cap for 1984/85
    First partial cap in place 1985/86
    No cap in place, first 6 months of 1986/87
    Cap in place last 6 months of 1986/87
    Contract re-opened March 1987 because of perceived "excess utilization"
    Partial caps in place 1987/88 and 1988/89; cap adjustment lag tightens

---

period since 1983/84. The B.C. Medical Association managed to negotiate a 40% increase over two years in 1981. In the second year of that agreement there was a fee rollback of 5 to 7%. There were essentially fee freezes in 1984/85 and 1985/86. In fact, there were virtually no increases of any substance until the late 1980s, and there was a further fee rollback in 1987/88.

The second major policy thrust has been directed at the supply and distribution of physicians, and again most of you will be well aware of the fact that there was a "billing numbers" policy commencing in 1983, then off, then on again, and finally permanently off (or as permanent as anything can be in this business) in the fall of 1988. During the periods when the policy was 'on', the issuance of new 'rights' to submit claims to the Medical Services Plan was slowed, and those 'rights' that were issued came accompanied by geographic restrictions.

The most recent initiative of the B.C. Ministry of Health has been attempts to cap utilization, to go beyond controlling fee levels and to attempt to control the total outlays for medical services. This too has had a very checkered history. The first time it came up in negotiations was in 1983/84. In 1984/85, the Association managed to convince the Ministry that no cap was necessary; in fact, as you will see in a moment, what is really quite interesting about that is that it seems to have been the year in which there was the slowest growth in utilization. There have since then been a series of partial caps, partial because they have really been quite complex agreements which have provided scope for population growth and for increases in utilization for other and undefined factors, and in addition have usually involved some sort of sharing of any utilization above and beyond negotiated targets. The period has also been marked by the fact that, because of the annual process of negotiation, there have been instances where for periods of time, although a cap was intended, a cap had not been negotiated.

Progress on the project has been slowed by the massive job of data processing and manipulation required to get to the point where we can actually look at some aggregate data. We started with about 400 million payment records, covering just over a 10-year period. We first allocated every payment record to its appropriate month of service. We then adjusted for the fact that some months are longer than others, and so we developed a protocol for standardizing the working days in every month so that we could compare payments and utilization on a standardized monthly basis. Finally, we developed a method of adjusting for price changes by attempting to value all items billed throughout the period 1979/80 to 1988/89 at a single point in time, April 1, 1988. This involved some detailed work by individuals in the Ministry of Health to provide estimates where items no longer existed in 1988/89.

PRELIMINARY RESULTS

We invested considerable energy in the process of fee deflation. In the end it turned out not to make a great deal of difference. In Table 2 we present three indexes. The first index is what the Health Information Division, Health and Welfare Canada, provides through its payment schedule comparison. We've called that a linked index. It essentially takes the reported increases provided by each province, and we have simply compounded them through that period. The second is a 1979 basket Laspeyres index, based on fee items that existed throughout the period in B.C. The third index is a Paasche index using 1988 actual or imputed fee levels for all items (1988 was the 'base year'). The estimation of the Paasche index in this manner was a major undertaking. It turns out we would not have been much worse off using either of the simpler indexes. The point where the extra effort may become important is when one starts deflating specific types of practice and types of service.

Table 2

ALTERNATIVE APPROACHES TO FEE INDEX CONSTRUCTION
(April 1, 1979 = 100.0)

	1988/89 Value
Health Information Division Health and Welfare Canada "Linked" Index	172.18
Laspeyres Index based on items that existed throughout period	170.40
Paasche Index, all items	170.58

In Table 3 we report Paasche fee indexes by types of practice. These results may explain some of the inter-specialty conflict in B.C. and other provinces over relative fees and incomes. Over these nine years, fees for general practitioners increased an average of 85%. The average increase for all fee items was 71%, very close to the growth in the Canadian consumer price index. Some of the diagnostic specialists did rather less well than that. Much of the inter-specialty controversy over this period has centred on general practitioners' claims that their incomes are falling behind those of their specialist peers. On the basis of the results here, it seems safe to suggest that any such erosion is not tied to relative 'mistreatment' by the process of allocating fee measures.

Table 3

FEE INCREASES BY PHYSICIAN TYPE OF PRACTICE
(April 1, 1979 = 100.0)

	1988/89 Values
General practice	184.68
Medical specialties	165.11
Surgical specialties and anaesthesiology	160.15
Radiology	160.40
Pathology	152.11
Other types of practice	159.73
All types of practice	**170.58**

Table 4 reports the change in utilization per capita by type of practice of physician alongside the fee indexes from Table 3. The smallest increase in fees (except for that for other types of practice, which is a grab bag), which is for pathology, is associated with really quite remarkable increases in utilization. The largest increase in fees – for general practitioners – is associated with very slow (at least relatively speaking) increases in utilization. We cannot infer anything about causality from these results, but this is an interesting observation at this point.

In the short time remaining I would like to present two final tables. Table 5 is very simply an attempt to portray the reason that one has to go to the effort of trying to look at services by date of service rather than by date of payment. You will notice in particular that in 1982/83, which was the year of the fee rollback in B.C., increases in total expenditures by the Ministry were 23%, but the actual increase in expenditures for services provided in that year was a much smaller 18%. There are less dramatic differences in each of the other years.

Table 4
FEE AND UTILIZATION CHANGES
1979/80 to 1988/89

	1988/89 fee index	Constant $ expenditures per capita Average % change
General practice	184.68	1.37
Medical specialties	165.11	3.98
Surgical specialties and anaesthesiology	160.15	2.60
Radiology (including ultrasound)	160.40	4.47
Pathology	152.11	6.08
Other types of practice (physical medicine, medical microbiology, osteopathy, nuclear medicine)	159.73	10.06

Table 5
YEAR OF PAYMENT VS. YEAR OF SERVICE

Year	Total expenditures (Yr pmt) ($)	Change (%)	Total expenditures (Yr serv) ($)	Change (%)
1979/80	369,497		375,202	
1980/81	428,259	15.90	439,750	17.20
1981/82	530,144	23.79	553,186	25.80
1982/83	651,727	22.93	651,511	17.77
1983/84	733,843	12.60	739,255	13.47
1984/85	752,404	2.53	747,787	1.15
1985/86	779,339	3.58	783,396	4.76
1986/87	833,103	6.90	828,941	5.81
1987/88	875,904	5.14	874,653	5.51
1988/89	931,905	6.39	945,061	8.05
% Change				
1979/80 - 1983/84		18.71		18.48
1983/84 - 1988/89		4.8		5.03
1979/80 - 1988/89		10.83		10.81

Finally, in Table 6 we provide the aggregated results of our deflation. Columns 1 and 2 show actual per capita expenditures and the year-over-year changes. There is clearly a sharp break in the B.C. experience between 1983/84 (the end of the 'high fee growth' era) and 1984/85 (the beginning of the 'fee control and expenditure targets' era). This shows up even more dramatically in the final two columns, which represent the per capita utilization experience over this period. The differences between columns 2 and 4 represent changes in fee levels.

Table 6
UTILIZATION TRENDS
1979/80 to 1988/89

Year	Expend per capita (Yr serv) ($)	Change (%)	Expend per capita at 1988 prices (Yr serv) ($)	Change (%)
1979/80	143.5		244.8	
1980/81	163.2	13.75	253.7	3.65
1981/82	200.2	22.65	264.1	4.10
1982/83	232.8	16.30	280.2	6.10
1983/84	261.5	12.32	285.8	2.00
1984/85	261.6	0.05	285.4	-0.15
1985/86	272.0	3.98	294.3	3.13
1986/87	285.6	4.98	305.4	3.77
1987/88	296.7	3.88	311.9	2.11
1988/89	314.3	5.93	314.3	0.76
% Change				
1979/80 - 1983/84		16.19		3.95
1983/84 - 1988/89		3.74		1.92
1979/80 - 1988/89		9.10		2.82

In 1984/85, there was an actual decline in utilization, or constant dollar expenditures per capita. In 1987/88 and 1988/89, as the attempts to cap expenditures became more binding, utilization trends seem to have fallen. 1986/87 was the year in which the first six months had no cap and also the year in which utilization during the last six months allegedly increased to such an extent that there was a contract "re-opener" that forced a fee rollback the following year. During 1985/86 there was a two-month window in the billing numbers policy.

These data alone do not provide a means to pair particular policies with particular 'utilization effects'. Our intent is to examine the data more closely, by type of practice and type of service and to use physician supply as well as population denominators. We eventually hope to be able to use multivariate analyses to ascertain the effects of particular policies or sets of policies on trends in per capita utilization and levels of service provision per physician.

NOTE
* edited transcript of talk by Morris Barer

WHO HAS SEEN THE WIND? EXAMINING THE EVIDENCE AND EXPLORING THE POLICY OPTIONS PERTAINING TO THE EFFECT CHANGES IN PHYSICIAN SUPPLY HAVE HAD ON INFLUENCING MEDICAL UTILIZATION AND COSTS IN ALBERTA

Richard H.M. Plain
Department of Economics
Department of Health Services Administration and Community Medicine
University of Alberta

INTRODUCTION

The purpose of this paper is to provide an overview and summary of the major trends characterizing the utilization and costs of medical services in Alberta. Attention is focused on the results of a "natural" experiment which occurred when the population ceased to grow and the supply of medical practitioners continued to expand at a high rate. An analysis is also carried out of health care spending and utilization within an economic boom as compared to a period with little economic growth.

The first part of the paper provides a brief overview of the major demographic and economic trends in the Alberta economy between 1971 and 1989[1], the second deals with the major medical utilization and cost trends in the province, and the third with the major medical economic policy issues.

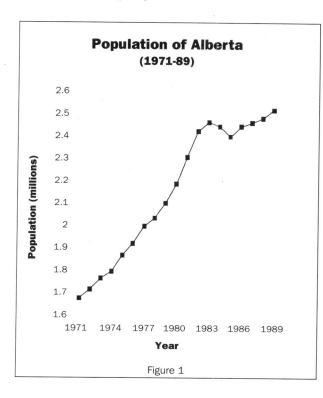

Figure 1

MAJOR DEMOGRAPHIC AND ECONOMIC TRENDS IN THE ALBERTA ECONOMY DEMOGRAPHIC DEVELOPMENTS

Figure 1 depicts the growth in the Alberta population between 1971 and 1989. Between 1975 and 1981, in the midst of the economic boom, the Alberta growth rates were 3 to 4 times the national levels. From 1981 onwards the picture changed dramatically. The total population of Alberta actually fell in 1984 and 1985. The rate of growth in the population rose to a level in excess of the national rate in 1986, fell to less than 1% in 1987 and 1988, and slightly exceeded the national rate in 1989. The rate of change in the Alberta population over the period can be characterized as one of high growth during the boom years – the equivalent of 85% of the current population of New Brunswick or approximately 70% of the current population of Saskatchewan or Manitoba was added between 1971 and 1981 – followed by a period of stagnation and modest recovery at the end of the 1980s. Stagnation is the appropriate term to describe the period (1983-87) when the total population of Alberta remained relatively unchanged – actually a slight decline of 2,236 people was recorded.

Shifts in the Age Composition of the Population

Table 1 provides estimates of the Alberta population categorized by age and sex. The 'child' dependents category is composed of all children 14 years of age or younger, the so-called 'elderly' dependents category of all individuals 65 years or more, and the 'working-age' group of all individuals 15 to 64 years of age. The following points should be noted:

(1) The total percentage of dependents was approximately 17.3% lower in 1989 than in 1971; however, the percentage of child dependents fell by approximately 25.9%, while the percentage of elderly dependents increased by 20.5%;

(2) The percentage of the population within the working age group increased by approximately 11.0% over the period;

Table 1
PERCENTAGE OF THE TOTAL ALBERTA POPULATION
IN THE CHILD, ELDERLY, AND WORKING AGE CATEGORIES

Year	Child (%)	Elderly (%)	Total Dependents (%)	Working Age (%)	Total (%)
1971	32.1	7.3	39.4	60.7	100
1972	31.2	7.3	38.5	61.5	100
1973	30.3	7.3	37.6	62.5	100
1974	29.4	7.4	36.8	63.2	100
1975	28.5	7.3	35.8	64.2	100
1976	27.7	7.4	35.0	65.0	100
1977	26.8	7.3	34.1	65.9	100
1978	26.2	7.4	33.6	66.4	100
1979	25.5	7.4	32.9	67.1	100
1980	24.9	7.3	32.2	67.8	100
1981	24.4	7.2	31.6	68.4	100
1982	24.2	7.2	31.4	68.6	100
1983	24.2	7.3	31.5	68.5	100
1984	24.2	7.6	31.8	68.2	100
1985	24.2	7.9	32.1	67.9	100
1986	24.0	8.1	32.1	67.9	100
1987	23.9	8.3	32.2	67.8	100
1988	23.8	8.6	32.4	67.6	100
1989	23.8	8.8	32.6	67.4	100

Source: Annual Reports of the AHCIP

(3) The shift in the proportion of the population within the working age and total dependents groups in the late 1980s gradually led to a population age mix approaching the 2/3 - 1/3 split existing in the late 1970s; and

(4) The period of stagnation (1983-87) was characterized by a 13.7% rise in the elderly portion of the population as the more mobile and younger members of the work force were more likely to move out of the province and older members of the population to remain.

MAJOR MACROECONOMIC VARIABLES:
INCOME, OUTPUT, EMPLOYMENT, AND PRICES

Table 2 provides estimates of the growth in output and personal income per capita, and the industrial composite of average weekly earnings (inclusive of overtime) expressed in terms of constant 1981 dollars.

Table 2
GDP AND PERSONAL INCOME PER CAPITA AND
AVERAGE WEEKLY WAGES
(in constant 1981 dollars)

Year	Real GDP per Capita ($)	Change (%)	Real Personal Income per Capita ($)	Change (%)	Real Average Weekly Wages ($)	Change (%)
1971	16,497	-	8,069	-	331.22	-
1972	17,422	5.6	8,676	7.5	342.33	3.4
1973	18,977	8.9	9,428	8.7	341.36	-0.3
1974	19,868	4.7	10,206	8.3	343.03	0.5
1975	19,763	-0.5	10,749	5.3	359.41	4.8
1976	19,963	1.0	11,190	4.1	380.24	5.8
1977	20,138	0.9	11,224	0.3	385.24	1.3
1978	20,584	2.2	11,708	4.3	372.90	-3.2
1979	22,095	7.3	12,370	5.7	380.19	2.0
1980	22,230	0.6	12,952	4.7	384.62	1.2
1981	22,627	1.8	13,702	5.8	390.39	1.5
1982	20,809	-8.0	13,526	-1.3	393.02	0.7
1983	19,976	-4.0	12,948	-4.3	366.31	-6.8
1984	21,197	6.1	13,492	4.2	364.84	-0.4
1985	21,989	3.7	14,006	3.8	358.61	-1.7
1986	21,940	-0.2	13,898	-0.8	349.95	-2.4
1987	22,550	2.8	13,668	-1.7	336.78	-3.8
1988	24,355	8.0	14,487	6.0	337.04	0.1
1989	24,133	-0.9	14,575	0.6	337.51	0.1

Source: Alberta Bureau of Statistics, "Economic Accounts", and "Alberta Statistical Review", First Quarter, 1990.

Figure 2 depicts the movement of real GDP per capita throughout the period. It is important to note that while central Canada enjoyed excellent economic growth from the end of the sharp recession in 1982, Alberta, like certain of the other regions in the nation, experienced troubled times. This is exemplified by the fact that the level of real GDP per capita in the province remained virtually unchanged between 1981 and 1987 and was only 6.7% higher in 1989 than in 1981. This is a remarkable change from the high growth era where real output per head in the province increased by approximately 37% between 1971 and 1981. Real personal income per capita also rose during this decade. It increased by approximately 70% from 1971 to 1981, declined and gradually recovered to reach a temporary high in 1985, followed by a further slide and a recovery. The point to note is that real personal income per capita in Alberta was still at its 1981 level in 1987. Real average weekly salaries peaked in 1982 and declined until 1987; a slight increase was experienced in 1988. Overall, real average salaries appear to have fallen by approximately 14.1% between 1982 and 1989; however, significant revisions in survey methodology in 1987 cast some doubt on the precise magnitude of the fall in the latter part of the period.

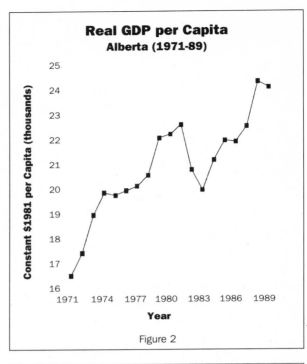

Figure 2

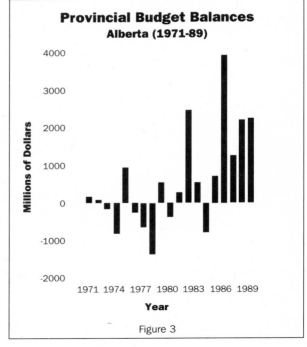

Figure 3

Table 3 provides an overview of the level of inflation, unemployment, and the provincial government budget balance[2] between 1971 and 1989. Alberta enjoyed exceptionally low levels of unemployment through the middle 1970s until the end of 1981. From 1982 and 1989 inclusive the Alberta unemployment rate was 2 - 2 1/2 times greater than the rates prevailing throughout the majority of the 1970s. High levels of inflation were experienced from 1974 to 1982, followed by relatively modest rates ranging between 2.7 and 4.5% for the majority of the remainder of the 1980s.

Table 3

UNEMPLOYMENT, INFLATION, AND THE PROVINCIAL GOVERNMENT BUDGET BALANCE
(1971-89)

Year	Annual Change in the CPI (%)	Rate of Unemployment (%)	Provincial Government Budget Balance ($M)
1971	-	5.7	149
1972	4.5	5.6	77
1973	7.8	5.3	-183
1974	10.4	3.5	-826
1975	10.7	4.1	934
1976	8.0	4.0	-236
1977	9.1	4.5	-661
1978	9.0	4.7	-1,355
1979	8.9	3.9	538
1980	10.2	3.7	-399
1981	12.5	3.8	279
1982	10.8	7.7	2,465
1983	5.8	10.6	556
1984	2.7	11.1	-795
1985	3.2	10.0	716
1986	3.3	9.8	3,923
1987	4.2	9.6	1,254
1988	2.7	8.0	2,203
1989	4.5	7.2	2,254

Source: P. Boothe, "Time-Consistent Data for Alberta's Public Finances 1969-89", Department of Economics, Research Paper No. 90-8.

The state of the provincial budget balance (expenditures minus revenues) over the period is depicted in Figure 3. The 1970s (with the exception of 1975) are characterized by mild deficits and moderate to quite significant surpluses; the surplus in 1978 amounted to approximately $1.4 billion. The 1980s were quite a different story. Deficits, incurred in every year except 1984, ranged from approximately one-quarter to slightly under $4 billion in 1986 – a record breaking level.

MACROECONOMIC ASPECTS OF THE ALBERTA MEDICARE PLAN
NOMINAL AND REAL TOTAL MEDICAL SERVICE EXPENDITURES

Table 4 provides a breakdown of the nominal and real medical service expenditures per capita made by the Alberta Health Care Insurance Plan from 1971 to 1989 inclusive. In 1989, nominal and real per capita medical insurance expenditures amounted to approximately 4.6 times and 1.6 times their respective 1971 levels.

Table 4
NOMINAL AND CONSTANT DOLLAR MEDICAL SERVICES EXPENDITURES PER CAPITA IN ALBERTA
(1971-89)

Year	Nominal Medical Service Expenditures per Capita ($)	Annual Change (%)	Real * Medical Service Expenditures per Capita ($)	Annual Change (%)
1971	54.76	34.5	119.05	–
1972	55.49	1.3	118.62	-0.4
1973	56.22	1.3	119.88	1.1
1974	59.02	5.0	122.94	2.5
1975	64.88	9.9	129.16	5.1
1976	72.64	12.0	130.18	0.8
1977	81.41	12.1	134.49	3.3
1978	84.28	3.5	130.30	-3.1
1979	92.46	9.7	134.10	2.9
1980	101.13	9.4	134.25	0.1
1981	115.66	14.4	136.36	1.6
1982	136.22	17.8	136.22	-0.1
1983	172.55	26.7	150.17	10.2
1984	194.64	12.8	161.76	7.7
1985	206.81	6.3	171.87	6.3
1986	221.03	6.9	183.69	6.9
1987	239.21	8.2	188.55	2.6
1988	245.60	2.7	192.13	1.9
1989	253.16	3.1	195.13	1.6

Source: Annual Reports AHCIP (1970-87)
* Deflated by the Alberta Medical Benefit Index Health Infromation Division, Ottawa, 1990

Figure 4 shows markedly higher levels of per capita spending on medical services in the 1980s than in the 1970s. Between 1971 and 1979 nominal medical services spending per head rose by approximately $37.70 (68.8%) as compared to $137.50 (118.9%) from 1981-89. In constant dollar terms these increases amounted to $15.05 (12.6%) in the 1970s and $58.77 (43.1%) in the 1980s.

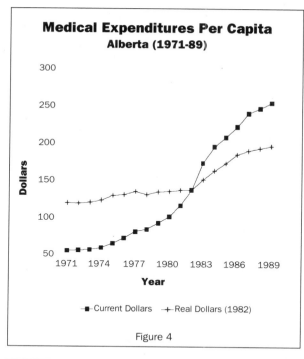

Medical Expenditures Per Capita
Alberta (1971-89)

Figure 4

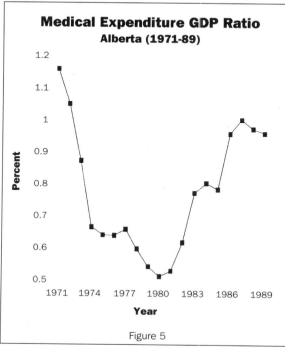

Medical Expenditure GDP Ratio
Alberta (1971-89)

Figure 5

Medical Expenditures in a Depressed Economy

The marked increase in real per capita medical spending in the 1980s is quite surprising given the extremely poor performance of the Alberta economy for most of that period. It has been shown that real GDP per capita was unchanged between 1981 and 1987, unemployment was high, real wages were falling, high levels of provincial budget deficits were being incurred, and little population growth was being experienced. It is instructive to focus on medical spending within this period. Between 1981 and 1987 real per capita spending on medical services increased from $136.36 to $188.55 ($52.19, or 38.3%), while nominal per capita spending, which includes major fee schedule adjustments during the early 1980s, increased by $123.55, or 106.8% (Table 4).

The absolute magnitude of these increases in medical spending across the period amounted to $322,174,182 in nominal and $149,699,928 in constant dollar terms.

Movements in the Medicare Expenditure GDP Ratio

Not unexpectedly, the combination of poor economic growth and sharply rising medical care costs is reflected in a rapid rise in the ratio of medical expenditures relative to GDP. Figure 5 shows that the medical care industry in Alberta doubled its share of total economic activity within the provincial economy between 1980 and 1987. Medicine expanded markedly during a period in which the rest of the small business sector experienced high levels of bankruptcy, foreclosures, and a contraction in profits, gross revenues, and employment and investment opportunities. The rapid fall in the medical expenditure ratio occurring in the 1970s reflects the effects of a high rate of growth in GDP and a relatively moderate rate of growth in medical expenditures. The point to note is that the Alberta economy turned from a high growth performer in the 1970s to a very low growth performer in the 1980s; the medical sector, however, grew relatively rapidly in both periods, particularly in the 1980s.

DEMOGRAPHIC CHARACTERISTICS OF MEDICAL EXPENDITURES IN THE 1970s AND 1980s

Table 5 shows that medical expenditures on females have accounted for the greatest proportion of AHCIP spending between 1973 and 1989. The proportion of the spending directed towards females has become slightly more accentuated over time. The female component of the total population was just slightly less than 50% of the Alberta population in both 1973 and 1989; however, the percentage of real medical care expenditures rose from 59.2% in 1973 to 60.6% in 1989. The bulk of this increase occurred between 1981 and 1987 when the economy was performing so poorly. This increase is partially associated with the shift in the composition of the population resulting from the greater out-migration of males vis-à-vis females during a period of recession and slow economic growth.

Table 5
DISTRIBUTION OF TOTAL REAL MEDICAL EXPENDITURES AND POPULATION BY SEX

	Expenditures		Population	
	Female	Male	Female	Male
Year	(%)	(%)	(%)	(%)
1973	59.2	40.8	49.5	50.5
1974	58.8	41.2	49.5	50.5
1975	59.0	41.0	49.3	50.7
1976	59.1	40.9	49.3	50.7
1977	58.9	41.1	49.2	50.8
1978	58.8	41.2	49.2	50.8
1979	59.1	40.9	49.1	50.9
1980	59.3	40.7	49.0	51.0
1981	59.5	40.5	48.9	51.1
1982	59.7	40.3	48.8	51.2
1983	59.8	40.2	49.1	50.9
1984	60.0	40.0	49.3	50.7
1985	60.2	39.8	49.7	50.3
1986	60.1	39.9	49.7	50.3
1987	60.4	39.6	49.7	50.3
1988	60.6	39.4	49.7	50.3
1989	60.6	39.4	49.8	50.2

Source: Annual Reports of the AHCIP Deflated by the AHCIP Benefit Index

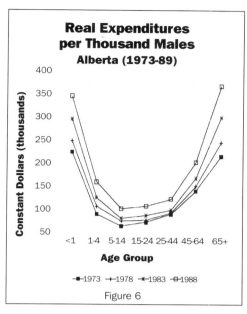

Real Expenditures per Thousand Males
Alberta (1973-89)

Figure 6

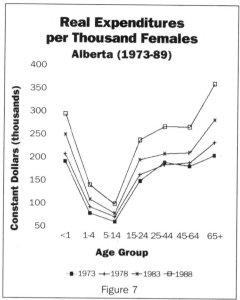

Real Expenditures per Thousand Females
Alberta (1973-89)

Figure 7

Figures 6 and 7 provide an overview of the upward shift in the constant dollar value of the medical services rendered per 1,000 males and females categorized by age group at regular five-year intervals from 1973 to 1988 inclusive. The following points should be noted:

(1) The intensity of the medical servicing of both sexes was markedly higher in the 1980s than in the 1970s for all age groups;

(2) The level of real total medical expenditures per 1,000 population is markedly higher for females than for males throughout the period under consideration; however, this does not hold true for all age groups. For example, real medical spending on males under 5 and those 65 and over tends to be greater than on females in the same age groups; and

(3) The total level of spending on females may be higher than on males; however, the average annual increase in real expenditures per 1,000 was approximately the same for both sexes – slightly in excess of 3% for 1973-79 and 4% for 1980-89.

Identifying the Medical Expenditure Drivers

What changes in the major factors determining the costs of operating a medical care system are responsible for driving up the costs of medical care in Alberta? A number of variables have only a limited role in explaining variations in medical utilization and costs. Demographic and physician supply variables, on the other hand, play a major role in explaining major changes in real medical spending and utilization within the Alberta health care system.[3, 4] The 1980s have been identified as a period when the rate of growth in population fell markedly relative to the prosperous 1970s. Indeed, it is possible to identify a period within the 1980s (1983-87) when the total population of the province remained unchanged. It is extremely useful to examine medical spending closely within this time span, since it provides investigators with a "natural experiment" in which the population is held constant and a large number of physicians are added to the system.

The Change in Medicare Expenditures in Alberta 1983-87

During the four years from 1983 to 1987 the number of medical practitioners participating in the provincial plan increased by 19.7%[5], total population remained virtually
unchanged, and total nominal spending increased by $163,738,036, or 38.6%. Nominal
per capita spending rose from $172.55 to $239.21 (38.6%), while real per capita spending
rose from $150.17 to $188.55, or 25.6% (Table 4).

It is important to note that during this period the provincial government continued
its long standing policy of paying all the bills submitted by fee-for-service practitioners
to the AHCIP without setting a budget with a fixed dollar limit which would restrict or
inhibit the level and rate of payments to the profession within a given fiscal year.[6] In
addition, the overall rate of increase in fees was negotiated with the profession (for all
practical purposes, the medical association set the individual fees); however, the increase
in expenditures generated by the increase in the volume of services or the selection of
higher cost, more lucrative procedures was borne solely by the government.

Decomposing the Average Annual Rate of Change in Medical Costs in the 1983-87 Period[7]

Figure 8 and Table 6 indicate that fee increases accounted for approximately 29% of
the average annual 8.5% increase in medical expenditures from 1983 to 1987 inclusive.
Although there was no growth in population, the number of physicians participating
in the medical care plan
increased by 4.6% per annum.
Servicing intensity (services
per physician) grew at 4.2%
per annum – a level tying in
with the extremely high servicing rates prevailing
between 1981-87. With no
growth in population and a
high rate of growth in physician supply, it is not surprising that the number of
patients per physician fell by a
record amount (-2.9% per
annum). It is of interest to
decompose this decline in the
patient to physician load into
its two components, namely, a
4.4% fall in the population to
physician ratio coupled with an
offsetting mitigating factor –
an annual rate of growth in
the ratio of discrete patients
relative to the total population
of approximately 1.6%.

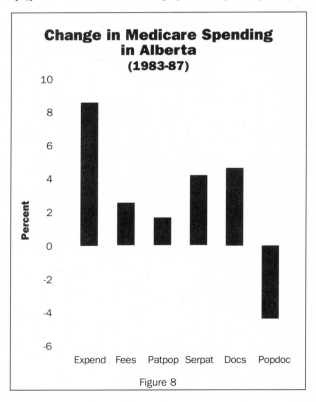

**Change in Medicare Spending
in Alberta
(1983-87)**

Figure 8

Payments per physician by the AHCIP are gross medical sales to the benefiting physician. During 1983-87 the high rate of growth in physician supply coupled with a zero population growth acted as a depressant on the average rate of growth in physician revenues[8] despite the fact that a greater proportion of the population used physician services and those who did received more services. The growth in Medicare earnings (medical insurance payments per practitioner) dropped to 3.7% per annum – an all time record low compared to the other time periods shown in Table 6. The interesting aspect of the marked expansion in the medical industry from 1983-87 is that the growth in the industry's sales revenue was positive and not negative in the face of the almost 20% increase in the number of new firms entering a depressed economy within a four-year time span. This suggests, other things being equal, that the medical industry has substantial supply-side demand generation capabilities.

The Alberta version of the Canadian medical insurance plan not only protected the present generation of Alberta doctors from the vicissitudes of the market place that had been experienced by their pre-Medicare predecessors (no chickens and eggs were paid in lieu of medical fees in the two sharp recessions in the 1980s), but it also allowed a medical boom to take place in an economy facing record high levels of unemployment, falling real wages and personal income, and rising levels of public debt. Maintaining a boom within the medical industry in the midst of a province-wide recession is a scenario future provincial policy makers may be quite eager to prevent.

Table 6

AVERAGE ANNUAL RATES OF CHANGE IN MEDICARE VARIABLES IN ALBERTA FOR SELECTED TIME PERIODS

Variable	1973-81 (%)	1981-87 (%)	1983-87 (%)	1973-89 (%)	1973-79 (%)	1980-89 (%)
Expenditures	13.3	14.4	8.5	12.5	11.9	12.8
Fees	7.7	7.2	2.5	6.7	6.7	6.4
Patient to population ratio	0.8	1.4	1.6	0.9	1.0	0.9
Services per patient	1.3	4.2	4.2	2.3	0.9	3.2
Physicians	2.9	4.8	4.6	3.6	2.5	4.4
Population to physician ratio	0.5	-3.5	-4.4	-1.3	0.5	-2.7
Services per physician	2.6	1.8	4.2	1.8	2.5	1.2
Patients per physician	1.2	-2.2	-2.9	-0.5	1.5	-1.9
Expenditures per physician	10.0	9.2	3.7	8.6	9.3	8.0
Services per capita	2.1	5.6	5.8	3.2	1.9	4.1
Expenditures per patient	8.7	11.6	6.8	9.1	7.6	10.0
Population	3.4	1.1	0.0	2.3	2.9	1.6
Expenditures per capita	9.5	13.1	8.5	10.0	8.7	11.0
Patients	4.2	2.5	1.6	3.2	4.0	2.5
Services	5.6	6.7	5.8	5.5	5.0	5.7

Source: Annual Reports of AHCIP 1973-89

Figure 9 focuses on the role played by the growth in population as well as on some of the other variables shown in Figure 8. This type of breakdown, although useful, is misleading when it is the only specification used to identify the factors accounting for increases in Medicare costs. The important role physicians play in affecting medical care spending is not highlighted, and the important links between physician supply and medical costs and utilization are missed. If the role of physicians in impacting medical care utilization and costs is not spelled out explicitly, the lead actor is missing from the Medicare play.

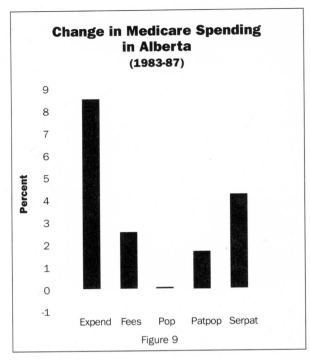

Figure 9

Decomposing Medicare Costs During the "Boom" and the "No Growth" Periods[9]

We next compare: (1) a boom period (1973-81) where a high rate of population growth prevails and the growth in the physician stock almost matches the growth in population; and (2) a so-called "no economic growth era" (1981-87) where some modest population growth is attained and the rate of growth in the supply of physicians is maintained at a record high level. Figure 10, derived from Table 6, provides a visual representation of the change in costs. The following points should be noted:

(1) The population to physician ratio fell rapidly through-

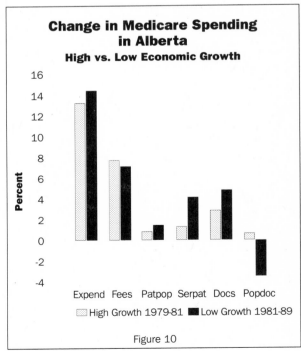

Figure 10

out 1981-87 because of a low rate of population growth and a high rate of growth in the supply of physicians. During the boom period the ratio actually rose slightly (approximately 0.5% per annum) as a result of the relatively higher rate of growth in the population vis-à-vis the stock of physicians. The population to physician ratio exhibited great stability during the high growth period (1973-81), varying by only 5% (832 to 794). In the low growth period the ratio ranged from a high of 833 to a low of 670 people per physician – a variation of approximately 24%;

(2) The rate at which the population was medicalized (the rate at which the patient to population ratio grew) during the "no growth era" was almost 75% higher than during the economic boom when the rate of growth in physician supply was markedly lower;

(3) The rate at which the intensity of the servicing of patients grew was 3.2 times greater during 1981-87, when the rate of growth in physician supply was high and the patient and population to physician ratios were declining, than during the boom period when the population to physician and patient to physician ratios were rising because of the more moderate rate of expansion in the number of physicians joining the Medicare plan;

(4) The rate of increase in the number of services rendered per physician (the so-called physician productivity ratio) was approximately 44% higher in the boom period when physicians were scarcer than in the no growth period when the supply was expanding rapidly; and

(5) The rate of increase in fees was approximately 6.5% lower in 1981-87 relative to 1973-81; however, the average rate of increase in total expenditures was approximately 8% higher during the low growth period in the 1980s as compared to the boom period. It is important to remember that real per capita spending on medical services in Alberta increased by 13.7% between 1973 and 1981, when the rate of growth of the population and the stock of physicians within the province was virtually balanced, and by 38.3% between 1981 and 1987 in the high physician growth low population growth period.[10] Indeed, it can be shown that between 1975 and 1982 real per capita spending on medical care was virtually stable, with only a 5.5% increase in costs.

HEALTH CARE ECONOMIC POLICY CONCLUSIONS[11]

The theme of this conference is *Restructuring Canada's Health Services System: How Do We Get There From Here?* The objective of this paper was to examine certain of the health care economics data garnered from almost 20 years of experience in operating a medical care insurance plan in the Province of Alberta to determine whether these data provided insights which could be used to formulate health care economic policies that would be of use in dealing with current problems and/or initiating long run reforms to the system.

STABILIZING REAL MEDICAL EXPENDITURES PER CAPITA AND THE POPULATION TO PHYSICIAN RATIO

The first lesson to be drawn is that it is possible to stabilize the aggregate population to physician ratio and the levels of real per capita expenditures on medical care and run a medical care system which is considered to meet the needs of the population and is popular with the public and acceptable to the overwhelming majority of the profession. The period between 1974 and 1982, which encompasses 40% of the time a publicly funded system has been operated within the Province of Alberta, provides concrete support for the contention that stable population to physician ratios and stable real per capita expenditures are attainable goals which can be made an integral part of a new macroeconomic medical care policy for the province.

What happens if no policies are developed to stabilize the industry in a nation with a high rate of growth in physician manpower? The second major lesson to be learned from the Alberta experience is that unless a province adopts an active policy which limits the rate of entry of medical practitioners into its Medicare plan, the province can only hope that its economy's rate of growth will be high enough to keep its population to physician ratio and its real expenditures per capita constant. Once the economy falters or stagnates and the rate of population growth falls, the high rate of growth in the number of physicians entering the plan will perturb the equilibrium and trigger off a round of rising service intensities, increased medicalization of the population, and rising real medical costs per capita. The natural experiment occurring in the province between 1983 and 1987, when the physician supply increased by approximately 20% and the population remained relatively unchanged, illustrates this phenomenon.

How do we get from here to there in controlling the rate of increase in the number of physicians per 1,000 population and the real per capita costs of Medicare? Suggestions have included eliminating fee-for-service as a means of remunerating physicians, drastically reducing physician earnings, closing or reducing the capacity of a certain number of medical schools, and restricting billing numbers or the number of licences issued. Although some of these proposals have been tried, after approximately 18 years an effective medical manpower policy has still not been put in place. Medical costs per capita and the rates at which the population is being serviced continue to mount. If past experience is any guide, the manpower issue is not likely to be resolved voluntarily unless cuts in the real dollar level of federal transfers coupled with rising provincial budget deficits force one or more provinces to tackle the problem head-on. However, "getting from here to there" is likely to be more noisy and time consuming since the loss by the government of British Columbia of its court battle with organized medicine over the imposition of limitations on the issuance of Medicare billing numbers. At this point, most of the other Canadian provinces appear to be in limbo as far as controlling the number of new entrants into their plans is concerned. Until new strategies are devised to control the supply of medical practitioners, all a wary provincial treasurer and minister of health can do is to ensure that medical insurance plan budgets are fixed and that the existing members of the profession share in at least some of the fiscal pain created by the unnecessarily high production of medical practitioners within the nation. This may raise the interest if not the outright curiosity of the members of the profession living in provinces whose open-ended Medicare budgets have sheltered them from the consequences of the rapid growth in the number of new individuals entering their industry.

NOTES

1. The population measures used in this report consist of Alberta Health Care Insurance Plan (AHCIP) registrations, since these registrations are viewed as providing a better estimate of population changes in years when there was no national census. Alberta joined the national Medical Care Insurance Plan on July 1, 1969. Given the "normal" start-up problems faced by the plan, it is customary to base the earliest data series on the year 1971; however, it should be noted that a number of key medical economic series are based on the reforms to the AHCIP information system that were implemented in 1972-73, thus restricting the time lines of certain types of analyses.

2. A positive balance implies that government expenditures exceeded revenues. A negative sign denotes the existence of a surplus.

3. The price mechanism has been effectively banned as a means of restricting access to medical services in Alberta since October 1986. Before that time extra-billing was permitted, affecting access to certain services by certain groups of individuals in certain regions of the province. However, the vast bulk of medical services were not extra-billed and the majority of physicians did not engage in the practice. Although prices have played a limited role in affecting consumer access to medical services, it should not be forgotten that the supply-side response between prices and the quantity and mix of services provided by medical practitioners still exists.

4. A single equation double log regression consisting of real medical expenditures as the dependent variable and population, the number of Medicare physicians, and the patient to population ratio as the independent variables yielded estimates for 1973-89 of 0.48 for population, 0.80 for the physician supply variable, and 1.54 for the patient population variable – a proxy for the extensiveness with which the medical care system is used by the population within a given year. All the estimated coefficients were significant at the 1% level. $R^2 = 0.99$ and the Durbin Watson statistic = 2.1, indicating an absence of autocorrelation at a 1% level of significance. Each estimate is an elasticity which measures the percentage change in real medical care spending resulting from a change in a specific variable, holding all the other factors constant. In this simple model both the population and physician supply estimates are inelastic, while the patient population is elastic and markedly larger than either of the other two variables.

5. For the purposes of this study, it is sufficient to use the physician count recorded in the annual reports of the AHCIP. The ratio of part- to full-time physicians is relatively stable in Alberta; this is not true, however, in all of the other provinces. Refer to the report entitled *Full-time Equivalent Physicians: Interprovincial Comparisons,* National Health and Welfare, Ottawa, January 1990 for a thorough discussion and analysis of full- and part-time practitioners.

It should be noted that the selection of a full-time equivalent is a matter of judgment. Numerous investigators can create different physician manpower series depending on both the definitions and techniques employed. If a standard such as that proposed by Health and Welfare was adopted in Alberta, we would have a standard series which could be used in all reports and studies carried out within the province. Until that happens it is simpler, if it is believed the part- and full-time ratios are stable, to use the AHCIP numbers and allow different vested interest groups to generate their own manpower series from the AHCIP data.

The reader should rest assured that the large increase in the physician supply which occurred in the 1980s can not simply be explained away as a part-time phenomenon. The percentage increase reported by Health and Welfare for full-time equivalents in Alberta, which encompassed all the medical and surgical specialities as well as general practice between 1983 and 1987, amounted to approximately 16%, while the increase for all physicians, part- and full-time, amounted to 17.5%.

6. Extra-billing was eliminated in the fall of 1986, with an equivalent dollar level of compensation added to AHCIP funding.

7. The most useful way to decompose the percentage change in medical expenditures for the purposes of this paper is as follows:

Change in Medical Care Expenditures = Change in Fees + Change in the Ratio of Discrete Patients to the Total Population + Change in the Number of Medical Services Rendered to a Patient + Change in the Number of Physicians Billing the Plan + Change in the Population to Physician Ratio. This is abbreviated in the graphical presentation as: (i) Expend = Fees + Patpop + Serpat + Docs + Popdoc, where each term is defined as above and the change referred to is in percentage terms.

A number of other decompositions of the percentage change in total medical expenditures can be made. Two of the most commonly encountered ones are:
(ii)   Expend = Fees + Pop + Serpat + Patpop; and
(iii) Expend = Fees + Pop + Docpop + Serdoc, where Pop is the registrations recorded by AHCIP, Docpop is the annual percentage change in the doctor to population ratio, and Serdoc is the number of medical services rendered per physician.

8. Both the population to physician and the patient to physician ratios fell markedly.

9. The so-called boom period in the Alberta economy is truncated, confined to the period 1973-81, for the purposes of the medical care analysis, because earlier data to develop some of the key medical series listed in Table 6 were not available. The so-called "no growth" period simply refers to the 1981-87 period where real GDP per capita remained approximately the same between both end points.

10. The demarcation of the high and low economic growth periods is based on a consideration of changes as well as the actual level of real GDP per capita. Population growth does not precisely match the movements in real GDP. This means that in reality the high population high physician growth period ends in 1982, not in 1981. The Alberta population continued to grow for one year into the recession.

11. It is important to note that this paper has not attempted to forge any explicit links between the macro dimensions of medical manpower and health status outcomes. We cannot link these macro variables both because the requisite data base has not been developed and because agreement on the relevant indicators to be included in an aggregate health status index for Alberta has not been reached. Standard morbidity and mortality measures are not suitable substitute surrogates for health status.

REFERENCES

Evans RG: *Strained Mercy: The Economics of Canadian Health Care*. Toronto: Butterworths, 1984.

Government of Alberta: *Alberta Statistical Review, Third Quarter, 1990*.

Government of Alberta: *Alberta Economic Accounts, 1989*. Edmonton, Alberta: Bureau of Statistics.

Government of Alberta: *Annual Reports of the Health Care Insurance Plan, Alberta Health, 1971-89*. Edmonton, Alberta.

Health and Welfare Canada: *Full-time Equivalent Physicians*. Health and Welfare Canada, 1991.

Health and Welfare Canada: *Payment Schedule Increases, Medical Care Insurance Plans*. Health and Welfare Canada, 1987.

Horne J (ed.): *Proceedings of the Third Canadian Conference on Health Economics*. University of Manitoba, 1987.

PHYSICIAN REMUNERATION: FEE-FOR-SERVICE MUST GO, BUT THEN WHAT?

Charles J. Wright
Vancouver General Hospital

INTRODUCTION

The current fee-for-service system of physician remuneration causes gross inequity in physicians' remuneration from specialty to specialty, disproportionate recognition of procedures, undervaluing of counselling services, and disincentives to productivity in all activities other than clinical, such as medical education, planning, and both clinical and laboratory research.

The remuneration system must be re-examined in the light of increasing accountability and responsibility of physicians and in recognition of the inappropriate incentives which the current system encourages.

THE RELATIONSHIP BETWEEN METHOD OF REMUNERATION AND SERVICES

The issue of incentives is fundamental in the choice of a method of remuneration for physicians' services in a health care system.

Does an itemized fee-for-service system encourage the provision of services that are medically unnecessary? There are those who would respond that this is an insulting question suggesting unethical and unprofessional behaviour. On the other hand, the intuitive response is otherwise. Physicians may consciously augment personal income in this manner or the process may be entirely unconscious because of the lack of definition of what constitutes a "necessary" service.

Does a salaried or contractual payment system tend to discourage physicians' "productivity"? Again, there are those who would respond that this is an insulting question and others who would agree that it is not reasonable to expect physicians to work as hard under such a system as they would under fee-for-service. It is an interesting paradox that many physicians so strenuously deny the implication of the first question, but have no trouble in agreeing with the second, in spite of the fact that these two responses are entirely contradictory. In other words, there are physicians who would claim that the itemized fee-for-service system does not cause them to provide unnecessary services, but argue that a salaried system would cause them to slack off.

There has been much discussion about the effect of the remuneration system on the quality and quantity of services provided (Evans, 1984), but there is little information on the subject from experimental models. There is some evidence for the "target income" concept, namely that physicians in a fee-for-service system will design their practice and services rendered to generate income within a predetermined range (Rice, 1983), and there is now strong evidence on the question from a serendipitous experiment recently reported from Denmark. Krasnik and his colleagues (1990) examined the provision of services in Copenhagen before and after the introduction of a fee-for-service system with appropriate indexing of services and controlled data. They found a moderate increase in the number of consultations, a large increase in the number of diagnostic and treatment services provided, and a significant reduction in the incidence of referral to specialists and to hospital.

They also found evidence in support of the "target income" hypothesis. It is tempting to observe that that which is obviously true can sometimes be proven.

WHAT IS THE "NEED" FOR CARE AS OPPOSED TO THE "DEMAND"?

If it is considered that the fee-for-service system stimulates the provider to greater activity, this result would be desirable if the services being provided are necessary. Accusations that physicians are providing unnecessary medical services or "over-servicing" usually generate a vigorous reaction. An understanding of the difference between "need" and "demand" is necessary in this debate, and this will become the key issue in the evolution of clinical resource management (or utilization management, as it is often called). The *need* for health care should be determined by population demographics, biological and epidemiological features of disease, and the establishment of clinical management guidelines. On the other hand, the *demand* for health care relates to the cultural background of the population, patients' expectations, media hype and, as we have seen above, physicians' decisions concerning both disease management and generation of income.

The most difficult of the requirements for establishing need is developing a consensus on clinical management standards. This is often regarded as a very threatening activity, but more and more physicians are now realizing that the issue is one of quality patient care, not of restraint, interference, or external control. Quality patient care cannot even be defined without clinical management standards because of the huge range of controversies in clinical practice in almost every area of human disease.

QUALITY AND FAIRNESS

Quality patient care implies not only appropriate care when required but protection from iatrogenic disease. Experience has also taught that quality patient care in the long run requires protection of the individual physician's time, stimulation of continuing medical education, a team approach to health care, and incentives for teaching and research. Which method of remuneration is most likely to encourage these objectives?

The remuneration system should be fair and equitable for physicians. Given a fair commitment, reasonable industry, and useful activity in the health care system, it may be argued that a differential of 100% or even 200% in personal income among physicians is fair and equitable. It may not be argued that a differential of up to 1500% is reasonable, and yet this is the situation in which we find ourselves today with the procedurally-based fee schedules. The fact that the current system renders it possible for certain individuals in certain specialties to bill $1 million annually should be an outrage to the vast majority of physicians who earn less than 1/6 of that sum. In simple terms, the fee schedules are grossly unfair. The current egregious anomalies could not exist under any type of fee-for-time as opposed to fee-for-service system, even with adequate recognition of differences in skills, training, hours of work, effort, etc.

ALTERNATIVE REMUNERATION SYSTEMS

Alternatives to fee-for-service include salary, contract, sessional payments, and capitation fees. It is obvious that problems can exist with any payment system and the decision should be based on an attempt to incentivise desirable outcomes. What system is most likely to encourage health care service by need rather than demand, stimulate the development of clinical management standards, facilitate physician participation in resource management, foster teaching and research, and generate a team approach? The alternative methods are not mutually exclusive and each will have a place to meet local circumstances. Each of them avoids the perverse incentives created by the fee-for-service system in encouraging service by demand, emphasis on intervention, and a climate designed to encourage entrepreneurs rather than team players.

Potential benefits of letting go of the itemized fee-for-service system include equitable remuneration specialty to specialty, security of income and benefits, a less interventive approach to health care in general and, arguably, less iatrogenic disease.

NATIONAL GUIDELINES BUT LOCAL DESIGN

There are many different practice settings in which these objectives can be fulfilled. Any attempt to impose a national and uniform practice system is doomed to failure, since local initiatives may require a wide variety of different organizations including health maintenance organizations, community health centres, comprehensive health organizations, multi-specialty group practices, clinical practice plans, or partnership plans.

In eliminating fee-for-service as the model for physician remuneration, national legislation will be required to establish guidelines as a framework within which provinces can design mechanisms to meet local needs. These guidelines should mandate the following directions to the provincial legislative bodies:

1. There should be no direct payment for items of service.
2. All appropriate physician activities must be recognized, including clinical care, teaching, and research.
3. A relative value scale must be developed to deal with different types of specialty and subspecialty activity.
4. Service expectations should be defined.
5. Mechanisms must be developed for handling expenses of practice, insurance, pension, and benefits.
6. Physician involvement in the local management structure must be emphasized.
7. Reporting relationships between the group and the health facility, the university, or the ministry as appropriate must be defined.
8. A mechanism for periodic review of levels of compensation and benefits must be defined.

Within the framework of these national guidelines, there would be considerable scope for local initiative in the design and definition of groups, base income, system of incentives in the compensation package, management and reporting structure, communication, and participation systems for members.

THE PHYSICIAN AS CHANGE AGENT

Physicians have not always demonstrated great visual acuity for the writing on the wall. We have tended to be dragged after public opinion rather than leading it. It is important that we do not ignore the lessons of Saskatchewan in 1962, or Quebec in 1969, or Ontario in 1986. We do not seem to realize how the public currently views the perceived range of physicians' incomes and the entrepreneurship that generates them. We are having difficulty with the trend towards accountability. We tend to find the concept of clinical management standards threatening. We still tend to resent any external influence on what we should do and how we should do it. The fee-for-service system militates against the adaptability and the openness to change currently required to meet the challenges to the health care system. The provincial studies from Alberta, Saskatchewan, Ontario, Quebec, and Nova Scotia have all recommended revised remuneration systems for physicians. The provincial medical associations, which carry major responsibility for negotiating the remuneration system with the Ministries of Health, are manifestly incapable of any significant change away from the current system because of their constituency representative structure.

New Canadian legislation will be required to facilitate the provincial changes which will be necessary to maintain uniform accessibility and standards in the country. We must face up to the perversity of the incentives created by the current itemized fee-for-service schedule. As with other inevitable changes, we should read the writing on the wall, strive for the best arrangement possible within the changing structure, and accept the pressures to change as an opportunity for growth and development rather than as a threat.

NOTE
A subsequent version of this paper has been published as:
Wright CJ: The fee-for-service system should be replaced. *Canadian Medical Association Journal* 144:900-903, 1991.

REFERENCES
Evans RG: *Strained Mercy: The Economics of Canadian Health Care.* Toronto: Butterworths, 1984.

Krasnik A, Groenewegen PP, Pedersen PA et al: Changing remuneration systems: effects on activity in general practice. *British Medical Journal* 300:1698-1701, 1990.

Rice TH: The impact of changing medicare reimbursement rates on physician-induced demand. *Medical Care* 21:803-815, 1983.

DISCUSSION
Chair: Jim Tsitanidis
Manitoba Health

Participant

I'd like to ask Morris Barer whether there is any move within the Ministry towards date of service data collection on an annual basis, versus date of payment?

Morris Barer (University of British Columbia)

As far as I know – and I should actually defer to my Ministry colleague here – but as far as I know, because the Ministry's administrative systems are set up to pay claims, the claims payment data will still be processed by date of payment. Whether in fact there are any plans within the Ministry to provide annual processing on a date of service basis, I really don't have any idea. Do you, Nick [Haazen]? [inaudible response from Haazen.]

Okay, so there is now inside the Ministry the capability, simply because of utilization caps. In order to monitor what goes on with utilization, the Ministry has to have the capability to track monthly date of service-based information.

Going back 10 years, however, we still had to do all the processing ourselves.

Raisa Deber (University of Toronto)

Do you have any information as to which of these policies work? Which of these policies might be effective?

Morris Barer

What does "work" mean? I think it's really too early to be able to tell. We just haven't gone in far enough. You really have to look at this thing in much more detail, to adjust simultaneously for all the things that might have been going on, to be able to say anything. If in fact you've got a utilization cap, and you make it binding, it's going to work in terms of the narrow objective of controlling expenditure. What's happened, I think, in B.C. to date has been that utilization caps haven't been on for an extended period. Early on they were relatively loose, and because they were partial caps there was still room for a fair bit of slippage. Furthermore, they have to be negotiated again every year. In what we have seen so far, we cannot identify any particular effect that one could attribute to a billing numbers policy's being on or off, and there may be a variety of reasons for that. But at this point, it's really hard to know.

Don MacNaught (Health and Welfare Canada)

Isn't it true, Morris, that as a starting point, B.C. had the biggest problem in Canada, so deriving any generalized conclusions for the rest of Canada based on B.C.'s relative medical care bill is somewhat suspect?

Morris Barer

Well, it depends on what sort of conclusion you are trying to generalize. It is true that B.C. had the largest physician supply and the highest fees. That does not, I think, mean that you can't generalize if you are able to, in fact, ascertain at the end of this project that fee controls do or don't bite, that utilization caps or targets do or don't work, that having controls on physician supply does or does not have an effect on utilization within a particular supply range. While B.C. was the worst off, there were enough other provinces that were in relatively similar situations that I think at the end of this you will be able to generalize to some extent.

Peter Ruderman (Toronto)

I was just wondering if anyone in B.C. has attempted to look at a balancing off between the physician care and the hospital care and the way one might have been utilized or influenced by the other. It struck me over the years that compared to other provinces you have always had the leanest hospital system, with fewer nursing hours per patient and lots of other factors, and I was wondering to what degree nominal overutilization of physician care may really be doing automatically what many people have urged in other provinces as policy, which is moving away from inpatient care to ambulatory care?

Morris Barer

How long have I got? It is true that in B.C., along with all these medical policy initiatives, there has been a massive shift away from acute care to longer term and extended care. As to whether the two things are related, I think you would actually have to go and talk to people in the Ministry. If you're hypothesizing a deliberate set of coordinated policies, I'm not sure. I think you really would have to talk to people in the Ministry who were active at the time.

Peter Ruderman

I'm giving you a research question.

Morris Barer

Thanks, Peter, I don't have enough of those.

Michael Alberti (British Columbia Ministry of Health)

Richard, I was interested in your comment that medical services were received by about 6% more people at the end of the period.

Richard Plain (University of Alberta)

Yes, we serviced them more intensively. The patient to population ratio increased more from 1983-1987 than it did from 1972-1982.

Michael Alberti

Given that at the start of the period there was a good medical infrastructure already in place, I was wondering if you knew anything about who made up this group of 6%.

Richard Plain

No. As I say, this deals with the system taken as a whole – the macroeconomic perspective – the great "whys" – these are good questions for later investigations.

Michael Alberti

And with this increase of 605 Medicare physicians, was there an improvement in the rural/urban split, or did most of these new physicians concentrate in the already well serviced areas?

Richard Plain

I can give you my impressions. We're still trying to devise new systems in Alberta to get more of our physicians from the urban out into the rural areas. The problem is still there. Whether patients are better off or worse off in terms of health status outcomes in the under- vis-à-vis the over-doctored areas is not known. But there are perceived shortages amidst all this plenitude of increased numbers of practitioners entering the provincial Medicare system. It is useful to note the comments of Roy le Riche, former Registrar of the College of Physicians and Surgeons, regarding attracting physicians to rural areas. If you're going to get a physician out in many of those areas, what you need to do is either ensure that a new graduate comes from a rural area or that he or she marries someone from a rural community.

Morris Barer

I guess you've noticed how fast British Columbians are. I've got a bunch of different questions, none of which you will be able to answer, but I'll ask them anyway.

Richard Plain

I appreciate this. I do penance in other ways, you know.

Morris Barer

Is there any sense yet from the data as to the extent to which the increased utilization came from more patients being seen, as opposed to patients being serviced more intensively? I don't know whether I missed something in what you said there. Number one. Number two, do you have any impression yet as to how the increased utilization distributed itself across age groups and/or across types of service? And number three, can you give us some sense of how the increase in physician supply distributed by specialty of physician?

Richard Plain

Yes, yes, and no. The first one – What would be really useful is that study that was done by Bob [Evans] and Pascoe and Roch in Manitoba. I have only the patient population ratio and servicing intensity data for the system as a whole. The Manitoba study would be an important follow-up to this study. With respect to the last one, in terms of the specialty breakdown, no, I haven't included that detail of analysis. This is still just the highly aggregated one. In terms of the age and sex specific question, I do have the nominal and real data. This is one of the issues I am looking at. I was glad to hear of your work on the indices, but we need age and sex specific indices. But if you do something crude like taking the aggregate index and just running it across all age-sex groups, I do have the constant as well as nominal dollar changes in each of the areas. In terms of the broad aggregates, there has been a slight shift to more female components in the nominal side in terms of servicing. But it's probably small and may not be significant.

Robert Evans (University of British Columbia)

My questions were twofold. The first one overlaps partly with your reply to Morris. Just to remind you that when we were looking at the Manitoba data during the 1970s, where there was a stable population and a rapid increase in physician supply, we did find most of the physician supply increase in Winnipeg. But the interesting thing was that while the volume of servicing per capita – the intensity of servicing – went up, the intensity of servicing per patient on each physician's rolls did not go up to anything like the same degree. Rather than each physician serving a smaller and smaller group of patients and servicing them more intensively, what happened was that the same physical flesh and blood person wound up on the rolls of a lot larger number of physicians. So that a *de facto* networking, or a sort of an implicit group practice pattern, seemed to emerge. I am quite serious about that. There was a higher degree of – depending on which way you look at it – patient sharing that went on, in order to fill in the larger number of physicians, so that it wasn't a more competitive market. If anything, it was a more integrated market where there were more physicians in place. And it would be very interesting to know if that finding persisted in Alberta, if that's a common situation or whether it was just peculiar to Manitoba. Because I think it would change significantly – it should affect significantly – our sense of how you get from here to there, in the sense of how you get from more physicians to more utilization. So that was my first query on the 'how you get from here to there' side.

The second one, which is, "How is it that you don't get from here to there?", why would you appoint as head of a committee to deal with this problem the dean of that medical school which is probably most at risk if one were to change one's manpower policy?

Richard Plain

Bob, neither you nor I had any hand in that appointment, did we?

Robert Evans

No, but this again is a general phenomenon that was documented by Lomas et al in that Ontario Economic Council study, that governments have consistently turned for advice on this subject to groups who, even a very amateurish political scientist could be fairly sure, would not give them the advice that they seem to want. Now this may be a question for our political science colleagues, rather than for naive economists: Why is the system so locked up that you consistently find this kind of pattern of seeking advice where you know you won't get it, and then winding up doing nothing? It's not consistent with the view that says that there really is a considerable amount of economic pain out there and that somebody really actually wants to deal with the problem. And I'd be interested in your reaction.

Richard Plain

In industrial economics, I guess we call it regulatory capture, but I would indicate that our existing deputy minister is the first civilian we have had for quite a while. The previous two deputy ministers were past presidents of the Alberta Medical Association and the Canadian Medical Association. In fact, in 1982, in that period where we had the most rapid escalation in fee adjustments, the head of the medical association became the deputy minister.

And I've been waiting for the president of the nurses' association to get her chance; however, no offers have been extended to her. I guess the current deputy minister is doing quite a good job. In part, though, it's a traditional thing. You know, it's fine for economists to make criticisms based on economic concerns over conflicts of interest; however, appointing a medical practitioner to a senior administrative post has been a traditional political response to try to tie the medical profession more closely with the provincial Medicare plan. One can't make a blanket statement that all medical personnel will act in the profession's rather than the public's interest. I don't want to leave the impression that the only good people are non-medical people. However, it is true that an individual's views on the policy front will tend to be seen through the eyes of the profession in which they have been trained. That's why it is very important to get a balanced input and why with outsiders participating, questions will arise which will require new consensuses to be reached and new policy options to be considered. Utilizing medical practitioners in senior administrative positions does not necessarily mean there is a conspiracy to do people in. I can think of a number of practitioners who have been quite major in reforming a number of areas.

Participant

I have a comment which may be a little bit unorthodox in this present context. Most of what you've looked at is based on physician supply and data intrinsic to payment, and so forth. I have a comment with regards to one of the data you indicated. Unemployment in Alberta went up from 3% to 11%. Could the additional stress associated with that have resulted in people in Alberta simply having more illness? And of course you can't tell that from physician payment data, but you might want to look at data extrinsic to this, for instance, the various Canadian health surveys, to see if there has been a higher reported level of illness. That, I think, might be worthwhile taking into account.

Richard Plain

Those are all part of it, along with the point I made that a slightly more aged population was left in the province as a a result of interprovincial migrations during the recession. There are a number of factors to be considered in explaining the phenomenon. There is no one single factor. But remember this: It's a 20% increase in Medicare physicians within the four-year period. So it isn't just a utilization increase explained by the fact that people have more time to see the doctor or that they are more psychologically distressed concerning their ability to acquire or hold a job. The system has been shifted on all fronts in a significant way. That's the interesting part about this experiment – a large scale shift on the supply side with no change in the total population.

G.H. Platt (Alberta Health)

I found your overheads very interesting, in that I think we're all aware that the majority of physicians are family physicians and you showed almost no change in intensity there or in the number of services. The change seemed to be with lab and X-ray and things like that. Would it not be simpler to just close the labs and the X-ray units rather than change the physicians?

Richard Plain

I'm sorry, it was the speaker before me who had the slides.

G.H. Platt

Apologies. Have you looked at that aspect in Alberta?

Richard Plain

What I've done is provide the large macro overview. The issue Bob [Evans] and a number of you have been raising: "What's true about the individual parts and components?"... can't be answered at this stage. I certainly have my opinions. Opinions are very nice, but I haven't finished massaging the numbers.

Participant

I want Charles Wright to know that I'm asking this from the perspective of being a physician. I'd like to ask you, "Do you think you can turn utilization around and make it a good word, rather than the four-letter word that your panel has painted it this morning?" This is not for you, sir, necessarily, but for other members of the panel to address as well. An issue too was raised here this morning, I think by the gentleman standing to my right, suggesting that utilization, the way we've seen it and the way it's being painted, may be short term pain for long term gain. In other words, could it in fact reflect a utilization in the community as a decompression of what would have been utilized in institutions had it not occurred?

Charles Wright (Vancouver General Hospital)

I'm not sure if you want an answer from me. I agree with you. That's why I would like the term "utilization management" to disappear. It has a bad history, which means control, suppress, cut, reduce, diminish – and that's not what we are talking about. We are talking about what I am calling clinical resource management. We're talking quality. We're talking guidelines for quality care.

Peter Ruderman

It is very interesting, but I think that perhaps it's time to reintroduce a little bit of economics into the discussion. Twenty years ago I found myself very busy exhorting the members of the Ontario Medical Association who, like you, really felt that there was some intrinsic value of a physician's work that could be remunerated, or identified successfully, and they too were playing at the time with [such concepts as] responsibility and skill and time, and so on – relative value scales – which really didn't get very far, because the reply of the economist is, in the first instance, that the "appropriate amount of money" – and I don't want to call it compensation or fee – is "whatever induces physicians to do their job or keeps them from leaving". That's true in other markets as well, and I don't think that if you want to be an apostle of the market economy you should go much beyond that. On the other hand, if you wish to leave the market economy, then we can open the whole thing up. And again, I would like to say that we are apparently on the verge of rediscovering what were the current issues of 25 to 30 years ago. That's the privilege of somebody in my age group, perhaps. But if you go back to James Hogarth's book (*The Payment of the*

Physician; Some European Comparisons, 1963), he was covering many of these issues. He noted, for instance, under the capitation systems in England, the principal abuse was over-referral. He would not at all be surprised to find, when they shift the system of payment in Denmark, that they suddenly discover they don't have to refer things anymore, because now they get paid for doing them. And so on. What I would urge is that everybody interested in this issue do some serious library reading of the material that came out between 1948 and 1968, before wasting too much time on what are apparently new directions, but are really very old.

Charles Wright

I agree with you, and of course none of that market economy debate has anything whatever to do with fee-for-item-service, as opposed to fee-for-time, or however the compensation method is derived.

Participant

I guess Peter had preempted my question in some respects. I notice in many of your prescriptions for the future that a lot of the design was all inputs as opposed to outputs, as opposed to what you compensate for. I didn't notice anything about outcomes or that kind of thing as a basis for designing a remuneration/compensation or payment system.

Charles Wright

That's a huge area and a problem one, you know, going back to the Arabic notion of either the patient gets better or the physician loses his right hand as a disincentive to bad productivity. We're a long way from being able to relate activity to outcomes, but I think as we get into clinical resource management, utilization management – we need a new phrase, and I don't know what it is going to be – but that area is the only way to go.

Robert Evans

I guess a couple of aspects of economics. One, to remind Peter of the general theory of the second best, that it is true that in an economy characterized by markets all over the place, and with all of the conditions of perfect competition holding, we might want to establish compensation in the way that he described – in such a way that it was just sufficient to get physicians to be prepared to supply their services and no larger. And I suppose that would mean that whatever the payment method that was used, we would want to try to drive the incomes of physicians down to the point where the number of applicants to Canadian medical school places was just equal to the number of places, rather than exceeding it by 4 to 1. First of all, I don't think that's politically feasible, Peter. But secondly, again coming back to the general theory of the second best, I think you'd have to convince the rest of us first that the whole of the rest of the economy was characterized by those competitive conditions. And I was trying to think of other industries – certainly not education, certainly not agriculture, certainly not anything else in health care – I was trying to think of other industries where those competitive conditions hold. And if we can't think of very many of them – in fact if we can't think of N minus 1 of them – then that kind of argument doesn't go through. On the other hand, this is after all an economics meeting and one shouldn't be too rude about economics, and I think we do have something to reply to the physician who said, "Does utilization have to be a four-letter word?" And the answer to that has clearly got to be "no", that what we're talking about is the modification of utilization at the margin, and I do like your phrase about clinical resource management because it seems to me that that is the issue we are getting at, that when people like Dick Plain fuss about the increase in utilization, they are not really, I think, getting into bed with the clinical nihilists who would say that the best utilization is none at all. All they are really saying is that the marginal adjustments to utilization – very large in the case that Dick was looking at – those marginal adjustments, which seem to be unrelated to anything to do with patient need, may therefore be suspected of being unnecessary and perhaps in the class of four-letter words. As for the question of, "Are Albertans sicker because they are unemployed?", the answer to that, it seems to me, is, "Yeah, they probably are, but is there a corresponding falling utilization during the boom period? Or were they sicker then because of the advantages of having lots of money and lots of partying and so on and so forth? So that whatever happens to you, economically or socially, your needs are going to go up?"

Charles Wright
I don't think that there was a question in there, so I will agree with you.

REPORTS AND COMMISSIONS: LOOKING FOR DIRECTIONS

A GREAT CANADIAN PRESCRIPTION: TAKE TWO COMMISSIONED STUDIES AND CALL ME IN THE MORNING

Douglas E. Angus
Community Health and Epidemiology
Queen's University

INTRODUCTION

During the past few years in Canada, as witnessed by the frequency of major research undertakings sponsored by governments and/or associations, there has been intensive interest in the delivery of health care services. With provinces allocating anywhere between 1/4 and 1/3 of their total budgets to this publicly-funded system, governments are concerned about their ability to continue to pay for hospital and medical services. Adding to this concern is the realization that increased funding of this system will not necessarily do too much to reduce further disparities in the health status of Canadians. It appears that major re-thinking of this system is required.

Furthermore, the people affecting (and affected by!) this system are experiencing varying degrees of anxiety and apprehension created by an increasing number of pressures and uncertainties, i.e., demographics, technology diffusion, human resources planning, changing public needs and expectations, and structural problems related to the sector's organization, funding, and reimbursement (particularly of health care providers). All these issues have a significant impact upon the management of human and financial resources and upon the choices of directions for health care facilities and services.

It is not surprising, then, that since 1983-84 there have been an increasing number of health care Commissions and Task Forces across Canada. It is primarily for this reason that a review of the major Commissions was undertaken, with the underlying goal of determining their implications for the acute care hospital sector.

OBJECTIVES AND SCOPE

More specifically, the objectives of this undertaking were to:
- identify the major Commissions and Task Forces in Canada since 1983-84;
- designate their relevance and importance to the Canadian health care system; and
- analyze significant findings and identify common themes and discernible directions and trends affecting the acute care hospital sector.

This review focuses on those Commissions and Task Forces which seemed "significant in scope"; this category was defined to include most Commissions. The author then judged which of the various levels of Task Forces, Committees, Advisory Groups, Panels, and other groups would also be included. The three Associations that funded the original project provided useful suggestions as well.

The remainder of this paper is divided into two components. In the first, each of the Commissions, terms, and mandates is highlighted. (More detailed information on the specific terms of references and major recommendations or findings is reported elsewhere (Angus, 1991)). In the next section, the major common themes, directions, and trends are analyzed for their implications for the acute care hospital sector in Canada.

MAJOR COMMISSIONS AND TASK FORCES

In highlighting the major characteristics of each Commission, we go geographically from east to west.

NEWFOUNDLAND

A. **Commission and term:** Royal Commission on Hospital and Nursing Home Costs, April 1983 - February 1984.

Composition: David B. Orsborn (chair), Paul Patey, M.D., Garfield A. Pynn.

Mandate: To hold an inquiry into the matters related to the reasons for increasing costs in hospitals and nursing homes and on the efficiency or otherwise of these institutions and to make recommendations for the improved efficiency and for the generation of additional revenue.

B. **Commission and term:** A Green Paper on Our Health Care System Expenditures and Funding, January 1986, no term specified.

Composition: J.F. Collins, Minister of Finance, Hugh Twomey, M.D., Minister of Health.

Mandate: To give detailed attention to health care expenditures and the means of financing them. This paper was prepared to give information and, of even greater importance, to stimulate discussion.

C. **Commission and term:** Advisory Committee on Nursing Workforce, June 1987, no term specified.

Composition: Joan Dawe (chair), Jeanette Andrews, Primrose Bishop, Heather Hawkins, Roy Manuel, Alice Murphy, Gladys Peachey, Ada E. Simms.

Mandate: To assess Newfoundland's nursing human resource requirements and examine issues regarding the recruitment and retention of nurses.

NEW BRUNSWICK

A. **Commission and term:** Commission on Selected Health Care Programs, January - June 1989.

Composition: E. Neil McKelvey, Q.C. and Sr. Bernadette Levesque, R.N. (co-chairs), Dr. Victor McLaughlin, Mr. Gilles Lepage.

Mandate: To review selected health care programs in the province and to report the findings and make appropriate recommendations related to the terms of reference.

B. **Commission and term:** Nursing Resources Advisory Committee, term unspecified.

Composition: Unknown.

Mandate and terms of reference: To study issues related to quality of worklife of nurses in New Brunswick and to develop recommendations and an action plan for improving quality of working life for nurses within the health care system.

NOVA SCOTIA

A. **Commission and term:** Nova Scotia Royal Commission on Health Care, term unspecified.

Composition: Mr. J. Camille Gallant (chair), Mr. George L. White (secretary/legal counsel), The Right Reverend G. Russell Hatton, Mr. Edward M. MacNeil, Ms. Sharon Marshall, R.N., Dr. Earle L. Reid.

Mandate: To examine the financing and delivery of health services in the province.

QUEBEC

A. Commission and term: Commission d'Enquête sur les Services de Santé et les Services Sociaux, January 1986 - December 1987.

Composition: Dr. Jean Rochon (chair), Harvey Barkun, Janine Bernatchez-Simard, Roger Bertrand, Jean-Pierre Duplantie, Norbert Rodrigue.

Mandate: To evaluate the operation and financing of the health and social services system in meeting its objectives.

ONTARIO

A. Commission and term: Minister's Advisory Group on Health Promotion, October 1984 - October 1987.

Composition: Mr. Steve Podborski (chair), Dr. Maurice Jette, Ms. Marilyn Knox, Mr. Norman Panzica, Dr. Andrew Pipe, Dr. Stuart Robbins, Ms. Nancy Shosenberg.

Mandate: To develop and recommend health promotion directions and strategies for the Province of Ontario.

B. Commission and term: Ontario Health Review Panel, November 1986 - June 1987.

Composition: Dr. John R. Evans (chair), Ms. Mathilde F. Bazinet, R.N., Dr. Alexander MacPherson, Dr. Murray McAdam, Sr. Winnifred McLoughlin, R.N., Ms. Rose Rubino, Dr. Hugh E. Scully, Prof. Greg L. Stoddart, Mr. W. Vickery Stoughton.

Mandate: To review and recommend a general direction for health in Ontario and to identify some specific issues to be examined further in order to strengthen, improve, and guide the evolution of health and health care in the Province of Ontario.

C. Commission and term: Panel on Health Goals for Ontario, November 1986 - August 1987.

Composition: Prof. Robert Spasoff (chair), Peter Cole, Floyd Dale, David Korn, Pran Manga, Victor Marshall, Frances Picherack, Nancy Shosenberg, Lorne Zon.

Mandate: To provide advice to the Minister...regarding health goals for Ontario. The goals are to be linked to appropriate data and stated in a way which will facilitate planning for their achievement.

D. Commission and term: Premier's Council on Health Strategy, term unspecified.

Composition: Hon. David Peterson (Premier) (chair), Elinor Caplan (Minister of Health) (vice-chair), Dr. Martin Barkin (Deputy Minister of Health) (secretary), Dr. Terry Sullivan (executive director), cross-section of members, numbering about 30.

Mandate: To develop a long term strategy for health in Ontario.

E. Commission and term: Conjoint Review Committee, June - July 1988.

Composition: Mr. David Corder, ADM, Ministry of Health (chair), included members/representatives of the Ministry of Health, Ontario Medical Association, Ontario

Council of Administrators of Teaching Hospitals, Ontario Nurses' Association, and Ontario Hospital Association.

Mandate: To review the operations of the designated hospitals with the aim of determining what factors have led to the deficit positions, why these have occurred, and how they have been managed.

F. **Commission and term:** Task Force on the Use and Provision of Medical Services, term unspecified.

Composition: Graham W.S. Scott, Q.C. (chair), Ms. Mary Catherine Lindberg, Dr. Adam Linton, Mr. Mark McElwain, Dr. David Peachy, Dr. Dennis Psutka, Dr. Walter Rosser, Dr. Gerry Rowland, Mr. Darrel Weinkauf.

Mandate: To help identify and quantify the factors responsible for the use and provision of medical services.

G. While not tied specifically to any of the above Commissions, the Ministry of Health and the Ontario Hospital Association each released reports which have some implications for future health care delivery. First is a Discussion Paper released by the Ministry of Health in April 1989, *Deciding the Future of Our Health Care*. The paper concentrated on six areas:

- enhancing the role and responsibilities of consumers;
- strengthening community-based care;
- maintaining the role of public hospitals, including psychiatric and university teaching hospitals;
- integrating private sector strengths and resources;
- improving quality assurance and treatment effectiveness; and
- strengthening the team of physicians, nurses, and other health professionals.

The second report is a Research Paper, *The Future Role of Hospitals in Providing Care: Issues to Consider*, released by the Ontario Hospital Association in September 1989. The Paper was put together to promote discussion and dialogue among trustees, hospital staff, and communities about their institution's future role both individually and within their region. Most of the issues can be classified into four broad areas: Hospital Services, Health Care Workers, Hospitals Within the Health Care System, and Moving Into the Future.

H. **Commission and term:** Health Professions Legislation Review, November 1982, term unspecified.

Composition: Alan M. Schwartz (coordinator).

Mandate and terms of reference:

- to determine which currently regulated professions should continue to be regulated;
- to determine which currently unregulated professions should be regulated;
- to update the procedures in the Health Disciplines Act, primarily to "fine tune" procedures introduced in 1974;
- to incorporate any substantive reforms or additions considered appropriate;
- to extend the structural and procedural reforms introduced by the Health Disciplines Act to all other health professions to be regulated;
- to develop a new structure for all the legislation governing the health professions; and
- to settle outstanding issues in several professions.

I. **Commission and term:** Task Force on the Implementation of Midwifery in Ontario, January 1986, term unspecified.

Composition: Mary Eberts (chair), Alan Schwartz (vice-chair), Rachel Edney, Karyn Kaufman.

Mandate and terms of reference: To make recommendations with respect to:
- how midwifery should be practised in Ontario;
- how midwives should be educated;
- requirements for entry to practice, scope and standards of practice, and governance of the profession;
- the setting in which midwives should provide their services; and
- optimal relationships between midwives and physicians.

MANITOBA

A. **Commission and term:** Health Advisory Network Steering Committee, ongoing from December 1988; Steering Committee and Task Forces to have about six month life spans.

Composition: Dr. Arnold Naimark (chair), Brian Gudmundson (executive secretary), about a dozen representatives of the health care sector.

Mandate: To obtain advice through cooperative deliberation among representatives of various facets of the health care community on organization, administration, and financing of six specific health aspects, through establishment of task forces on:
- teaching hospitals cost review;
- Winnipeg hospital-role definition;
- extended treatment bed review/re-examination;
- rural health services;
- northern health services; and
- health services for the elderly.

SASKATCHEWAN

A. **Commission and term:** Saskatchewan Commission on Directions in Health Care, July 1, 1988 - March 30, 1990.

Composition: Dr. R.G. Murray (chair), Mr. Walter Podiluk (deputy chair and executive director), Mr. Morris A. Anderson, Ms. Berva Farr, Ms. Maureen L. Kurtz, Mr. Ernest E. Moen, Bishop B. Morand.

Mandate: The Commission was given the mandate to:
- investigate the full range of issues affecting the quality, availability, accessibility, and cost of health care services, with particular consideration of the differences between rural and urban communities;
- identify and give priority to emerging and long-term issues affecting health care delivery; and
- recommend policy options to the government on:
  - ways to improve health care delivery and the efficiency of the system while maintaining quality and accessibility of service, and
  - management of future health care delivery needs, including funding and servicing, education, technology, and training requirements.

ALBERTA

A. **Commission and term:** Advisory Committee on the Utilization of Medical Services, September 1987 - September 1989.

Composition: Dr. M. Watanabe (chair), Ms. Connie Cook, Dr. Robert C. Cooper, Ms. Marilyn Croon, Dr. C. Bruce Hatfield, Dr. D.J. Junk, Ms. Sandra E. Larsen, Dr. Dennis H.J. Linden, Dr. G. Fred MacDonald, Dr. G.A. MacKenzie, Mr. Scott Rowand, Ms. Sharon E. Snell, Dr. Donald E. Young.

Mandate: To follow up on the recommendations of the 1985 Utilization Committee Report and to advise the Minister on ways to reduce or control increases in the use of medical services.

B. **Commission and term:** Premier's Commission on Future Health Care for Albertans, December 1988 - December 1989.

Composition: Mr. Louis D. Hyndman, Q.C. (chair), Dr. T.A. McPherson (deputy chair/executive director), Dr. Joy Calkin, Dr. Ruth Collins-Nakai, Mr. Gene Murrant, Father Pat O'Byrne, Mrs. Carol Sneddon, Mr. Bill Sturgeon.

Mandate: To recommend a course of action to ensure that Alberta's health care system continues to be the best in Canada well into the next century.

NATIONAL

A. **Commission and term:** Task Force on the Allocation of Health Care Resources, June 1983 -1984.

Composition: Ms. Joan Watson (chair), The Honourable Pauline McGibbon, Dr. John O'Brien-Bell, Dr. Leon Richard, Mr. Roy Romanow, Q.C.

Mandate: To examine the allocation of health care resources in the face of an increasing elderly population and the explosion of new technology.

B. **Commission and term:** Committee on the Health Care of the Elderly, 1984 - 1987.

Composition: Dr. Dorothy C. Ley (chair), Dr. Aviam Mark Clarfield, Dr. Gordon Ferguson, Dr. Murray McAdam, Dr. Mark Schonfeld, Mr. Alan Warren, Dr. Gerald Zetter, Dr. Stuart Hampton (corresponding member).

Mandate: To examine the health care system for those over 65 and to develop proposals to correct the existing inequities and inadequacies that result in an unacceptable medical and social milieu.

COMMON THEMES, DIRECTIONS, AND TRENDS

This part of the paper synthesizes the major issues and trends with some element of commonality across the country. Recommendations and directions proposed by various Commissions which could have major implications for the acute care sector are of particular interest and importance.

FACTORS LEADING TO COMMISSIONS

Although it is not earth-shattering to note that major health care reviews have occurred in Canada, it is particularly interesting to observe that, since 1983, a wave of them has thundered across the country. Like the proverbial snowball rolling down a snow-covered hill, the number and pace of these major reviews increased quite dramatically as the decade wore on. Why? What are the factors behind the establishment of so many Commissions and Task Forces?

Invariably, when the mandate and terms of reference of each Commission are examined, concerns are seen about rising health care costs (including funding and revenue, efficiencies, effectiveness, and utilization); dissatisfaction with the existing organizational structure of health care delivery; requirements for human resources (particularly nurses and physicians); technology; and quality and accessibility of care. Although the order or emphasis of these issues varies from one Commission to the next, there is no doubt that fiscal concerns represent the major underlying thread. "Fiscality" is inextricably linked to issues related to human resources, technology, and alternative approaches to health care delivery. It becomes clear that factors related to the organizational structures of health care delivery (including the search for alternatives), followed by cost concerns (containment, funding and revenues, efficiencies, effectiveness, and utilization), and human resources were the key elements which precipitated the review process across the country.

SYNTHESIS OF RECOMMENDATIONS

What significant findings and recommendations have emerged, and specifically, which ones could have a bearing on the existing acute care hospital sector? For ease of presentation, recommendations have been grouped into five major sub-headings: Financial Resources, Human Resources, Organization, Management, and Other Issues and Trends.

Financial Resources

A few reviews expressed concern over the decreasing rate of growth of fiscal transfers from the federal to the provincial governments, received primarily under the terms of the Established Programs Financing Act. By and large, however, most of the Commissions seemed to accept this situation as a "given" and instead recommended a number of initiatives that would enhance cost controls, funding and revenues, efficiencies, and cost-effectiveness. Important recommendations to note are those with respect to the following directions:

- reduction in the number of acute care hospital beds and establishment of freezes on capital construction plans, construction of new hospitals, and budget and salary/fee increases;
- development of incentive programs for hospitals to become more efficient, i.e., allowing them to keep certain (or all) portions of "surpluses" and insisting that they absorb deficits (unless those deficits have occurred for strong and unavoidable reasons, e.g., demographics, legislative changes beyond hospitals' control for such requirements as "pay equity", the necessity to accommodate new occupational groups, or other unforeseen circumstances);
- consideration for such revenue-increasing options as payroll taxes, income surtaxes, corporation capital taxes, or even deficit financing (but not to be given too serious a consideration!); the small emphasis on other ways to increase revenues is likely a reflection of the reality that there are very few open avenues in this regard;
- global budgeting or modifications to global budgeting using, for example, the case mix approach as a basis for allocating budgets;

- examination of private sector management techniques for possible directions to take to improve efficiency;
- increasing the number of outpatient clinics as well as home care and community support services, providing additional funds for health promotion and illness/injury prevention, and substituting in-home services for inpatient services. Unlike previous eras, these proposals are not recommended as "add-ons"; it is very important to note that many of the reviews recommended *reallocating* existing financial resources to these alternatives;
- although not seeming to have major direct impact on acute care hospital funds, many reviews have suggested the establishment of mixed systems of reimbursement/practice for physicians. Related to this is the suggestion that the definition of "basic insured services" be re-examined and that supplemental health insurance for people who wish to obtain coverage over and above these basic services be offered. At a macro level, one might expect some easing of pressure on provincial budgets if these options are adopted, which could indirectly work in the hospitals' favour;
- basing the size of hospital medical staffs on regional council plans (which are to be based on population health needs) and on "impact analyses" of adding more medical staff;
- more efficient and cost-effective use of nursing staff by such initiatives as reducing or eliminating non-nursing responsibilities, use of labour-saving and mechanical devices, and increased job sharing or other reduced work week options. There is overlap, here, with human resources and management considerations. There will be a short-run increase in costs to hospitals for these job enhancement conditions, but in the longer run, improvements in working conditions and morale could have positive impacts on hospital costs;
- possible substitution of lower cost generic drugs, or establishing of a "lowest-available price-product" system for pharmaceuticals.

Summary

It would seem that if many of the Commissions' recommendations are implemented, few (if any) additional acute care beds will be funded; global budgeting will become more refined, case-mix specific, and tighter; and resources will be shifted towards the development of alternative and (the hope obviously is) less expensive ways to deliver health care services.

At the same time, it appears that pressures on existing budgets will become even greater in the short run, primarily as a result of having to improve the working environment for nursing staff and to accommodate additional medical and related staff (e.g., midwives).

Human Resources

Because the system is so labour intensive, it is not surprising that there are human resources issues, particularly with respect to nurses and physicians. The industrial and interprofessional relations in the health care system are problematic because of such issues as the impact of specialization and skill complexity on role clarification, inappropriate use of professional skills, excessive staffing levels, potential job obsolescence, and career mobility. Since morale and working conditions are perceived to be major problems, many of the recommendations have been directed towards ameliorating these situations. The types of recommendations made in this regard were:

- establishing "targets" for numbers of physicians, or restricting physicians' billing numbers, ultimately impacting upon the amount of resources which are used in hospitals, particularly in light of the relationship between physicians and utilization/costs;
- examining reasons for staff turnover seriously and developing strategies for retention, e.g., job enhancement, provision of a safe and secure working environment;
- building much more flexibility into scheduling and making staffing and scheduling the responsibility of the unit/head nurse;
- development of acceptable nursing workload measurement systems for use in hospitals;
- expanding the role of nurses and involving nurses in planning and operating all services, programs, and facilities, as well as in committee work, e.g., through "hospital professional advisory committees";
- undertaking "impact analyses" to determine the effects on nursing requirements prior to agreeing on new/expanded programs and/or additional medical staff;
- compensating nurses on the basis of the clinical ladder concept and increasing salary ranges for nurses with managerial responsibilities;
- increasing job sharing or other reduced work week options for nurses; and
- addressing such other important aspects as:
  - development of support systems for nurses, e.g., with respect to stress, conflict, and time management;
  - enhanced benefits such as extended maternity leave, sabbaticals, and deferred income;
  - continuing education needs – making scheduling flexible and providing financial support;
  - development of child care services in facilities;
  - elimination of nurses' non-nursing responsibilities; and
  - enhancing role and status of nurses, e.g., having nurses play a major role in multi-disciplinary patient care/teaching rounds.

Summary

Many of these recommendations overlap with those suggested for financial and management issues and in the short run could mean increased costs for hospitals. Yet, based on the existing situation with respect to the nursing working environment, it is likely that many of these recommendations will have to be implemented. There is no doubt that this will place additional pressures on budgets, management time, and organization. It would seem, however, that not dealing with these problems in the immediate future could result in more serious longer-term difficulties. One is reminded of the "Pram Oil Filter" commercial...the garage mechanic suggests that it's better to pay a little now rather than having to pay a fortune later!

Organization

While much of the underlying emphasis of the Commissions was related to organizational issues, the Quebec review probably best described the organizational concerns and limited vision in the existing system. Its message is that the system is plagued by counter-productive competition among the various interest groups for the limited resources available. More attention is paid to the *means* as opposed to the *objectives*. Furthermore, the approach is sectoral and limited in scope, while the health and social problems with which we have to contend are complex. What is needed to offset this sectoral and unproductive system is an intersectoral approach based on objectives. As a result, many reviews made some very visionary and far-reaching recommendations related to directions and organization of the system which, no doubt, will impact upon the acute care sector. Among them are the following:

- provincial-level planning which specifies shared goals, targets, and strategies for health and social services. Part of this process includes redefining the mandates of hospitals, resulting in a more relevant classification of acute care facilities. If expected results and performance of the health care sector have not been adequately defined, then translation from capital planning to health service planning is hampered significantly;

- a major shift in emphasis from illness and treatment to health promotion and disease prevention which is based on a multi-sectoral approach, e.g., by establishing medical services centres which could allow and encourage medical practices to adopt an interdisciplinary professional health team approach to providing primary care. It was also suggested that the population take more responsibility for their own health;

- development of community-based/innovative alternatives to defer admission to or facilitate rehabilitation from institutional care, as well as the establishment of a continuum of care with the necessary links;

- accountability for achieving predetermined results from resources allocated;

- retaining "macro" planning at the provincial level, while having administration and management (including financial) of health *programs* take place with regional health authorities, councils, or boards. Funding would be decentralized via health and social "envelopes". The emphasis would shift to new forms of organization and management; to increased local planning, management, accountability, and funding envelopes; and perhaps even to health care "budgets" for each provincial resident;

- "pilot projects" to address different delivery models, nursing models, and physician practice/reimbursement systems. These alternatives should be carefully evaluated in relation to the existing system;

- increased funding for home support and services. There could be user fees for some home care services; and

- other "organizational" changes, including:
  - establishment of physician practice guidelines;
  - delegation of functions from physicians to nurses;
  - development of a mixed reimbursement system for physicians;
  - defining and clarifying institutional roles; and
  - accommodating additional occupational groups (e.g., midwives) in the institutional setting. Provincial legislation would have to be modified for this to occur.

Summary

It is obvious that these organizational recommendations are linked closely with the financial and human resources issues. The theme of strategic redirection of the system is clear. In addition, much more attention will be paid to improving planning guidelines and treatment protocols in an effort to correct service maldistribution and inefficient utilization, situations which overlap with improving management of and within the system. Rational planning (as opposed to institutional rivalry), efficient and appropriate use of hospital beds, and more controlled introduction of sophisticated technology and equipment are underlying goals of this organizational restructuring.

Management

The Commissions observed the number of concerns related to management, planning, and information support. Management could be strengthened by the application of supporting information, evaluation, and relevant research. Evaluation is a key component in these requirements. Poor links between the collection and use of health status, clinical, and accounting data are affecting the quality of health sector management and planning. Some of the recommendations to improve management of the system are:

- cross-representation on Medical Advisory Committees and management boards of hospitals;
- active involvement of physicians and nurses in the management of hospitals;
- using accepted MIS guidelines to establish comprehensive utilization management systems in hospitals which involve not only hospital executives but also physicians and nurses;
- monitoring performance by making utilization reviews a regular component of management practice (multi-disciplinary) and basing these reviews on statistics in addition to peer review. Development of systems to collect, transfer, store, and update individual health data was suggested;
- managing hospitals, nursing homes, and other facilities in the same geographic area under a multi-unit management concept, in concert with the regional planning concept;
- explicit delegation of responsibilities defined in the regulation of health professionals; and
- allowing hospitals the flexibility to trade-off programs and services as part of the changed emphasis in organization.

Summary

Such recommendations have implications for the organization within a hospital and, along with the requirements for MIS guidelines and appropriate computer technology, translate into resource requirements. As with the recommendations related to enhancing nursing work environments, the long run benefits likely would offset the necessary increase in short-term expenditures. It is also quite likely that governments would attempt to derive much of the funding necessary to improve management and working conditions from within the system itself. The underlying objective is to make hospital management more accountable.

Other Issues and Trends

Elderly

There is no question that the impacts of an increasing elderly population could be significant for the acute care sector, *if nothing else is done.* As was noted in the Watson Task Force, "...promotion of better health will not necessarily reduce health expenditures. It might simply allow us to live long enough to develop the infirmities of old age. This is why it is essential to act to improve the manner in which we care for the elderly" (Watson, 1985:127).

Small Population Base

Trying to provide services to a widely dispersed population will add to the trick of trying to control provincial health expenditures which, in turn, likely will be passed on to the regional health authorities and, ultimately, to the hospitals to resolve. Other priority groups with which to contend are caregivers, single parent families, the disabled and handicapped, the terminally ill, Natives, and immigrants.

Technology

Most of the Commissions underscored the need to "get a handle" on technology diffusion. The feeling is that no new technology should be introduced unless there is demonstrated need and cost-effectiveness has been considered. This concern obviously has been felt, for early in 1989 a technology assessment centre was established in Quebec, and soon to be launched is a national office for the assessment of health technology.

Shift Away From Inpatient Care

The Ontario Hospital Association in its paper on "The Future Role of Hospitals in Providing Care" has stated: "...the shift from inpatient to outpatient care will lead to further evolution of the definition of the hospital. The hospital whose identity and value is largely a function of the number of beds it has will be threatened by the shift away from inpatient care. The hospital whose identity and value is linked more closely with the services it provides will view this shift as opportunity. It is incumbent upon the hospital to move into the future by asking itself, 'What do we want the hospital to be?' It is also the responsibility of the hospital industry to answer this question in relation to the trends and influences that exist in society today" (Ontario Hospital Association, 1989:40). These trends and influences have been dealt with in most of the work by the Commissions.

OVERALL SUMMARY AND CONCLUSION

Various financial, organizational, social, and political pressures have obliged many provinces to review the cost of health care during the past decade. This review process has gathered tremendous momentum across Canada since 1983, and its overall effect likely will be a significant change to the health care sector during the 1990s.

A review of these Commissions and Task Forces revealed commonality in the issues identified and in the general strategies being recommended and implemented to take Canada's health system well into the 1990s (and perhaps even into the next century!). In many provinces, we can find organizational restructuring, health planning, and funding innovation.

The basis for these reforms is a concern to rebalance and redirect the system in three ways: towards greater emphasis on disease prevention and health promotion, towards community-based care alternatives, and towards greater accountability.

ACKNOWLEDGEMENTS

The original research for this paper was done under contract for the Canadian Medical Association, Canadian Hospital Association, and Canadian Nurses Association. I am grateful to these organizations for their assistance and for allowing me to disseminate the results of the analysis and synthesis more broadly.

REFERENCES

Angus DE: *The Review of Significant Health Care Commissions and Task Forces in Canada Since 1983-84.* Canadian Hospital Association, 1991.

Brunton W: *Provincial Health Systems Reviews: Synthesis and Future Directions,* unpublished (mimeo) for the Health Policy Division, Health and Welfare Canada, 1989.

Canadian Centre for Policy Alternatives: *Medicare: The Decisive Year.* Proceedings of the Conference on Medicare: The Decisive Years, November 12-13, Montreal, Quebec, 1984.

Collins JF, Twomey H: *A Green Paper on Our Health Care System Expenditures and Funding.* St. John's: Government of Newfoundland and Labrador, 1986.

Dawe J (chair): *Report of the Advisory Committee on Nursing Workforce.* St. John's: Government of Newfoundland and Labrador, 1989.

Eberts M (chair): *Report of the Task Force of Midwifery in Ontario,* submitted to the Hon. Murray J. Elston, Minister of Health. Toronto, 1987.

Evans JR (chair): *Toward a Shared Direction for Health in Ontario.* Report of the Ontario Health Review Panel. Toronto, 1987.

Gallant JC (chair): *The Report of the Nova Scotia Royal Commission on Health Care: Towards a New Strategy.* Halifax: Nova Scotia Royal Commission on Health Care, 1989.

Hyndman LD (chair): *The Rainbow Report: Our Vision for Health.* Report of The Premier's Commission on Future Health Care for Albertans. Edmonton, 1989.

Lavoie-Roux T: *Improving Health and Well-Being in Quebec: Orientations.* Québec: Ministère de la Santé et des Services Sociaux, 1989.

Ley DCH (chair): *Health Care for the Elderly, Today's Challenges, Tomorrow's Options.* Ottawa: Canadian Medical Association, 1987.

Manitoba Health Advisory Network: *Newsletter,* Numbers 1, 2 (1989) and 3 (1990). Winnipeg: Manitoba Health.

Manitoba Health Services Commissions: *Report of the Health Services Review Committee, Volume I: Summary and Recommendations.* Winnipeg: Government of Manitoba, 1985.

McKelvey EN (chair): *Report of the Commission on Selected Health Care Programs.* Fredericton: Government of New Brunswick, 1989.

Ministère de la Santé et des Services Sociaux: *Objective: A Health Concept in Quebec.* Report of the Task Force on Health Promotion. Ottawa: Canadian Hospital Association, 1986 (translation of original report in French, *Objectif: Santé* (1984)).

Murray RG (chair): *Future Directions for Health Care in Saskatchewan.* Report of the Saskatchewan Commission on Directions in Health Care. Regina, 1990.

New Brunswick Nurses Resources Advisory Committee: *Action Plan on Quality of Worklife Issues of Nurses in New Brunswick.* Fredericton: Government of New Brunswick, 1988.

Nova Scotia Royal Commission on Health Care: *Issues and Concerns: Summary of Public Hearings and Submissions.* Halifax: Nova Scotia Royal Commission on Health Care, 1988.

Ontario Hospital Association: *The Future Role of Hospitals in Providing Care: Issues to Consider.* OHA Research Paper. Toronto: Ontario Hospital Association, 1989.

Ontario Ministry of Health: *Report of the Conjoint Review Committee on 23 Hospital Operational Reviews.* Toronto: Ministry of Health, 1988.

Ontario Ministry of Health: *Deciding the Future of Our Health Care System.* Toronto: Ministry of Health, 1989.

Ontario Premier's Council on Health Strategy: *A Vision of Health, Health Goals for Ontario.* Toronto: Ontario Premier's Council on Health Strategy, 1989.

Ontario Premier's Council on Health Strategy: *From Vision to Action, Report of the Future Health Care System Committee.* Toronto: Ontario Premier's Council on Health Strategy, 1989.

Orsborn DB (chair): *Report of the Royal Commission on Hospital and Nursing Home Costs to the Government of Newfoundland and Labrador.* St. John's, 1984.

Podborski S (chair): *Health Promotion Matters in Ontario.* A Report of the Minister's Advisory Group on Health Promotion. Toronto, 1987.

Premier's Commission on Future Health Care for Albertans: *Interim Report, Caring and Commitment.* Edmonton: Premier's Commission on Future Health Care for Albertans, 1988.

Premier's Commission on Future Health Care for Albertans: *What You've Said,* Newsletter Special Edition. Edmonton: Premier's Commission on Future Health Care for Albertans, 1989.

Quebec Ministry of Social Affairs: *Quebec's System of Health and Social Services.* Quebec: Government of Quebec, 1985.

Rochon J (chair): *Commission d'Enquête sur les Services de Santé et les Services Sociaux.* Québec, 1988.

Spasoff RA (chair): *Health for All Ontario.* Report of the Panel on Health Goals for Ontario. Toronto, 1987.

Stevenson Kellogg Ernst & Whinney: *Funding and Incentives Study.* Health Care Systems Committee. Toronto: Ontario Premier's Council on Health Strategy, 1989.

Watanabe M (chair): *An Agenda for Action.* Report of the Advisory Committee on the Utilization of Medical Services. Edmonton: Government of Alberta, 1989.

Watson J (chair): *Health – A Need for Redirection – A Task Force on Allocation of Health Care Resources.* Ottawa: Canadian Medical Association, 1985.

REPORT OF THE PHARMACEUTICAL INQUIRY OF ONTARIO: AN OVERVIEW

J. Ivan Williams
Clinical Epidemiology Unit, Sunnybrook Health Science Centre
University of Toronto

Frederick H. Lowy
Centre for Bioethics, University of Toronto

Wendy Kennedy
Risk/Benefit Management of Drugs Project
Canadian Public Health Association

Michelle Chibba
Ontario Optometrists Association

PHARMACEUTICAL INQUIRY OF ONTARIO

The Pharmaceutical Inquiry of Ontario was established on May 26, 1988 to examine the role and influence of the government of Ontario with respect to prescription drugs. The Inquiry addressed those factors that would enable the use of public funds and government influence to:

a) promote the *availability* of high quality drug treatment,

b) facilitate the appropriate *access* to drug treatment, and

c) achieve the *cost-effective* use of drugs.

The Inquiry held 18 days of hearings throughout the province and received over 180 briefs and oral presentations. The recommendations of the report are contained in the report *Prescription for Drugs,* which was released to the public in August 1990 (Pharmaceutical Inquiry of Ontario, 1990).

The members of the Inquiry were:

Frederick H. Lowy, MD (chairman), director of the Centre for Bioethics at the University of Toronto and former dean of the faculty of medicine and chairman of the department of psychiatry at the University of Toronto.

Michael Gordon, MD, medical director of Baycrest Centre for Geriatric Care, head of the division of geriatrics at Mount Sinai Hospital, and associate professor of medicine at the University of Toronto.

Martha Jordan, RN, staff development coordinator at Rideaucrest Home in Kingston; member of the Ontario Nurses' Association, the Registered Nurses' Association of Ontario, and the Gerontological Nursing Association of Ontario.

Richard Moulton, MD, family physician and educator of family physicians in Fort Frances, Ontario, associate professor in the department of family medicine at the University of Western Ontario, and board member of the Ontario Medical Association; founding member of the Kenora-Rainy River District Health Council, past-president of the Canadian Association of Medical Clinics, and past-chairman of the Ontario Medical Association committee on drugs and pharmacotherapy (the committee that runs the adverse drug reaction program and provides *The Drug Report).*

Reva Spunt, MSW, social worker and coordinator of gerontological services at North York General Hospital, with a private practice (Seniors' Resource and Consultation

Services) directed toward the development of services for the elderly in the community.

Jake J. Thiessen, PhD, specialist in pharmacokinetics, professor and graduate studies coordinator in the faculty of pharmacy of the University of Toronto, and chairman of the Drug Quality and Therapeutics Committee of the Ontario Ministry of Health.

Donald C. Webster, BSc, founder and chairman of Helix Investments Limited (a venture capital company); director of a number of public companies and of the Canadian Schizophrenic Foundation and the Canadian Psychiatric Research Foundation; member of the Premier's Council of Ontario; past director of the National Research Council of Canada and the Royal Ontario Museum.

William Robert Wensley, MSc, Registrar for the Ontario College of Pharmacists (the licencing and regulating body for pharmacy in Ontario); teacher in the faculty of pharmacy at the University of Toronto; former member of the Ontario Council of Health and the Drug Quality and Therapeutics Committee (advisory bodies to the Minister of Health).

All members were actively involved in attending hearings, reading briefs, drafting position papers, and writing the report.

DRUG EXPENDITURES IN ONTARIO

In 1988, sales of prescription drugs in Ontario were estimated at $1.2 billion. Of that amount, the Ontario Drug Benefit (ODB) plan paid $360 million and the public hospitals $230 million; public expenditures accounted for the remaining 49%.

The ODB plan has grown rapidly in both absolute and relative terms. The Ontario Ministry of Treasury and Economics stated that the plan had experienced an average annual increase of 20.4%, making it "one of the fastest growing health programs over the period [1978-1988]" (Economic Outlook and Fiscal Review, 1988). The percentage of the health care dollar going to the ODB was 2.6 in 1978/79 and 5.0 in 1988/89. The per capita expenditure on drugs is higher in Ontario than in any other province, and Ontario is one of the few jurisdictions in western industrialized countries where the relative expenditures on drug costs have increased markedly (Scheiber, 1987). In 1988/89 the total paid for the ODB program was $630 million in 1988 dollars. Table 1 summarizes these expenditures.

Table 1

EXPENDITURES AND CLAIMS, ONTARIO DRUG BENEFIT PROGRAM, 1988-89

Expenditure	Amount	Claims
Prescription drug costs	$354,884,500	32,022,900
Upcharge or surcharge	35,488,400	
Dispensing fees	188,803,200	
Non-prescription drug costs	50,774,300	3,348,600
Total	*$629,950,400*	*35,371,500*

Drug manufacturers were paid $405.7 million for drug products. The surcharge or upcharge was paid to pharmacists, who retained about half of this amount for the drugs that were sold directly without charges for distribution costs. For the drugs sold indirectly, the pharmacists paid wholesalers about $14,195,400 in fees and retained $3,548,800. The gross income to pharmacists in fees and upcharges was about $210.1 million, or about 1/3 of the ODB costs.

There was a 308.5% increase, in constant dollars, in the ODB plan from 1976/77 to 1988/89. The component parts of this increase were studied so that their relative contributions to the ODB costs could be identified. For example, if the number of claimants was allowed to increase while the average claims for prescribed and non-prescribed drugs per claimant, average drug costs per claim, and average dispensing fees per prescription were held at 1976/77, there would have been a 74.3% increase in ODB costs in constant dollars.

Even though the coverage under the program has been expanded for those receiving general welfare, social assistance, and home care, the increase in the number of aged individuals has been the driving force. At both ends of the time period, they comprised 60% of the claimants and accounted for 80% of ODB costs. The demographic projections of the number of aged individuals through the year 2011 indicate that, even if all other costs are constrained successfully, the ODB costs will double again.

The most important component, contributing 50.1% to the overall increase in the plan's costs, was the average number of claims of prescribed drugs per claimant. This component could be accounted for by increases in utilization of physician services and prescribing activity, changing health status of claimants, or quantities of the drug prescribed.

The average cost of prescribed drug per claim contributed 48.1% to the overall increase and can be attributed to increases in the price of drugs, changes in the drugs prescribed, or the introduction of new and more expensive products.

There are multiplier effects as well. If one allows the number of claimants, the average number of claims for prescribed drugs per claimant, and the average cost of drug per prescription to increase to 1988/89 levels while holding other components constant, these three components, independently and together, contribute a 294.5% increase – 95.5% of the overall 308.5% increase – to the ODB plan.

The average number of claims for non-prescribed drugs and the average costs of non-prescribed drug per claim remained relatively constant over the time period. The dispensing fee for the ODB claims is negotiated between the Ontario Pharmacists' Association and the Ministry of Health (MOH). Increases in the ODB dispensing fee have been held to increases in the CPI. Taken together, these latter three components account for the remaining 5% of the overall increase in ODB plan costs.

Apart from the ODB program, the Ministry of Health also provides drugs and over-the-counter products through the Ontario Government Pharmacy Medical Supplies and Services. The government pharmacy is a centralized purchasing and distribution function of the MOH which services provincial psychiatric hospitals, correctional institutions, and facilities for the developmentally handicapped.

The MOH funds clinics for drugs and confidential treatment and counselling of persons with sexually transmitted diseases. Drugs for the management of tuberculosis and leprosy are provided through public health units. There are outpatient, hospital-based programs to provide human growth hormones, cyclosporin, and drugs for AIDS, cystic fibrosis, thalassemia, and other health problems. The MOH funds drugs for use in ambulance services under two programs, basic life support and advanced life support.

The ODB provides coverage for about 15 to 20% of Ontarians. About 60% of Ontario residents are covered by private health insurance plans obtained through the workplace, with Green Shield Prepaid Services Inc. and Blue Cross being the two largest companies. The remaining 20% or so of the population pay cash for their drug products and are without drug plans. In a study of access to coverage, Hurley (1990) identified a number of groups that may face financial difficulty in obtaining prescription drugs: "individuals with extraordinary drug expenses, those requiring special drugs, those only employed part-time, and other subgroups who do not qualify for the ODB program or for private third party coverage".

The Social Assistance Review Committee (Transitions, 1988) recommended that the Family Benefits and General Welfare Assistance programs be extended to the "working poor" and to government social assistance program recipients who may not be eligible for ODB. Municipalities share in the costs of the special assistance and supplementary aid, and there is considerable variation amongst cities as to the coverage provided. This recommendation was implemented in October of 1989, and at the time of the writing of the report the impact of the Supports To Employment Program (STEPS) on coverage was unknown.

KEY RECOMMENDATIONS REGARDING PRICE, ACCESS, AND EFFECTIVENESS
THE PRICING OF DRUG PRODUCTS FOR THE ODB FORMULARY

The Inquiry commissioned Paul Gorecki of the Economic Council of Canada to study the purchasing and distribution of drugs in Canada (Gorecki, 1990). After reviewing the advantages and disadvantages of the Best Available Price (BAP) (the price of the drug at the factory gate) versus Actual Acquisition Cost (the price recommended by the manufacturer), the Inquiry concurred that the ODB should continue to have manufacturers submit their Best Available Price for drug products listed in the ODB Formulary. The BAP for standard dosage and packaging should be as low as the lowest price for which the drug is sold in Canada. The members agreed that ODB should continue to pay the lowest BAP listing for interchangeable products. The patient can either accept the lowest price drug or pay the difference between the BAP and the price of the brand name prescribed.

Had the Actual Acquisition Cost been recommended, the model would have been similar to that of British Columbia, where the pharmacist dispenses the brand name product prescribed and is remunerated according to the price submitted by the manufacturer. There is debate as to whether British Columbia pays less for specific drug products than Ontario, but the question is nearly impossible to answer without understanding the choices of drugs prescribed for the patients' specific health problems. The Inquiry was convinced that the BAP served the purpose for which it was intended.

The Patented Medicines Prices Review Board estimated that the increases in the prices of drugs were about 2% above CPI until January 1989, when the board's guidelines were promulgated. Since then, the price increases have been below CPI. There was a marked increase in ODB drug prices between 1986 and 1989. To offset the long term impact of the increases, the Inquiry recommended setting the drug prices for the January 1991 Formulary at December 1986 Formulary listings plus increases up to CPI. If the listings in the latest Formulary were below the 1986 listings plus CPI, the lower drug prices would be listed in the new Formulary. To control the impact of price increases further, the Inquiry recommended that between January 1991 and January 1994 increases in drug prices be limited to the 1991 listings plus 50% of CPI.

In an analysis of the prices of generic drugs, it became evident that the savings in price increased as the number of interchangeable drug products increased. The price for the first generic drug product was set at about 75% of the brand product price. It tended to remain at that level until the second interchangeable drug came on the market, at which point the Best Available Price dropped to between 40% and 60% of the original brand product.

The Pharmaceutical Manufacturers' Association of Canada noted that the manufacturers of generic products were subject neither to the initial development and research costs for innovative drugs nor to the price control mechanisms as manufacturers of patented drugs, and hence had an advantage in the pricing of their products. The Inquiry generally agreed with the points made and recommended that a new generic drug product be introduced into the Formulary at a price no greater than 60% of the price of the brand product for which it was interchangeable.

ACCESS AND DRUG PLAN COVERAGE

Jeremiah Hurley, a health economist at McMaster University, agreed to undertake a study of the access of Ontario residents to drug plans and the question of copayments by consumers (Hurley, 1990). He estimated that in 1987 1.5 million Ontarians were insured under Blue Cross and Green Shield plans and another 4 million or so were insured by 137 other insurance companies providing health benefits in the province. Since the insurance companies do not maintain databases on the numbers of individuals covered under their specific plans, Hurley's best estimate was that at the time of his study 1.4 million residents were without third party drug coverage by either ODB or a private plan.

These residents fell into two major groups: (1) individuals, either in families or unattached, whose incomes were low but above the eligibility limits for family benefits or general welfare assistance; and (2) individuals with extraordinary drug costs, particularly those with chronic diseases or disabling conditions, who were not covered by disease-specific plans provided by the government, workers' compensation, family benefits, or social welfare. There was some overlap between the two groups, but the numbers were unknown.

Working with data from Statistics Canada, Hurley estimated that in 1987 18% of Ontario households – families and unattached individuals – had annual incomes below $15,000. After subtracting the households receiving family benefits and general welfare assistance and the households headed by individuals 65 years of age and over whose incomes were less than $15,000, he estimated that there were about 138,000 low income households ineligible for public assistance or coverage for drug costs. Assuming an average of 3.5 individuals per household, this would translate to about 500,000 Ontarians.

In its interim reports, the Inquiry recommended that coverage be extended to persons with cystic fibrosis and thalassemia, and these recommendations were implemented by the Minister. There were also submissions for extending the coverage to other groups with chronic and disabling disease.

In the 1986 census, questions were asked about disabled household members. The results of a follow-up Statistics Canada health and activity limitation survey suggested that there were about 675,000 disabled individuals between the ages of 15 and 64 years (The Health and Activity Limitation Survey, 1989). After subtracting individuals with coverage and low income individuals, we estimated that there were between 60,000 and 190,000 individuals who should be considered for coverage in addition to the 500,000 low income individuals not covered by old age and social assistance. The costs would likely range from the average annual ODB costs for general welfare assistance recipients

($107) to those for recipients of family benefits ($337). The estimated costs for extending coverage ranged from $59.2 million to $232.5 million a year, with an estimated mid-range of $150 million.

Even extending the ODB's coverage, there would still be 700,000 to 800,000 individuals in the province without drug coverage. Possible options would be to cover them under ODB as well or for the government to sponsor a plan with private insurance companies to provide coverage to persons unable to secure plans through their place of employment. Given the apparent lack of interest in these options, the Inquiry gave them minimal consideration.

The Inquiry considered the issue of copayments for ODB recipients who do not receive social assistance payments. Sixty percent of the seniors in Ontario would be liable for such copayments. Ontario is one of four provinces/territories that provide drug coverage without cost-sharing in the form of copayments and deductibles. The other jurisdictions require deductibles, coinsurance, or a fixed charge per prescription to be paid by the consumer not receiving social assistance.

It was also clear that most Ontarians share in the costs of their drugs under the private insurance plans. Blue Cross indicated that the average prescription cost in 1988 under its plans was $23.13, of which the consumer paid $1.59, or 7%. The per prescription price to the subscriber of Green Shield ranged from 0 to $5.00, with an average of 49.5 cents.

Hurley reviewed the literature and estimated the impact of copayments on drug use. He estimated that drug use would drop from 10-20% with a copayment of $2.50 per prescription and that drug use would drop between 10% and 40% for each additional 50 cents added to the copayment. A cap on expenditures would limit the liabilities of the consumer for any given year.

After weighing the trade-offs among drug coverage, consumer responsibilities for the costs of drugs, and government expenditures on health care, the Inquiry recommended that ODB beneficiaries not receiving social assistance pay $3.00 to $4.00 per prescription with an annual cap on expenditures of $250. We estimated that the average copayment costs for seniors would be between $65 and $90 a year, with no more than 10% of the recipients reaching the $250 cap.

It should be noted that physicians tend to write prescriptions for ODB beneficiaries to last 30 days. If larger quantities were prescribed, the number of prescriptions would be reduced and the consumer would receive the same amount of medication at a lower cost.

OTHER RECOMMENDATIONS
THE DRUG QUALITY THERAPEUTICS COMMITTEE AND THE FORMULARY

The Drug Quality and Therapeutics Committee (DQTC) decides which drug products should be listed on the ODB Formulary and which drug products can be interchanged. Drug manufacturers prepare submissions for listings, and once a drug is listed it stays on the Formulary. If a brand product is not listed in the Formulary, generic drugs that are interchangeable with it are also not listed.

Drug manufacturers have viewed the Formulary as unnecessary. Their stance is that once the drugs have been licensed by the federal government, no further reviews should be required. There are particular complaints about the time and costs required to make submissions and about the delays in decisions and listings.

The Special Authorizations (SA) Program, which was started in 1974, permitted a physician to obtain authorization from the Ministry for prescribing a drug not on the list, but deemed necessary for the health of the patient; ODB would then cover the cost of the drug. Drug manufacturers found that SAs could be used to bypass the approval process for listings in the Formulary and undercut the market for any available interchangeable products. There are 2,500 drug products listed in the Formulary, and by 1988 some 1,600 drugs had been approved as SAs. The costs of the Special Authorizations Program, which included oxygen and allergens, came to 8% of ODB expenditures.

The Inquiry recommended that this program be discontinued and that the SA drugs be reviewed and approved for either regular or limited use in the Formulary. The DQTC was to define the conditions under which limited drugs were to be prescribed. These recommendations were made in an interim report and implemented by the Minister of Health.

The Inquiry further recommended that the hand of the DQTC be strengthened. According to these recommendations, the DQTC would review all drug products on the Formulary and discontinue listings for those that were no longer deemed effective. Furthermore, criteria on cost-effectiveness would be considered in deciding whether to recommend a drug for listing. Lastly, the DQTC would establish a mechanism for the quick review of new drugs considered major therapeutic advances.

DISTRIBUTION OF DRUGS TO THE PHARMACIST

Bills 54 and 55 introduced changes in the ODB Act in 1986 that established the Best Available Price and mechanisms for negotiating dispensing fees, and that required pharmacists to provide more information to the consumer on the availability of lower-cost substitutes and to list the drug price and dispensing fee separately on the prescription receipt. The amendments also allowed for a 10% surcharge on the price of the drugs "to cover distribution costs and differences in purchasing volume". The Ministry viewed this 10% surcharge paid to pharmacists as the monies allowed to cover the costs of distributing the drugs from the manufacturer or wholesaler to the retailer. The pharmacists came to view this as part of the professional income to cover costs of inventory and carrying the drug products listed in the Formulary.

It quickly became apparent that certain drug manufacturers would sell and distribute the drugs directly to the pharmacist without charging for the distribution costs, thereby allowing the pharmacists to keep the entire 10% surcharge. If pharmacists purchased the drugs from wholesalers, however, they typically paid 8% of the drug costs for distribution.

There was, understandably, a marked shift from indirect sales through wholesalers to direct sales, and in 1989 it was believed that 50% of the drugs were sold and distributed directly by the manufacturers. For the most part, generic drug manufacturers sold directly and innovative drug manufacturers sold through warehouses. It also became apparent that direct sellers were offering "back door" incentives such as discounts, free products, and bonuses in cash and goods and services; these incentives were strictly illegal.

The Inquiry recommended that drug companies not be allowed to include distribution costs in the price of their products and that the surcharge be eliminated for drugs sold directly to the pharmacist. The goal was to make the mode of purchase and delivery revenue neutral to the pharmacist.

Wholesalers are essential for the prompt and orderly distribution of drugs to pharmacists in all parts of the province. There are three major wholesalers of drug products, two of which provide a full range of services. Wholesalers in Ontario must register with the Ontario College of Pharmacists and in 1989, 40 had done so. Most of these firms are small operations that are owned by pharmacists and provide a limited range of service. The Inquiry recommended that minimum standards be established and enforced in the registration of wholesalers before pharmacists could receive reimbursement for distribution costs of drugs dispensed to ODB beneficiaries.

The Ontario Government Pharmacy and Medical Supply Services purchases, warehouses, and distributes drugs, vaccines, and medical and laboratory supplies in Ontario government agencies and facilities and public health units across the province. This agency provides most drugs for the provincial psychiatric hospitals and non-prescription drugs for homes for the aged, nursing homes, and other facilities. The Inquiry heard numerous complaints as well as some positive comments about the government pharmacy. After a limited review, the Inquiry recommended that an outside group conduct a comprehensive management and operational audit of the services and examine alternatives for assuming responsibility for purchasing, warehousing, and distributing drugs. More specifically, it was recommended that psychiatric hospitals be allowed to use the purchasing plans of the Ontario Hospital Association.

THE PRESCRIBING OF DRUGS

The Inquiry focused on recommendations for improving rational pharmacotherapy. Included were recommendations for emphasizing good prescribing practices, the integration of pharmacology and pharmacotherapy in the curriculum, the critical appraisal of drugs, and the treatment needs of the elderly during the undergraduate and postgraduate training of physicians. It recommended that each medical school establish a Department of Clinical Pharmacology to work towards these ends.

The Inquiry recommended effective programs in continuing medical education, innovative post-marketing studies involving large numbers of general practitioners, and the development of drug utilization review programs. Specifically, the Inquiry recommended pilot projects to test unbiased, non-commercial detailing of drug products, as outlined in the research by Soumerai and Avorn (1986).

At the provincial level, the Inquiry called for a centre for the study and improvement of drug prescribing, to be jointly funded by the Ministry and the industry. Organized medicine was to take the lead in the development and updating of prescribing guidelines that would be published and distributed to all physicians. The Inquiry called for extension of formularies in hospitals and into other health care settings, the use of generic names in writing prescriptions, restricted use of drugs, and the substitution of less costly alternatives for expensive medications.

THE DISPENSING AND ADMINISTRATION OF DRUGS

The responsibilities of the pharmacist encompass two sets of functions: (1) patient-related activities, such as consulting with patients, prescribers, and other health professionals; and (2) product-oriented activities, such as acquiring, storing, labelling, packaging, dispensing, and record keeping. The professional dispensing fees remunerate the pharmacists for the product-oriented activities, but not the patient-related ones.

The Inquiry recommendations were designed to strengthen the information and consultation activities with patients, prescribers, and other professionals. These recommendations were directed toward the education and clinical training of pharmacists, maintaining patient medication profiles, the introduction of "smart cards" that include identification of diagnoses and prescribing doctors, and expanding the clinical responsibilities of the pharmacists in the community.

The Inquiry concurred with manpower studies that have suggested that a new faculty of pharmacy be established and that the current faculty at the University of Toronto be reduced in size. The Inquiry also called for joint instruction of pharmacists with other health professionals. Lastly, the Inquiry recommended that a doctoral program in pharmacy be established.

ESTIMATING THE COSTS AND SAVINGS OF THE RECOMMENDATIONS

The members of the Inquiry attempted to estimate the costs and savings that would have resulted had these recommendations been enforced during the 1988-89 fiscal year. We could estimate the effects of the recommendations that related directly to the costs of the ODB program. Other recommendations, however, such as those related to physicians and pharmacists, rational prescribing and dispensing, monitoring of drug use, and the role of pharmaceutical products in health care, were global in character and their economic impact, either in terms of costs or benefits, could not be estimated.

Table 2 shows the estimated savings and costs of the recommendations of the ODB.

Table 2

SAVINGS AND COSTS OF RECOMMENDATIONS REGARDING THE ONTARIO DRUG BENEFIT PROGRAM, 1988-89

Recommendation	Added savings (millions)	Cost (millions)
Eliminate special authorizations	$14.7	
Constrain price increases for prescribed drugs	29.5	
Modify distribution costs	21.5	
250 day supply limit for prescription renewals	18.8	
Copayments for elderly not receiving social assistance	111.2	
Extend ODB coverage with copayment to low income and disabled persons		$95.0
Total	*$195.7*	*$95.0*

About 55% of the savings would come from the introduction of copayments and would be attributable in part to the payment itself and in part to the decrease in utilization. The manufacturers would lose on constrained prices, the elimination of SAs, and the reduced uses of drugs by seniors making copayments. The pharmacists would lose revenues from the altered surcharges, reduced prescription fees because of 250-day rather than 30-day supply limits, and reduced fees resulting from decreased use of drugs associated with copayments. The savings would be approximately twice as great as the costs of extended coverage for low income and disabled persons.

The expanded scope of activities of the DQTC would double its operating costs from $170,00 to $350,000 a year. The doctoral program in pharmacy would cost about $950,000, but the monies would be reallocated from existing budgets of the University of Toronto and its teaching hospitals.

It would cost about $3 million to operate a second faculty of pharmacy. The need for additional monies for start-up costs and capital expenditures would depend on the resources of the university where the faculty would be located.

The introduction of a clinical preceptor year to the existing program at the University of Toronto would cost about $1.2 million a year in operating costs. No savings could be expected from the reductions in class size.

The total of these identified cost increases would be about $5.32 million. The net savings of the recommendations would be in the vicinity of $95 million a year. This would presuppose that the trade-offs explicit in the recommendations are deemed politically feasible and acceptable. For example, if the introduction of copayments was not deemed acceptable, there would be a relatively small but net increase in the costs of the ODB program.

The Inquiry has achieved its objectives of setting forth recommendations that would enhance availability of and access to quality drug treatment, while at the same time leading to a more cost-effective, rational use of pharmacare services in the province. At the same time, it has attempted to "level the playing field" and protect the interests of the key participants in the provision of pharmacare as well as those of Ontario's residents.

REFERENCES

Economic Outlook and Fiscal Review: Ontario 1988. Toronto: Ontario Ministry of Treasury and Economics, 1988.

Gorecki P: Getting it right: an evaluation of alternative systems of the organization of the Ontario prescription drugs distribution system. In: *Prescriptions for Health: Research Reports.* Toronto: Ontario Ministry of Health, 1990.

The Health and Activity Limitation Survey: Subprovincial Data for Ontario. Ottawa: Statistics Canada, 1989.

Hurley J: An examination of access to prescription drugs in Ontario and an evaluation of selected cost-sharing policies. In: *Prescriptions for Health: Research Reports.* Toronto: Ontario Ministry of Health, 1990.

Pharmaceutical Inquiry of Ontario: *Prescriptions for Health: Report of the Inquiry into the Acquisition, Dispensing, and Prescribing of Pharmaceutical Medications.* Toronto: Ontario Ministry of Health, 1990.

Scheiber GJ: *Financing and Delivering Health Care: A Comparative Analysis of OECD Countries.* Paris: OECD Social Policy Studies No. 4, 1987.

Soumerai SB, Avorn J: Economic and policy analysis of university-based drug detailing. *Medical Care* 24:313-331, 1986.

Transitions. Report of the Social Assistance Review Committee. Toronto: Ontario Ministry of Community and Social Services, 1988.

REDEFINING THE GLOBE: RECENT CHANGES IN THE FINANCING OF BRITISH COLUMBIA HOSPITALS

Dominic S. Haazen
British Columbia Ministry of Health

BACKGROUND

The Institutional Services department of the British Columbia Ministry of Health (BCHA) is comprised of three major programs – Hospitals, Continuing Care, and the British Columbia Ambulance Service – as well as support services.

These three programs were brought together within the overall umbrella of Institutional Services to ensure coordination in providing and financing a continuum of care services from pre-hospital care, through acute inpatient and ambulatory services, to chronic and long term care services.

Within Institutional Services, the mandate of Hospital Programs is to ensure the Provincial Government receives value for funds expended and that the people of British Columbia receive the best possible and affordable hospital-based care in coordination with other health care services.

This implies several important policy objectives:

Equity – in the distribution of funding to hospitals and the access to services throughout the Province;

Integration – and coordination of hospital services with other types of health care services;

Efficiency – in the provision of health care services by the Province's hospitals, and in the hospital system as a whole;

Quality – health care services that are effective in treating or managing illness or coping with chronic or debilitating conditions.

This paper examines how recent changes in the mechanisms the Ministry of Health uses for funding hospitals in British Columbia have been directed at achieving these policy objectives.

The paper is divided into several parts. The next sections provide a historical perspective on the funding methods for British Columbia hospitals; a description of the change in the basic approach to funding from a workload-based approach to one based on the population served by a hospital and its role in the community; an outline of other initiatives designed to encourage innovation, integration, and accountability; and a description of the next steps in the process and a vision of where all this is taking hospitals in British Columbia.

HISTORICAL PERSPECTIVE

Until 1981/82, hospitals were funded on a per diem basis, whereby each unit of work that was done was reimbursed by the Ministry of Health. This created certainty on the part of hospital administrators, but resulted in problems for Ministry staff, not to mention the Minister of Finance. For example, in 1980/81 a Special Warrant or supplementary funding allocation, in addition to the amount voted of the Estimates, of $189 million (or 24% over the budgeted amount) was required.

Clearly this was unacceptable from the Government's point of view. Therefore, in 1981/82 the funding of hospitals was changed to a "global" basis, whereby hospitals were given an initial allocation each year and told to provide the required services within this allocation. Generally, the allocation was increased each year only for inflationary growth.

THE QUARTERLY REVIEW PROCESS

To recognize increases in utilization, a quarterly review process was implemented. During this review, a hospital could make a case for additional funding based on workload growth, and the Hospital Programs Regional Teams would examine this case in the light of the relative efficiency of the hospital in relation to its peers and the relative need of the facility when compared to competing priorities. Invariably, regardless of the case made, the financial position of the hospital (working capital, projected year-end, etc.) became a major consideration.

As well, the often limited amount of funding available meant that decisions were frequently postponed both to provide more certainty as to available funding and to ensure that the workload situation and other variables did not change. In the meantime, however, hospital administrators were faced with the need to cope with increasing demands with no assurance of more resources and a Ministry policy that frowned on operating deficits.

The natural response was to attempt to limit service growth by closing beds or adopting other "blunt" coping mechanisms. When the various elements were finally lined up and the discretionary funding made available to the "appropriate" hospitals, it was often too near the year-end to address the utilization issues. To add insult to injury, the hospital was likely to end the fiscal year in an operating surplus situation, thereby incurring the wrath of the medical and nursing staff which had borne the brunt of the coping mechanisms earlier in the year.

Nowhere were the drawbacks of this approach more obvious than in the winter of 1987, when a special commission toured the Province to hear submissions on the distribution of an additional $20 million in operating funding for hospitals. By the time the smoke had cleared and the final allocations were made, the hospital that precipitated the study ended the year in a substantial and embarrassing surplus position. In response, the next BCHA Annual General Meeting passed a "thanks but no thanks" resolution, asking for a better method of allocating funds.

In addition to the great deal of uncertainty generated by this funding approach, there was also a significant mismatch between the incentives provided to hospital administrators and the behaviour desired by the Ministry. It did not take administrators long to figure out that the only way to get more money out of the Ministry was to "pump up the volume" and then scream loud and long. This obviously ran contrary to the Ministry's desire to have hospitals and other health care providers (especially physicians) manage utilization growth.

In April 1988, there was a major shift of senior management staff in the Ministry of Health. Within Institutional Services, there was a new Assistant Deputy Minister and two new Executive Directors, including one for Hospital Programs. The new management team took as one of its key initial tasks a reform of the funding system for hospitals.

THE POPULATION/DEMOGRAPHIC FUNDING APPROACH
RATIONALE FOR THE POPULATION/DEMOGRAPHIC MODEL

The development of a more appropriate funding model required reference to both Hospital Programs' mission statement and its key policy objectives. Any new approach to funding would have to provide appropriate recognition of hospital and community needs as well as incentives for hospitals to provide the appropriate amount of high quality care to meet these needs.

Population growth and the aging of the population stood out as the most obvious measures of need, particularly since the Ministry was using both these factors to argue with Treasury Board for additional hospital operating funds. Thus, by moving closer to a population/demographic basis, the Ministry both moved toward using more objective criteria based on need and improved the consistency between its micro funding decisions and its macro funding requests. There is a general feeling in the Ministry that this has helped to increase the acceptance of population/demographic pressure as a legitimate funding issue, thereby reducing at least some of the uncertainty with regard to the Ministry's budget.

At the facility level, it was believed to be imperative to provide each hospital administrator, as soon as possible in the new fiscal year, with a fairly clear picture of the total fiscal resources that would be available during that year, so that appropriate actions could be taken and administrators could be held more accountable for the operation of their facilities.

This was addressed first by making the allocation available earlier in the year, and second by incorporating as many adjustments as possible – including the population/demographic funding – in the initial allocation.

With respect to the selection of variables to be included in the model, the Ministry wished to make the maximum use of data sources that were both available and generally recognized as being objective, especially those related to actual utilization. Thus the hospital morbidity database (HMRI) became the key source of data; the only other major variable used was population over time by age, sex, and local health area. In the absence of an objective "standard" for utilization, the British Columbia age/sex specific utilization rates were used.

The underlying rationale here is that there seemed to be no compelling reason that an "average" individual in one region of the Province of a particular age and sex should require more or less hospital care than one of the same age and sex residing in another region. This assumption will be revisited below.

DESCRIPTION OF THE MODEL

As shown in Figures 1A and 1B, the utilization of hospital services varies considerably by age and sex. These provincial utilization rates for the five levels of care – acute/ rehabilitation, long-term care in an acute care institution, intensive care, inpatient surgery, and day-care surgery (extended care is not included in the model, since growth is handled through the explicit funding of new beds) – are used to apply to the population growth by local health area (LHA) (roughly, school district) by age and sex. Figure 2 shows the change in population over the years used. The result (Figure 3) is the change in services in weighted patient days (WPD) required by level of care attributable to both population growth and aging (since age-specific utilization factors are used).

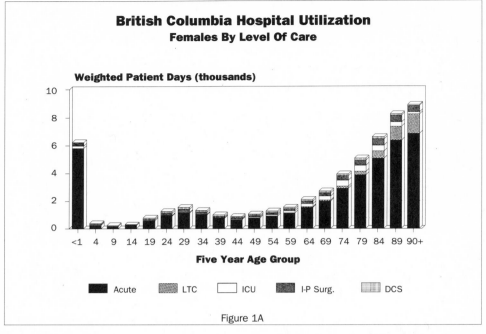

Figure 1A

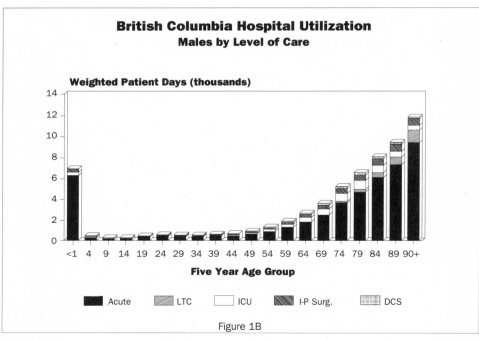

Figure 1B

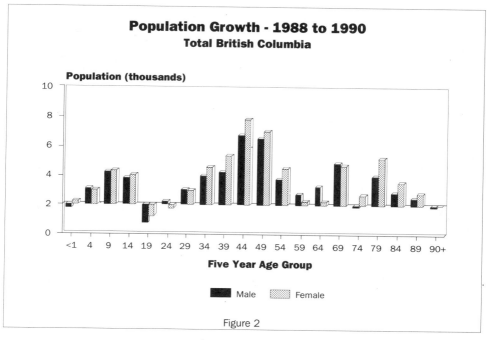

Figure 2

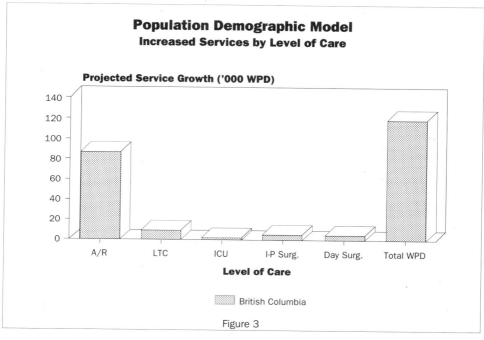

Figure 3

The next step is to allocate these indicated increases in service "needs" to each hospital based on existing referral patterns for each level of care. For example, if a hospital provided 40% of the acute/rehabilitation services to an LHA, it would get credit for 40% of the indicated increase in acute/rehabilitation days for that LHA. Once this is done for each level of care, the totals are aggregated into one figure for each hospital using the weighted patient day weightings.

Some time ago, a study was done within the Ministry to determine the relative resource requirements for average units of different types of care, including the five levels of care used in the model. Each of these types of care was equated to an average acute/rehabilitation day. Thus, a day in an intensive care unit was equated to 3.5 acute/rehabilitation days, a surgical suite visit (inpatient or day surgery) to 1.65, and so on. This allowed a wide variety of different types of care to be consolidated into a single workload measure: the Weighted Patient Day (WPD).

The final step of the model is to adjust the resulting increase in weighted patient days (Figure 4) by hospital by each facility's cost per WPD to provide a rough proxy for the higher acuity of some weighted patient days in relation to others across the Province. The available funding is then allocated to each hospital in relation to its "slice of the pie" of the adjusted service growth (Figure 5).

RESULTS TO DATE

This model was used for the second time in the allocation of hospital contributions for the 1990/91 fiscal year, and a number of refinements were made in this latest iteration. The model is currently used to allocate only the incremental amount (close to $60 million over the last two years) available for population and utilization growth. Hospitals have been required, in their budget submission which demonstrates to the Ministry how they intend to use their funding allocation (in terms of finance, workload, and staffing), to accommodate all new acute beds and new programs (with the exception of Provincial referral services) within their population/demographic allocation.

These changes have generally been well received within the hospital industry. Although some concerns have been expressed about certain aspects of the model – either the numbers used or the application of the model in terms of policy – these have not been either substantive or great in number. There appears to be general agreement with the philosophy underlying the model and the basic fairness of its application.

Implicit in this approach to the model is the assumption that the base funding for each hospital is appropriate. This is obviously not true for all hospitals, and Hospital Programs has undertaken to examine the funding base of each hospital over a three-year period, beginning in 1989/90, to ensure that it is appropriate. In determining "appropriateness", Ministry staff are increasingly relying on information regarding the role and nature of the facility, as well as the population served by that facility, rather than strictly using productivity or workload comparisons. These latter indicators will be used primarily to suggest strategies for coping with the funding level rather than to determine the level itself.

OTHER CHANGES TO THE FUNDING SYSTEM

Coincident with the introduction of population-based funding, several other changes were made to the funding system for hospitals. The introduction of the Hospital/Community Partnership Program and the Hospital Innovation Incentive Program attempted to address

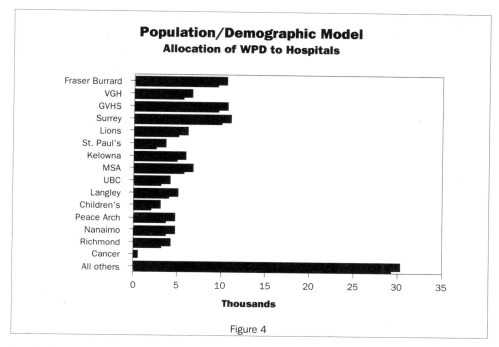

Figure 4

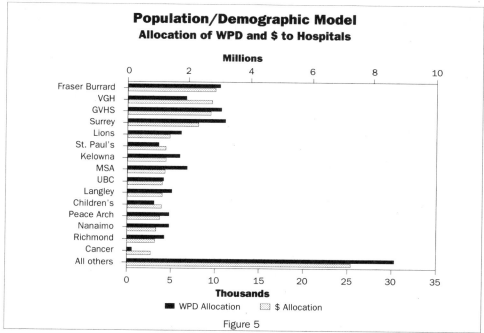

Figure 5

the need for hospitals to reach out to the community to provide the best care in the best setting and to look inward to ensure that the necessary services were being provided in the most efficient manner.

In addition, there have been policy changes that increase the flexibility of hospitals to use operating funds for capital purposes, revisions to equipment funding policies generally to improve both local decision-making and accountability, and a major revision to the Hospital Accounting Policies which should ensure that hospital financial statements fairly represent the resources used to provide health care services.

Two final examples of the Ministry's new approach to funding include a particular emphasis on addressing leave management issues and new policies stressing the need for each hospital to have a functioning utilization management program. Each of these initiatives is briefly described below.

HOSPITAL/COMMUNITY PARTNERSHIP PROGRAM

A great deal of attention has been focused in recent years on the need to move care into the community as much as possible. An ongoing problem, however, relates to ways hospital administrators can be encouraged to pursue this objective. In many locations in British Columbia, there has been considerable difficulty in getting hospital administrators to talk to administrators of other types of care facilities, let alone community-based service providers.

The Ministry felt strongly, in large measure because of the early results of the Victoria Health Project, that the integration and continuity of care could be enhanced by encouraging interaction between various service providers.

To facilitate this interaction, the Ministry set aside in each hospital's 1989/90 budget allocation an amount equal to 1/2 of 1% of the Hospital Programs operating grant. The "catch" was that to obtain this funding, the hospital, in cooperation with one or more community organizations or service providers, must put forward a joint proposal to a committee within the Ministry composed of senior management from both the institutional and community-based divisions of the Ministry. The overall objective of these proposals was to "improve health care while controlling the utilization of hospital services". The purposes for which funds could be requested included:

1) programs to assist in utilization management of hospital services, and
2) programs to prevent disease, promote health and generate healthy public policy.

Upon approval of a specific program, the Ministry provides funding for a 12-month period on a one-time basis. An evaluation component is an essential aspect of each proposal, and once this evaluation is completed, its results are used to make a permanent funding decision.

The 0.5% amounted to some $8 million in 1989/90; the amount was increased in 1990/91 to $ 12.4 million, or 0.75%. Over time this total could increase to up to 2%, as long as appropriate programs continue to be generated.

To date, a total of 149 proposals have been received (more than one per hospital), with a total cost of $13.1 million. Of this total, 50 programs, valued at $4.3 million, have been approved. A substantial proportion of the balance are still under review, while a number of others are awaiting available funding (some hospitals have submitted proposals valued in excess of 0.75% of their operating grant).

The programs funded range from $1,500 for a cholesterol clinic at a small Diagnostic and Treatment Centre to over $500,000 for a geriatric psychiatry outreach program at a major metropolitan teaching hospital. Quick response programs, various types of outreach programs, and palliative care programs are the ones being proposed most often, although the amount of innovation and creativity shown by the hospitals is quite impressive.

One unique feature of this program is that where funding is needed by other community service providers as part of a program, arrangements are made to transfer the necessary funds to those providers (generally through their funding source in the Ministry). Upon a successful evaluation, the base funding will be transferred. Hospitals have shown very little reluctance to engage in these types of arrangements, since they are sure that the funding will stay in their community to provide needed health services.

HOSPITAL INNOVATION INCENTIVE FUND

Hospitals often complain that they may have ideas that could improve the efficiency of their operations or otherwise lead to cost reductions, but the discretionary funding is not available to pursue these ideas. Moreover, any funding that does become available is almost immediately snapped up for patient care enhancements.

To address this concern the Ministry, starting in 1989/90, made available a revolving fund of up to $4 million, which would make interest free loans to provide the "seed funding" to pursue these ideas. Each proposal must be supported by a business case which outlines a payback schedule. Once the proposal is accepted and the loan made, repayment is made automatically by the Ministry through adjustments to the hospital's grant payments. Because these funds are made available through "financing transactions" in the Government's books, hospitals have no discretion as to whether to repay the loans.

To date 13 projects, totalling $850,000, have been approved, with payback times ranging from 13 months to three years.

OPERATING FOR CAPITAL POLICY

One of the hallmarks of hospital financing in British Columbia, as in other parts of Canada, has been the sharp distinction between government funding provided for operating and capital purposes. This tight control on capital is often credited with keeping hospital costs somewhat under control, especially in relation to the United States.

However, there are increasing concerns in the hospital sector that the controls on capital are not only limiting cost growth brought about by proliferation of new equipment, but are also strangling the hospitals' ability to ensure orderly replacement of necessary equipment.

Recognizing these concerns, the Ministry has relaxed its policies regarding the separation of operating and capital funds, so that hospitals with excess working capital in their operating accounts can apply to the Ministry to use these funds for necessary equipment purchases. This policy is relatively new, although several quite substantial requests have been made.

CHANGES TO EQUIPMENT FUNDING

Changes have also been made in the funding procedures themselves for hospital equipment. Previously, over 900 individual equipment requests were processed each year by the Ministry's Equipment Grants Secretariat. Of these, roughly 90% were for items costing under $100,000. Add to that the variety of cost sharing formulas for local contributions to different types of equipment, and the need for Regional Hospital District involvement in each request, and the need for reform can readily be appreciated.

Beginning in 1990/91 several major changes were made. First, the existing cost-sharing formulas for diagnostic, non-diagnostic, and construction-related equipment were replaced with a single 60-40 cost-sharing formula for shareable equipment. As well, both non-shareable equipment and provincially funded referral centre equipment are 100% funded by the respective bodies.

The second change required all hospitals to submit annual rolling five-year equipment plans, with fairly detailed specifications for the first year. The first year plan is divided into one list for high-tech equipment, equipment for new programs, and items over $100,000, and a second list which includes all other items. The plan generally and both lists are reviewed with the Regional Hospital District and then forwarded electronically to the Ministry and discussed with the Regional Teams. Hospital Programs then vets the second list and, upon approval, hospitals are able to purchase any item on that list without further reference to the Ministry.

To facilitate this, each hospital received a funding allocation based on its size grouping, function, and the number of beds of different types it operated. This represents a total allocation, and the Ministry share is 60% of this total. The remaining share must be obtained from local sources, including Regional Hospital Districts. In 1990/91 a total of $25 million province-wide was allocated using this approach.

This change should achieve several objectives. First, it should reduce considerably the ongoing paperwork burden of the hospitals, the Regional Hospital Districts, and the Ministry. Second, and perhaps most important, it will put the onus on the hospital to plan adequately for its capital needs and will also provide the flexibility to set priorities within those needs. For example, a hospital may have an allocation of $500,000 and an approved list totalling $800,000. The hospital can then proceed to set its priorities to purchase any group of items on that list to a total of $500,000.

Finally, it should introduce both more equity and more certainty in the way the Ministry allocates its available equipment funds and, it is hoped, provide a basis for developing strategies to increase those funds over time. The combination of a set allocation formula and regular, credible five-year plans should allow the Ministry to make appropriate representations to Treasury Board regarding the importance of funding growth in this area.

The Ministry has developed capabilities for monitoring and reporting which allow hospitals to transmit the required information to the Ministry electronically using the same system as is used for monthly reporting. The Ministry portion of the grant will be paid in several instalments during the year, with the payment of each instalment being contingent upon appropriate reporting and accounting for the previous amount.

HOSPITAL ACCOUNTING POLICIES

A final area in which Ministry-initiated changes will influence the financing of hospitals concerns proposed changes to hospital accounting policies. The *Hospital Insurance Act* provides the Minister of Health with the authority to specify the accounting policies to be used in hospitals. The fact that the existing policies had not been reviewed or amended for some time, together with the recent changes to the CICA Handbook regarding accounting for non-profit enterprises, indicated that this was an opportune time to review these policies.

The process for revising these policies included the circulation of a draft set of policies to a number of people in the field and a number of meetings with an industry group of hospital administrators and finance executives. As well, written submissions were requested; a number were submitted and subsequently reviewed internally within the Ministry.

A further element has been the completion of a review of purchasing practices in British Columbia hospitals by an outside accounting firm. This review made a number of recommendations that relate to hospital accounting policies.

Based on this input, the revised accounting policies include the following key elements:

a) **MIS Guidelines** – The concept has been endorsed, as well as the need for each hospital to develop the capacity to provide reports in a format compatible with the Guidelines. A specific due date is not specified, nor are the internal coding requirements prescribed.

b) **Fund Accounting** – The new policy mandates the use of integrated fund accounting for external reporting, because of the feeling within the Ministry that the use of capital assets is an integral part of the provision of health care services and this should be appropriately reflected in the hospital's financial statements.

c) **Depreciation** – The reporting of depreciation in the operating statements of the hospital and policies for recording of assets, amortization of capital grants, and establishment of fixed asset accounting systems are all included in the new policy. To ease the burden on hospitals, the recording of all existing assets will not be required. The new policy also includes the appropriate thresholds for capitalizing equipment and minor renovations.

e) **Accrual Accounting** – Full accrual accounting is supported, including the accrual of vacation and sick/severance pay.

f) **Accounting Cycles** – A move to a 13-period, 28-day accounting cycle with a common payday for all facilities is mandated to ensure common periods for the collection of statistical, staffing, and financial information.

These various initiatives will assist hospitals in meeting the financial imperatives they face by providing increased internal flexibility in the allocation of resources, as well as increased scope for innovation and improved planning and priority setting. These changes also attempt to recognize the true nature and importance of the hospital "business" and to ensure that funding and accounting policies reflect the need to approach hospital management in a more business-like manner.

A VISION FOR THE FUTURE

This section examines the next steps in both the demographic-based funding methods and the other financing initiatives and concludes with an overall vision for hospital financing in British Columbia.

POPULATION/DEMOGRAPHIC FUNDING

As noted, a major effort in the near future will be to "level the playing field" for all hospitals, so that their total funding base adequately reflects their role and size and the catchment population they serve. This will require a great deal of attention to the specific construction of "peer groupings", as well as further refinement of the measures to be used to assess equity in funding. Another aspect will likely be a more precise definition of the roles of and programs to be offered by different types of facilities.

It is also hoped that further refinements can be made over the next few years to incorporate more needs-based indicators and to develop better measures of "acuity" in the allocation process. In this regard, the Ministry is examining the possibility of using Resource Intensity Weighting (RIW) factors, although a number of practical and methodological considerations must be addressed before these can be used.

With respect to other needs-based indicators, some work has already been done examining the impact of socio-demographic, geographic, and health status factors on a regional basis, and research is proceeding in this area. To date, factors such as standardized mortality rates, education level, native percentage of the population, distance from a major population centre, and composition of the workforce have all been shown to be correlated with age-sex adjusted utilization rates, although there are also significant collinear relationships among a number of these variables.

It is expected that as the base funding is adjusted and equalized to reflect these refinements, it should be possible at some time in the future to provide the total funding allocation based on population needs and the role/size of each facility.

OTHER FINANCING INITIATIVES

In the near term, efforts will be directed at improving the flexibility of individual hospitals to meet their care delivery needs in the most cost-effective manner. This will likely include further refinements to the capital equipment funding methods to integrate operating and capital planning and decision-making processes at the hospital level more closely, as well as further expansion of programs that promote innovation and alternative care delivery methods.

However, the Ministry is also likely to continue to play a significant role in bringing industry-wide issues and concerns to the attention of hospitals and in facilitating collective action to deal with these issues. Examples currently under development include a thrust to improve leave management practices in hospitals and an increased emphasis on the implementation of utilization management programs in hospitals. In both cases, the Ministry will be taking a key role in providing advice and incentives to individual hospitals or groups of hospitals.

THE LONGER TERM VISION

Over the longer term, British Columbia is clearly moving towards a system of hospital finance that provides resources to hospitals consistent with their roles and the types of services they are expected to provide to their catchment population, and then gives hospital boards and administrators the maximum flexibility to provide this necessary care. Concomitant with this, however, will also be an increased level of accountability for providing efficient, effective, and appropriate care.

The concept of the hospital global budget will be substantially redefined from being an expenditure target within which hospital operations must be carried out to being a key component of each hospital's overall plan to provide this necessary care. But it will be only one component – staffing, workload, capital and program plans will gradually assume an importance equal to that of the fiscal plan or framework.

Balancing the budget will become only one aspect of the Ministry's evaluation of a hospital's performance. A balanced budget with poor quality care or inappropriate services will be grounds for appointing a public administrator as much as will a large budget deficit. In many ways, the Ministry has already made substantial strides in this direction.

One key element of this vision is an information base that supports both the Ministry and hospitals in assessing efficiency, effectiveness, and appropriate, high quality care. Many of the basic data are already available, although attention must be paid to appropriate systems for analyzing and distributing these data in the form of meaningful information.

Taken together, the initiatives described above and the longer term vision should provide the hospital board and administration with the wherewithal to provide the right care to the right persons in the right setting and should also ensure that those who do not do so have very few excuses.

DISCUSSION
Chair: Rashi Fein
Harvard University

I had lived in the United States with a misguided view of why you had a successful – it seemed to us, and relative to us, obviously – successful health care system and we didn't. My view, sitting in Boston, was that we had an awful lot of health economists and you didn't. I was clearly mistaken. There are a lot here. There may be an *ex post* and *ex ante* problem. Maybe you should get the health economists after you've put the system in place. In any case, however, I can return to Boston and tell my friends that they need not fear that if we in fact institute something more rational than what we have in the United States, they will be unemployed. Clearly, there are still things to study, and clearly no matter how good your data bases may be in relation to ours, they can always be improved upon, studied further, with new indices developed, etc.

I am correct in saying that each of the three speakers took the 15 minutes not in an effort to avoid questions, but because, as we all recognize, they had a lot of material to present. And it strikes me that perhaps it would be appropriate for any of you who want additional details to search out our three speakers now or at additional coffee breaks.

I do want to make one comment. That's the prerogative of the chairman. I want to take a minute to contrast what seems to me to be what this meeting's like and what a similar kind of session in the United States might be, because it's perhaps a non-trivial observation. It may even be interesting in addition and is worth your thinking about. You are wrapped up in a health care system that is being studied because you believe deeply it has some problems and can be improved upon. You may lose some perspective in that involvement with your own health care system. So let me take a second to remind you of what a U.S. meeting of this kind might be.

The coffee conversation and the coffee break would involve individuals trading stories about how they may have been able to solve, or whether others know how to solve, a particular health insurance problem for one of their relatives. That is, I would have been out there saying to colleagues, "You know, last week I had a problem with my daughter, who is a part-time employee for a firm that doesn't offer health insurance for part-time employees, and is a part-time graduate student in a university that says, 'Because you're part-time, you cannot use the student health service', and she has what we call a pre-existing condition." And I would have said to friends, "Do you know what I ought to do?" At the more general level of the program, remember that a U.S. health care meeting would spend lots of time on making hospitals more efficient, lots of time on pharmaceuticals, lots of time on cost containment and budgets, and an awful lot of time on, "How do we achieve a system in which at least everybody has a fair shot at access?" You're not even talking about that. And I congratulate you for that. Remember that your problems are real, but remember you've got a lot to be proud of.

THERE'S
NO
PLACE
LIKE
HOME

COST-EFFECTIVENESS OF HOME CARE*

William G. Weissert
Department of Health Services Management and Policy
Institute of Gerontology, University of Michigan

When Rashi Fein was talking about comparisons with the U.S., I was reminded of a line of one of our minority leaders of the U.S. Senate who used to say, "A billion here and a billion there, and pretty soon you are talking about real money." I noticed all your problems have only 6 zeros, so there is hope for you. Think about it as a rounding error on the rate of inflation in the U.S. healthcare problem, and it puts it in some context you can live with.

I am here to talk about cost-effectiveness of home care, and really to focus more on where that has led me, which is on the issue of, "How do you make it more efficient so that it has a prayer of becoming cost-effective?" So the question is, "Why would you study home care?" And since I'm from the States, the real reason is to save money. But on the outside chance we might be asked to present our results in Canada sometime, we also look at outcomes, or at least we give some lip service to them.

Now if you want to save money on home care, the obvious idea is that what you are trying to do is to substitute home care for institutional care. And so you say, "We're going to take this person out of hospital or out of the nursing home," or more likely, "We're going to try to avoid getting them in there by giving them home care services, and although we'll spend some more money on home care services and some outpatient costs, we'll save more than that by keeping them out of a hospital or out of a nursing home." I am going to give you the results not of one study, but of 27 studies (Figure 1). About half of them were con-

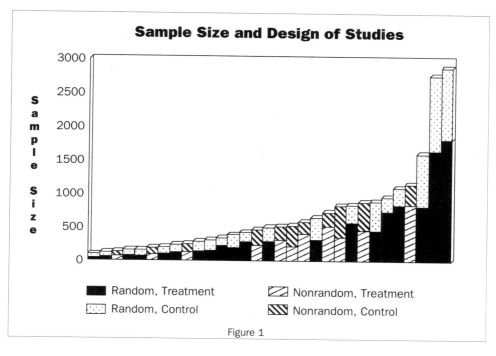

Figure 1

trolled experiments, where we randomly assigned people to either extra home care benefits or to a control group. Both groups got our Medicare and Medicaid program, but the treatment group got extra home care – much broader eligibility and availability of services. And then we had some studies that were quasi-experiments, where we had a group that was getting home care and we compared them to another group. In Figure 1, the bars with the darker colour at the bottom come from the randomized studies; the sample sizes are on the left. And what you see is that we've had studies ranging in size from about 30 patients in each group on up to several thousand in the treatment group and the control group. This is the pattern of these 27 studies. If you counted the studies that I showed you, there are actually 31 of those columns, and the reason is that several of the studies had two or three treatment arms, to which we gave different combinations of home care services.

When I talk about home care, our definition in the States includes home health, homemaker, home health aide, chore services, friendly visitor, meals on wheels, and a whole range of services that we lump under the rubric of home care. On the other hand, if you ask people, "Where did the money go? You offered 25 services; what did people use?", the answer is homemaker services. So to some extent, although our studies cover all services (therapeutic included), people tend, when you offer them a choice, to focus their options on homemaker.

These studies started back as early as the 1960s (Figure 2). Again, these were all controlled experiments or quasi-experiments. And it went along, with a couple starting every couple of years, until the mid 1970s. Several colleagues and I did some randomized experiments where we controlled and looked very carefully at costs, which had not previously been done. And what we found was that home care not only did not save money, it substantially increased outlays and it had little or no effect on health status outcomes.

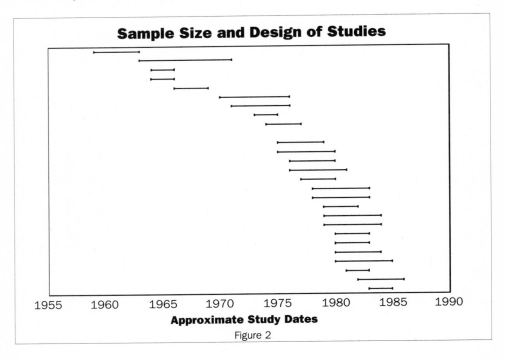

Sample Size and Design of Studies

Approximate Study Dates

Figure 2

There were two results. First of all, people called me a variety of unflattering things. And then several other studies were funded, including some very recent ones to the tune of $50 million each, to try to refute what I had found, and I am happy to say – not happy because of the results, but happy that at least, after being pilloried, I was not driven out of the field – that I was proven right by these studies, to the extent that one can prove something is right. That is, they all came to the same conclusion. So here are the average results of these 27 controlled experiments and quasi-experiments (Figure 3).

Let me start with the bottom line here, and that is that the treatment group – those who got the extra home care services – cost more than the control group. The good news out of this synthesis was that the size of this difference was not as large as we had seen in some of the individual studies. It's around 15%. When you offer home care services the net, after everything shakes out, is it adds about 15%, maybe 17% or 18%, to net costs.

Why does it do that? One of the big reasons, and really the biggest disappointment, is that although home care does save nursing home use – it avoids people going into nursing homes – the problem is that most people who use home care aren't on their way to a nursing home. That's why the rate of expenditures on nursing homes is so small. What we found is that despite the fact that we were using the latest assessment tools and crack teams of multi-disciplinary assessors, and we studied only patients who lived through the assessments that were so exhaustive (that's a joke), we were wrong about 4 times out of 5 when we said, "Yes, this is a patient who will benefit from home care because they are at risk of going to a nursing home." Most people who use home care are not at risk of going to a nursing home. In the control group, they don't go to a nursing home. So whether they get the treatment or not, they tend to stay out of a nursing home. If they get the treatment,

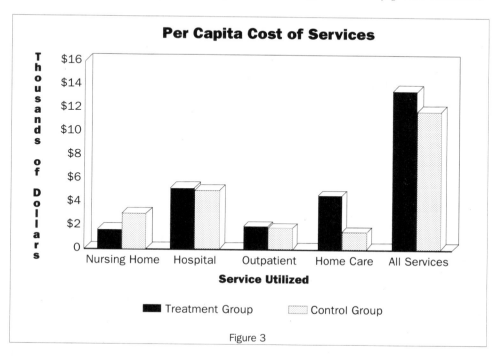

Figure 3

then it does reduce their nursing home use, but unfortunately it is a relatively small portion of them that are getting the benefit, and it doesn't reduce the nursing home use of *all* of those who would go in.

Hospital costs actually go up slightly with home care. Some go up and some go down – go up in some studies and down in others – but the net is a slight increase associated with home care use instead of a reduction. That is terrifically bad news, of course, because you are looking to save money, and in fact you wind up spending more on the hospitalization. Outpatient costs run about 2% higher for the treatment group than the control group, and it is actually surprising that it is not more than that, because you would expect outpatient costs to go up. On the other hand, home care costs go up astronomically. As I have said, the control group here was not locked in a room – these were people who were eligible for our rather stingy benefits in home care under Medicare and Medicaid. So some of them are getting some home care. For example, you can get home care under Medicare if you are actively in a rehabilitation plan, you have rehabilitation potential, you are homebound, and you are receiving at least one skilled service.

What home care does, and this is important to understand, is that it radically increases the amount of home care used. I don't know exactly how many people are actually enfranchised by our home care, but it is a smaller portion than we set out to serve. We thought we were going out with these services to enfranchise a lot of new users. What we actually did was to add a lot of use. I am inclined to believe that health care is just like everything else, in that it experiences diminishing returns to scale. The more of it you give, the less benefit you get. And so as the amount of home care used goes up radically, I think you get less benefit for each additional unit. One of the ways that you might think about saving money is to cut down on that additional amount of home care use. The bottom line is about a 15% to 18% increase in cost.

I did mention that I would pay some attention to outcomes. We actually studied outcomes quite exhaustively (Table 1).

We looked at survival and found no effect. People don't live any longer because they get one of these home care services, or many of them. And they don't function any better in terms of their activities of daily living and a variety of other measures of physical functioning. Across these 27 studies, we have used just about every scale you can think of, including the Townsend Scale and the Katz ADL Scale and Breslow, and lots of others.

Table 1
OUTCOMES STUDIED

- Survival
- Physical functioning
- Mental functioning
- Life satisfaction
- Informal caregiving
- Informal caregivers':
  - Stress
  - Burden
  - Life satisfaction

We even had people come up with some inventive things. One of the things that surprised me, looking at all the different measures, was that one of the studies looked at the ability to wash the inside of a window. Home care does not improve that, in case you are wondering. In fact, there were half a dozen studies in which the use of home care was associated with declining physical functioning ability. We think what happens is that the aide doesn't wait long enough for the individual to do it and takes it over. And if you are measuring things behaviorally, a function that has been taken over is one that is lost. We see half a dozen times where that has happened, in good studies, not trivial ones. Mental functioning was not affected by home care in these 27 studies. Life satisfaction was affected. In the treatment group, the patients experienced about a 6% increase, that is, about 6% of them increased their life satisfaction or declined at a slower rate in the course of the study. Caregivers' life satisfaction – about 9% of them increased. That is the good news, although that's a pretty small increase. The bad news is that it doesn't last very long. Even though you continue treatment, the effects on the patient go away in six months, and the effects on the caregiver go away in about nine months, and in terms of stress and burden on the caregiver – the things that we really expected to be relieved – we saw no difference. Caregivers still felt as stressed by their chores and as burdened as they had before, although they felt somewhat higher life satisfaction. One bit of good news was the following: There was a great fear in the United States that if you gave people paid-for home care, it would drive out informal unpaid care. And what we saw was it did that only to the tune of about 2%. Informal care giving dropped by only about 2%, and it tended to be reordered somewhat. Informal caregivers gave up medically oriented therapeutic tasks and did more of the routine aid tasks, but they were not likely to just walk away from it.

This has led me to question whether there is any further work for an analyst who is interested in proving that home care is not cost-effective. And I actually turned down a large grant to do one more study like that recently and told them instead, "I already know the answer to that. How about we work on how to get it cost-effective?" And so that is what I am currently engaged in, and that is what I would like to finish this talk with today. I think that we can make home care cost-effective, or come awfully close to it, and we have to do that by working on both the cost and the effectiveness (Table 2).

Table 2
HOW TO MAKE HOME CARE LESS EXPENSIVE

- Increase Risk
  Use risk assessment scales combined with clinical judgment to improve screening accuracy
- Reduce Hospital Admissions
  Replace "extra" hospitalization resulting from home care aide observations with lower cost interventions
- Reduce Outpatient Costs
  No reason to believe that such reductions can or should be achieved
- Reduce Home Care Costs
  Duration, intensity, outliers; operate at capacity
- Improve Outcomes
  Match patients, services, and care objectives

I think in terms of effectiveness, one of the things you have to do is a better job of screening – I am going to call it targeting because that is the word we use in the United States. We have to do a better job of screening individuals so that we are serving more people who would go to a nursing home. Instead of 1 out of 5, it needs to be 1 out of 3, or something like that. And if you could get that number up by doing better jobs of estimating risk of institutionalization, then you'd have a better chance of saving some money on nursing home costs.

In about half the studies hospitalization went down, and it went down sometimes by as much as 18%. But in the other half it went up by, again, as much as 18 or 19%. One possible explanation is random variation around the mean, but those are pretty big numbers for that, so I am inclined to think that what's happening is that some people are being diverted from hospitals and others are being sent there. I don't think there is any reason to expect that we are going to see a reduction in outpatient costs. This is an outpatient setting, and I think you are going to see those go up, and you ought to expect that. I do think it is possible to reduce the duration, the intensity, of home care and have no adverse outcome impacts. And I think that a well-managed program would do a better job of avoiding some of the very costly patients who got into our home care programs and probably could have been served more efficiently and perhaps more effectively in institutional settings. We also find that most of our home care programs operate below capacity. Now that may not be a problem here, but it is in the United States. They operate at 1/2 to 2/3 of capacity, which makes the unit costs go through the roof. And I think the way you avoid that is with better studies of demand – better demand estimates – and more efficient management of the care so that you're delivering services under one management instead of multiple ones. The other thing I think we have to do is that instead of giving everybody that gets home care basically the same package – we have care planning teams who do all kinds of things, but patients pretty much wind up getting things that seem to be unrelated to their characteristics and quite expensive – so my suggestion is that we try to do a better job of saying, "What exactly would this patient be at risk of developing if we didn't do home care?", and let us focus our efforts on that specific problem.

On the business of trying to focus on people who are at risk of going into a nursing home, we have done studies, and others have, and Evelyn [Shapiro] has done these and synthesized them here. This is a study we did recently – we are just completing it in fact – based on our 1985 National Nursing Home Survey and our National Health Interview Survey, which we merged together to give us all of the elderly people in the United States, and we said, "Well, what are the characteristics that distinguish people in nursing homes vs. those in the community?" And what we find is that dependency in toileting, eating, bathing, dressing, mental disorder, all of these things, very largely increase the odds that someone is in a nursing home. For example, someone who is toileting-/eating-dependent is 144 times more likely to be a resident in the nursing home than someone who is not toileting-/eating-dependent (Table 3) (Weissert and Cready, 1989b). With age, each increase in year of age adds seven-tenths of a percent to the probability of being in a nursing home.

The important thing here is not so much the individual traits, but the multiplicative effects of these things. We have tended to look at patients and say, "Gee, they are toileting- and eating-dependent. We know that increases their risk of institutionalization."

When you do multivariate analysis like this you see that what really increases risk is having lots of these things wrong. My suggestion is that what we ought to be doing is letting our clinical teams make their judgment, then we should put the patients' characteristics into a simple algorithm, come up with a predicted probability of institutionalization, which may or may not be right but you can compare it to your clinical judgment and say, "Gee, there is an instance here where I have got two different probabilities, one is clinical, one is based on my algorithm, and they don't agree and I want to go back and take another look." I think if we did that we would do a much better job of targeting people at risk. God forbid that I would ever be subjected to this if I want to get into home care. But I wouldn't mind having it taken as part of a clinical decision making process. We've put this thing into software for a PC and you can punch the characteristics of the patient in and get a prediction which will be wrong, but it will make you feel good that you have it.

Reducing hospital admissions – this is my research agenda for the next couple of years, or at least a major piece of it. I am convinced that there are things going on here that I don't yet well understand, but I have enough hunches I hope to get funded. I think there is something going on that we've seen in some studies called the Discovery Effect. We send an aide or a case manager out to the home. You have a very old patient who is suffering multiple disorders. She sees the patient. She says, "My God, what terrible shape she is in!" She calls the doctor. She tells him all about how terrible the patient is. He is not on the scene, he is busy. He admits the patient. He finds out she really hasn't changed that much from the last time she was admitted, but you now have a hospital admission and it is expensive. Our thinking is that there may be ways to forewarn the physician with some algorithms, some questions, some additional questions he can ask, based on predictions of who it is that is likely to have one of these discovery effect admissions, and he may be able to get enough additional information to make the decision. I fantasize that he actually might go out there and take a look, but I know that will not happen.

Table 3

RISK OF INSTITUTIONALIZATION: LOGISTIC REGRESSION RESULTS

Variable	Odds Ratio
Toilet/eat dependent	144.02
Bathe/dress dependent	33.78
Mental disorder	14.15
Injury	11.82
White	4.48
Not married	4.31
Poverty	4.14
Nursing home stay	3.97
Respiratory diagnosis	1.97
Midwest residence	1.88
Male	1.23
Age	1.07
Living children	0.37

• all significant at p<.001, except male

I looked in these studies at the rate of hospitalization that resulted in death and at the characteristics of those patients (Table 4).

Table 4

CHARACTERISTICS OF HOME CARE PATIENTS WHO WERE HOSPITALIZED AND DIED

- Sum of activities of daily living (ADLs)
- Perceived poor health
- Beddays in past two months
- Number of conditions
- Some care sites

There is a very high proportion of the patients who were going into the hospital to die. We've got enough debate going on over this issue of right to death with dignity and things like that that I don't need to step into it. But it does make sense to me to ask the question, "If you know that the prognosis for the patient is death, why do you have to put a hospitalization in the process? Why can't you do a little bit of advance planning with the family, write a living will, think about a direct admission to a skilled nursing facility or to a hospice setting instead of going to the hospital to die, or going through the hospital to the skilled facility?" Again, I think there is an avoidable hospitalization, and the thing is that with the relatively small difference in cost between nursing home and home care – the control group and the treatment group – you don't have to avoid very many hospitalizations before you're getting close to being cost-effective. I think that there is some variation that is just associated with physician style of practice that we might be able to change.

I mentioned that one of the major sources of increased cost is the very high increase in home care use. Figure 4 asks the question, "Does the difference in the high rates of home care use among patients make any sense?" The solid black bars represent people who used the top fourth, that is, they used about $7,000 per year of home care. The other set of bars represent people who used the bottom fourth, about $700, or 1/10 as much care. I don't know how good your naked eye is, but mine fails to detect differences in these two groups. This is not multivariate analysis. I have done multivariate analysis, and it doesn't change much from this. Patient characteristics don't appear to be playing as much of a role as you would like. You ask yourself, "How long have we been doing home care? What kind of algorithms do we have for it? Compare that with some of our clinical, more acute-related kinds of interventions, and do we really know exactly how much home care somebody needs to accomplish something?" I think the answer is that we don't and we need some much better planning, starting with the assumption that if a patient is going to benefit from home care it is likely to be in the early part of the stay and not in the later part, and everything I have looked at would suggest that. You might be asking the question, "Wouldn't it better, if you have scarce resources, to allocate them to new patients, relative to older patients, and as the patient is in home care longer begin to look for less costly substitutes, like friendly visitor visits to substitute for aide visits, alarm response systems and other technological innovations to try to reduce the cost associated with home care?"

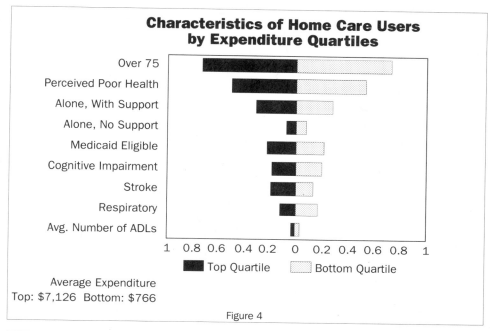

Characteristics of Home Care Users by Expenditure Quartiles

Over 75
Perceived Poor Health
Alone, With Support
Alone, No Support
Medicaid Eligible
Cognitive Impairment
Stroke
Respiratory
Avg. Number of ADLs

1 0.8 0.6 0.4 0.2 0 0.2 0.4 0.6 0.8 1

■ Top Quartile   ▨ Bottom Quartile

Average Expenditure
Top: $7,126 Bottom: $766

Figure 4

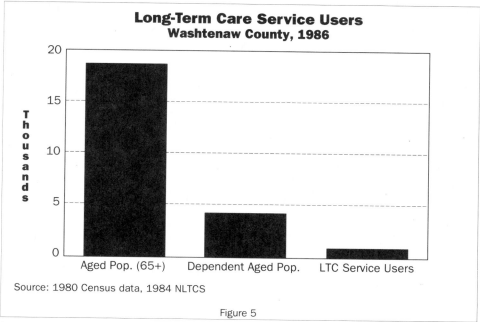

Long-Term Care Service Users
Washtenaw County, 1986

Thousands

20
15
10
5
0

Aged Pop. (65+)   Dependent Aged Pop.   LTC Service Users

Source: 1980 Census data, 1984 NLTCS

Figure 5

I mentioned that one of the costs of home care comes from the fact that programs operate below capacity in most cases. In the county around Ann Arbor, Michigan, the aged population is about 18,000 or 19,000 people (Figure 5). The dependent population as we projected it using synthetic estimation techniques is about 4,000 people. Only about 700 of those people are using formal home care services. If you start off another daycare centre or home care services, thinking that there are thousands of people waiting for you, you are in for a shock, at least in the United States. You'll find that after the first meeting of pent up need in the first few months, you'll have a hard time meeting your quota. This is simply a comparison of our projection of ADL [Activities of Daily Living] dependency and IADL [Instrumental Activities of Daily Living] dependency, using national data, for which we obtained a very good fit to our models. (Note: ADL dependency means that human help is needed in bathing, dressing, transferring, toileting, continence, or eating, and IADL includes activities like walking, telephone use, cooking, and meal preparations.) We then used this to make projections down to the county level, which would be a useful thing to do for Ontario. Estimating how many people are out there gives you some basis for planning. We are now trying to convert these things into demand estimates, not just prevalence.

If you look at the groups that we serve in home care, I think that we can focus on some subgroups who have different kinds of outcome objectives. Some of these outcomes would be to:
- shorten hospital stay
- avoid rehospitalization
- achieve rehabilitative potential
- avoid nursing home admission
- shorten nursing home stay
- improve patient life satisfaction
- improve caregiver life satisfaction

We can try to focus our efforts more specifically on the needs of these groups, instead of serving everybody as if they were the same.

NOTE

* edited transcript of talk. An earlier version of this paper was delivered at the U.S. Department of Veterans Affairs Eighth Annual Symposium on Geriatrics and Gerontology, St. Louis, Missouri, September 14, 1989, and is published in the proceedings of that symposium (Weissert WG: Community-based long term care: a prospective budgeting strategy for achieving cost effectiveness. In: Romeis JC, Coe RM (eds.): *Quality and Cost Containment in the Care of the Elderly.* New York: Springer Publishing Company, Inc., 1991, chapter 13). Figures 1, 3, and 4 appear in that chapter and are used here by permission of the Springer Publishing Company, Inc., New York 10012.

REFERENCES

Weissert WG: Strategies for reducing home-care expenditures. *Generations* 42-44, Spring 1990.

Weissert WG, Cready CM: A prospective budgeting model for home- and community-based long-term care. *Inquiry* 26:116-129, (Spring) 1989a.

Weissert WG, Cready CM: Toward a model for improved targeting of aged at risk of institutionalization. *Health Services Research* 24:485-510, 1989b.

Weissert WG, Cready CM, Pawelak JE: The past and future of home- and community-based long-term care. *The Milbank Quarterly* 66:309-388, 1988.

THERE'S NO PLACE LIKE HOME

Discussant: Evelyn Shapiro
Department of Community Health Sciences
University of Manitoba

The use of the same generic terms in referring to home care or nursing homes in U.S. and Canadian studies can mislead the initiated because U.S. policies and the populations served differ substantially from those in Canada. Although time constraints preclude detailing the major differences, it is critical for us to be very careful in deciding which, if any, findings and conclusions of U.S. studies are applicable to Canada, especially when they look so alike because, for example, the proportions of elderly using home care services in any one year are remarkably similar.

This problem is compounded for us in Canada by three other factors. We have no agreed-upon terminology or national information system. Provincial home care programs continue to differ despite their ever-increasing similarity. Canadian research and, therefore, research reports on home care are scarce, with few economists having shown any interest in home care. I have therefore decided to focus on two themes:

1) home care use in Manitoba, based on data from the provincial program and from the Manitoba Longitudinal Study on Aging, and

2) key issues currently affecting home care.

Manitoba's Continuing Care program is a provincial, no-cost-to-consumer program which assesses persons requiring community or nursing home care, coordinates and delivers services at home, or places individuals in a nursing home. (Note the comment by Weissert et al, 1988 that "best results might be achieved by coupling home care with nursing home admission screening"). It serves persons requiring care on a short- or long-term basis. Eligibility does not require an M.D. referral or the specific need for a medical service. Nursing home care is insured, with persons paying a room and board per diem which is designed to leave those with minimum pensions some discretionary funds. Home care consumes about 3% of the provincial health care budget, a percentage which has remained almost constant despite the growth in the number of elderly who are the predominant consumers.

Table 1 summarizes annual data on home care caseloads, the ratio of total caseloads to the elderly population, and the ratio of nursing home beds to persons aged 75 or more every two years from 1982/83 to 1988/89. I am using age 65 or more as the reference population for home care because 77.1% of all persons served are the elderly (20.6% are aged 19-64 and 2.2% are under age 19) and age 75+ for nursing homes because over 80% of all nursing home admissions are aged 75 or more.

Table 1

HOME CARE CASELOADS, TOTAL SERVED/1,000 ELDERLY[1] AND NURSING HOME BED SUPPLY[2] 1982/83 TO 1988/89

	1982/83	1984/85	1986/87	1988/89
In program on March 31st	10,631	11,848	13,193	–[3]
New admissions	9,696	10,438	11,827	10,320
Discharges	9,202	9,479	11,409	–[3]
Total served during year	19,716	21,371	25,020	23,403
Total served/1,000 elderly	156.0	165.1	173.4	166.7
Nursing home bed supply/ 1,000 persons aged 75+	161.4	159.9	149.7	143.8

1 Source: Office of Continuing Care, Manitoba Health
2 Source: Annual Reports, Manitoba Health Services Commission
3 Data as yet unavailable

From 1982 to 1986 the total home care caseload/1,000 elderly increased from 156 to 173.4 as the nursing home bed supply ratio decreased from 161.4 to 149.7. Note that in 1984/85 and 1986/87, the numbers in the program at the beginning of the year increased, indicating a growth in those receiving long-term care. In fact, our own study (Shapiro and Tate, 1989) shows that from 1976 through to 1984, years with higher nursing home admission rates had statistically significant lower home care admission rates and vice-versa. 1988/89 shows a reduction in both home care caseloads and bed supply. It will be interesting to see what happens as bed ratios, currently at 140/1,000, continue to fall.

Table 2 examines the care equivalent of persons admitted to home care in 1988/89. Half required the equivalent of hospital care and about 30% the equivalent of nursing home care. However, for almost 20% of all service recipients, the services were a substitute neither for hospital nor nursing home care. These latter service recipients are not assessment errors but legitimate, usually low-cost, consumers whose situation and that of their families would otherwise become too stressful or totally untenable, provided that home care is acknowledged to be more than merely a substitute for institutional care (and there are compelling reasons for acknowledging this which I cannot go into now).

Table 2

CARE EQUIVALENT OF PERSONS ADMITTED TO HOME CARE IN 1988/89[1]

	N	%
Hospital	5,238	50.8
Nursing home	3,092	29.9
Neither	1,990	19.3
Total	*10,320*	*100.0*

1 Source: Office of Continuing Care, Manitoba Health

Table 3 presents the annual cost per person served in home care and in nursing homes in 1988/89. The nursing home cost of $22,051 includes only public expenditures. It therefore underestimates the cost because the per diem paid directly by the recipient is not included. The per person cost of the direct home care services placed in the home is $1,667. When the expenditures for the provincial administration and management office, the assessment and case coordination services, and direct services are all included, the cost is about $2,100 per person. It should be noted, however, that this also somewhat underestimates costs because some expenditures, such as medical supplies and equipment, are excluded.

Table 3

ANNUAL COST PER PERSON SERVED IN NURSING HOME AND HOME CARE IN 1988/89

Nursing home	$ 22,051 [1]
Home care services only	$ 1,667 [2]
Home care services + central administration, assessment, case coordination [3]	$ 2,102 [2,3]

1 Source: Annual Report, Manitoba Health Services Commission, 1988/89. Excludes non-government expenditures
2 Source: Office of Continuing Care, Manitoba Health
3 Excludes cost for Administrative Services Branch area for medical supplies/home care equipment

---

Clearly, home care is less costly than nursing home care, confirming earlier findings by the Manitoba/Canada Home Care Study (1982). Even if we deduct all the persons for whom home care is neither a hospital nor a nursing home bed substitute as if they would otherwise be in a nursing home, the per person cost ($2,627.56) is still substantially below the cost of a nursing home placement.

To round off the focus on home care, preliminary findings from a study now under way but confined exclusively to the elderly indicate that 5% of the elderly are admitted to the program each year and about 10% use services during the year. Bivariate analyses indicate that users are older, less healthy, less functional – both physically and mentally – and closer to death than non-users. Multivariate analysis discloses that the characteristics that significantly differentiate users from non-users are, in descending order: 1+ problems with the Instrumental Activities of Daily Living, being unmarried, 1+ problems with the basic ADL, Age 85+, Age 75-84, fair-bad self-rated health, living in Winnipeg as compared to the rest of Manitoba, being female, not having a relative in the same building, and 4+ self-reported health problems.

KEY ISSUES FOR HOME CARE

Several recent developments are accelerating a trend which began earlier and are increasing the pressure on home care to expand without a concomitant and proportionate expansion of resources. Briefly stated, these developments are:

1) growth in physician supply, coupled with governments' decision to reduce the ratio of acute beds/population. The result is that hospitals are demanding that community

care provide services to earlier and earlier discharges, i.e., to sicker and sicker people, and provide "high-tech" services at home;

2) increasing use of outpatient surgery. The result, especially for those procedures whose major clientele is the elderly (e.g., cataract surgery), is that more persons require care at home;

3) increasing numbers of elderly, particularly older elderly who are the main users of community care;

4) increasing efforts by governments to reduce the ratio of long-term beds/1,000 older elderly;

5) increasing prevalence of dementia as the size of the very elderly population increases, since the rate of dementia increases from about 3% to about 25% with advancing age; and

6) financial constraint. These fiscal constraints have become even sharper since the federal government recently reduced its EPF contributions and announced further reductions to the provinces in the future.

These six major developments, combined with the power and influence of the institutional sectors, are pushing community care into providing more emergency services, more medical services, more "high-tech" services and more 24-hour-per-day, 7-day-a-week services. The result is that, with budget limits as stringent as they are now and with expenditures per person rising, we are now beginning to hear questions such as:

1) Should we continue to serve frail elderly persons who need only minimal support services?

2) Should hospitals take over service delivery?

In respect to the first question, the amount of support services required is a function of the availability and capacity of informal resources. Therefore, what will we gain if we let the circumstances of the elderly and their caregivers who require minimal support deteriorate to the point where they require more or to the point where their families insist on institutionalization?

The answer to the second question is more complex. Four key factors reinforce the importance of maintaining the community-based model. First, the vast majority of people, including the elderly, do not enter a hospital during the course of a year, and most elderly enter the home care program from the community. Research shows that:

1) 70% of elderly home care admissions over age 75 enter from the community rather than from hospital;

2) 6-8% of the very recently hospitalized (8-30 days previously) elderly are admitted from the community, suggesting either that the hospital staff thought they would fare better than they actually did when they left hospital or that the staff was not sufficiently well-informed about their social situation at home;

3) with advancing age, home care serves increasingly as a nursing home bed, rather than a hospital bed, replacement program; and

4) about 1/4 of the long-term recipients of home care are non-elderly, disabled community dwellers. Furthermore, there are major advantages to encouraging the use of home care instead of nursing home admission for younger elderly who require light or medium levels of care because such admissions result in average stays ranging from about four to almost 17 years (Shapiro and Tate, 1988).

In addition, two recent systematic evaluations cast doubt on the assumption that hospital-bed replacement services could be provided more efficiently or most cost-effectively by hospitals than by the community-based program. In Montreal, the Verdun Hospital's "hospital-in-the home" program proved more expensive than in-hospital treatment, whereas Victoria's Quick Response Team, run by the community-care program, was cheaper than in-hospital care. Nevertheless, with only these two studies to go on, we would be wise to withhold final judgement on this issue until the results of further trials are in.

However, the hospital-based model has other serious disadvantages. It is medically oriented, an orientation not reflective of the needs of most home care recipients. It is high priced, both because it is medically oriented and because it is not necessarily geographically close to the homes of recipients. It is less likely to have adequate knowledge about the individual's home and family. Its acute care orientation and experience is not a good basis for understanding long-term community or institutional services.

However, the technological explosion will mean that serious consideration may have to be given by home care programs to using hospital resources to deliver highly sophisticated treatments at home. This consideration should, however, first take account of the following factors:

1) Is it cost-effective and safer to provide the treatment at home at all?

2) If it is, how can the delivery of hospital-based services be integrated into the community-based model so that the non-medical resources are not duplicated and the individual's care plan is coordinated?

ONE POSSIBLE RESPONSE

Giving serious consideration to emergent issues requires an established mechanism and an established process for joint planning at the highest level. However, the problem is that most provinces have not included representation from their community care program in the overall planning for health care. In some provinces, this occurs because community care reports to the Ministry of Community Services or to the Ministry of Social Services, whereas other health care sectors report to the Ministry of Health. In provinces that do not have this division of responsibility, community care, probably because it is not a major spender, is regarded as nice and maybe even necessary, but peripheral. Each province, in my view, should have some conjoint vehicle for:

1) reviewing what changes in treatment modalities require changes in the kind or amount of home care services delivered,

2) anticipating what effect changes in one care sector will have on another,

3) deciding whether a new type of service should be delivered, and

4) ensuring that serving a new sub-population does not jeopardize serving vulnerable elders.

REFERENCES

Manitoba Health Services Commission: *Annual Reports,* 1982/83, 1984/85, 1986/87, 1988/89.

Policy Planning and Information Branch Department of National Health and Welfare: *The Manitoba/Canada Home Care Study, An Overview of Findings.* Ottawa: Health and Welfare Canada, 1982.

Shapiro E, Tate RB: Is health care using changing? A comparison between physician, hospital, nursing-home, and home-care use of two elderly cohorts. *Medical Care* 27(11):1002-1014, (November) 1989.

Shapiro E, Tate RB: Survival patterns of nursing home admissions and their policy implications. *Canadian Journal of Public Health* 79:268-274, (July/August) 1988.

Stone R: Aging in the eighties. Age 65 years and over – Use of community services. Preliminary data from the Supplement on Aging to the National Health Interview Survey: United States, January - June 1985. National Center for Health Statistics. Advance Data from *Vital and Health Statistics No. 124.* DHHS Pub. No. (PHS) 86-1250. Public Health Service, Hyattsville, Md., Sept 30, 1986.

Weissert WG, Cready CM, Pawelak JE: The past and future of home- and community-based long-term care. *The Milbank Quarterly* 66(2):309-388, 1988.

DISCUSSION
Chair: Doreen Neville
Memorial University

Peter Ruderman (Toronto)

Could you perhaps put your heads together for our benefit and compare your definitions of what goes into the two home care programs, and differences in the percentage of cases originating on discharge from hospital, as explanations of why programs would appear to be more cost-effective in Canada?

William Weissert (University of Michigan)

Well, roughly half of the patients that we studied came from hospitals. It doesn't seem to make much difference whether they come from hospitals or not, although in terms of potential for reducing hospital use, of course, it's very important that they came from hospitals. Our definition of home care is so broad that it would be impossible I think, even in Canada, to come up with something that wasn't in it. But again, people tend to pick and choose what they use, and they use homemaker services more than anything else. About 70% of our dollars go into homemakers. Is that true for you?

Evelyn Shapiro (University of Manitoba)

About 67-70% of our population is getting homemakers.

William Weissert

I don't know about the cost-effectiveness aspect of it. I can tell you what we found – that it is, in simple terms, a false positive problem. You give a treatment to someone to solve a problem they don't have, and damned if it doesn't not work.

Evelyn Shapiro

I have a somewhat different answer. I think that you'll find that there is a very great variation in cost-effectiveness across Canada. I've given you only Manitoba data and so I can tell you about some of the things that we differentiate that are not differentiated elsewhere. We really differentiate very clearly between what I call "essential services" and what I call "aging in place" services. Some provinces don't do that. That is, we really do not provide aging in place services. Those are the services like yard work or whatever helps people stay where they are. We have the idea, being a poor province, that we have to be very careful, that those kinds of people have a choice. They can move into apartment buildings or senior citizens' housing, of which we have a fair stock. That's one thing. I think the second thing is we are very tight with professional service use. I know that in some places in Ontario you provide nursing services to many more people than we do. But that has been because you can't get home care unless you are eligible to get a skilled nursing service or a medical service of one kind or another. We don't have those provisions, so we use a lot less nursing, for example. And that substantially reduces the cost because medical services are the highest cost services.

William Weissert

Well, in some contrast to that, Vern Green, who I think is at Syracuse, the Maxwell School, has done some work on one of these studies that I am reporting on trying to look at what specific services were cost-effective. And he found that the skilled nursing service returned the most benefit for units of service, in terms of reduced hospitalization, and reduced nursing home use, and some other benefits. We don't include yard work or chore services in our definition, although in one study that I reported on here, they did do snow shovelling. In one instance, in a Wisconsin study that was also included here, there was a fellow who needed a cataract operation and he had six prize bulls and he wouldn't go without getting them cared for, so they gave him bull sitting services.

Michael Rachlis (Toronto)

Although I don't usually say this in front of large audiences, good medical care can certainly make a big difference in people's quality of life and the types of services, particularly hospital services, that they consume. And we know, of course, from the literature on the organization of medical services that there are very big differences in costs for other services, particularly hospital services, depending on how you pay physicians. So I was wondering in the studies you've reviewed, Dr. Weissert, have you looked at the type of medical care that was provided, and in particular how the medical care was paid for, and whether the medical care was directly associated or part of the home care program, or whether the program was just using family doctors as we tend to use in most provincial home care programs?

William Weissert

Well, of course the idea of randomizing is that we theoretically control for that. Now it turns out that randomization is not always the solution you think it is. When you randomize two groups you are supposed to get two identical groups, but then that assumes that you have very large numbers, and in most of these studies we didn't, so there may have been some differences in the medical care they received. And in quasi-experiments you are even less confident. But as a general rule, we did not find differences in the pattern of medical care between the treatment and the control group, which is why I limited my analysis to these kinds of studies, where we are controlling for these potential outside influences.

Michael Rachlis

In the experimental groups, who provided medical services? Was it a doctor who was employed by the home care agency, or otherwise associated with the home care agency?

William Weissert

Well, the medical components, as opposed to what we called home care, were invariably the same in the treatment and the control group. And that was usually a family physician of some type, although not always. And I have to say that we accuse physicians and providers, maybe wrongly, of not paying much attention to this population that doesn't have acute problems, looking at them only in their home care setting, so frequently we think there is less involvement of the physician than perhaps would be desirable although we find that home care has no effect on physician utilization.

Michael Rachlis

I'm not sure if you know exactly what I'm getting at, but I'm thinking specifically, for example, if you had a physician or a group of physicians associated with the home care program and they knew the people that were in the program, because it's been documented in a report in Ontario recently that physicians by and large don't see their patients who are receiving home care. So if they were in fact in regular contact with them or at least with the nurses providing direct care, if they were able to see a patient immediately at home, if they were called to see the patient, etc. – I'm just wondering whether or not that would make any difference. And I'd be happy to hear Evelyn speculate on that as well.

William Weissert

Well, I think the issue is that we weren't trying to experiment here with changing physician behaviour, we were trying to experiment with increasing home care use. In fact, one of the things I advocate is trying to change physician behaviour as part of the intervention, so I think you're talking more about a solution that we haven't yet tried.

Evelyn Shapiro

If the family or individuals feel that they are having a special problem, we tend to use their own personal physician, asking them to come to see the person. If we're not able to get their physician – we have some people in home care who have no physician – we tend to use our geriatric units for crisis intervention when appropriate, rather than using the hospital. And so, in effect, we will call the geriatric unit and they will send out one of their graduate students or one of the geriatricians. We are singularly blessed with enough geriatricians to perform this and other functions.

William Weissert

We don't have that problem.

Doreen Neville

I was interested, Evelyn, in your comments about having a certain number of people on your rolls for whom home care is not actually substituting for hospital/nursing home care. You said you didn't have time to go into it. We have a little bit of time now. Could you give us an example of what types of people these are? I think it's interesting in light of Dr. Weissert's comments about appropriate utilization of services.

Evelyn Shapiro

Well, obviously we're really talking about a small group. But we do have individuals who are elderly and who, for example, live with a very elderly spouse. An individual may be 87, his wife 85, and they are finding it very difficult to cope but they really don't need very much help. If the spouse has Alzheimer's, we may provide one half day, or two half days of social relief. We are not talking about expensive services, but they help the family carry on. Since the family is not asking for the person to be institutionalized, home care is not a substitute for nursing home admission.

But there are other situations in which the minimal service that a family is getting is enough to enable it to carry on, because otherwise it couldn't manage the situation. For example, a daughter may do the laundry and a son the shopping, and formal service such as a home helper may be added for one morning a week. Again, that's a very minimal service, but it may keep the person at home in the community unless there is further deterioration or some cataclysmic event occurs.

I think we do home care an injustice when we don't recognize that type of need as a legitimate need. It worries me that home care has been perceived only as a substitute, in the sense that if it's not acting as a substitute, then somehow it's not worth paying for.

Now, with more and more technology, we have people being cared for at home with equipment that not even nursing homes are allowed to have. It seems to me then that if home care is restricted more and more to this type of care and it absorbs all the money, what will happen to these people who really need a minimal amount of service. I am more and more often hearing the question, "Do these people who are getting only three hours a week of homemaker, or two hours every two weeks of homemaker, do they really need it?" Maybe we should be asking instead: "Should we be caring for people at home with needs for which the institutions aren't even allowed to provide?"

WHAT GAINS CAN WE EXPECT FROM HEALTH PROMOTION AND DISEASE PREVENTION, OR 'WHITHER OAT BRAN'?

EVALUATION OF FEDERAL HEALTH PROMOTION INITIATIVES*

Lavada Pinder
Health Promotion Directorate
Health and Welfare Canada

First of all, let me say that I have never spoken at a conference with such snappy titles for its sessions, e.g., "Yankee Influences: Playing in the Bush Leagues?" and "A Great Canadian Prescription: Take Two Commissioned Studies and Call Me in the Morning". I must confess that I find the expectation for wit and wisdom somewhat intimidating.

And I have another confession. At first I was a little insulted by the title of this session, "What Gains Can We Expect From Health Promotion and Disease Prevention, or 'Whither Oat Bran'"? Can this be a plot on the part of brainy health economists to trivialize health promotion, I asked myself? We in the field of health promotion are sensitive souls. However, when I noted that Michael Rachlis was on the panel I accepted the invitation immediately.

Now when I look at the title I quite like health promotion's being associated with oat bran. The association brings the word "ubiquitous" to mind – "omnipresent; present, or seeming to be present, everywhere at the same time". Oat bran is, or was, everywhere...in muffins, bread, cereals...there was even oat bran in oat bran. The cereal products industry was turned upside down in an effort to find new ways to introduce and package this key to health...this destroyer of cholesterol. It's a bit like this with health promotion. Health promotion is everywhere. The words are on the lips of politicians like a song...health professionals are "doing" health promotion...physicians have visions of fees for health promotion dancing in their heads...PARTICIPACTION has never been happier...and ordinary folks are buying diet books and going to Dancercise classes. There's even some health promotion in health promotion.

We all know what happened to oat bran. Studies have shown that the reason cholesterol levels were lowered was not because of oat bran itself but because of the fact that people ate so much of it they had little room for anything else. There's a lesson here for health promotion. If we can just keep everyone talking about health promotion, it can eventually take up so much of people's time they will not have a moment left over to be sick.

Now I must turn to my own topic and the realization that the title, "Evaluation of Federal Health Promotion Initiatives", is dull. It is out of step with the titles of other presentations. Initially, I felt it may have been made boring to reflect my status as a federal public servant. Having successfully come to grips, however, with oat bran, I now feel in the swing of things. In this spirit, I've decided to rename my presentation "The Evaluation Two-Step, or 'I'd like to be evaluated but my dance card is full'".

In my few remaining minutes (after one of the world's longest introductions), I will try to cover a couple of issues of importance to health promotion evaluation. The first has to do with the relationship between the evaluators and the evaluated. The second concerns health promotion realities which compound the natural tensions between the evaluator and the evaluated. Finally, so you will not go away with the impression that my life position is one of complete avoidance, I will comment on a recent evaluation of the health promotion program.

EVALUATORS AND THE EVALUATED

I liken the situation the evaluators and the evaluated find themselves in to a dance, because they are partners who so often step on one another's toes. The result is that their cries of anguish and despair are painful to the ear and they miss the opportunity to glide gracefully to fame and fortune.

I feel qualified to discuss this situation because, as a program manager, I have so frequently been locked in this embrace. More recently, as director of a fairly large federal program, I have tried to be more reflective. Another motivation is the fact that in the federal government there is no choice. In May 1981, the Office of Controller General of Canada at Treasury Board issued a "Guide to the Program Evaluation Function", and the Program Evaluation Policy of our Department says that most programs will be evaluated every five years. The Deputy Minister is the client for all evaluations. In other words, when the DM introduces you to someone and suggests you dance...you tend to get on with it.

The problem arises because the dancers hear a different tune. They have different views of the world.

In 1980 Scriven said, "Evaluation is the process of determining the merit, worth, or value of something. Evaluation in the broad sense is inescapable for rational behavior and thought. More narrowly defined, it requires a systematic, objective approach and often utilization of social science research methods."

In my experience most program managers are more comfortable with the first half of this definition than the last, and the reverse is true for evaluators. Initially there are always good intentions. Evaluators say things like, "We want you to work with us, so the evaluation will be useful to you." Program people say things like, "We want to know if our program works." In reality, there is a power struggle. The evaluator, in his or her ivory tower, is convinced that the evaluation will decide the future of the program. The program manager, with both feet firmly on the ground, is confident that the evaluation is only one piece of information to be considered along with the political and public stake in the program.

The relationships are not improved by a subtle and sometimes not so subtle mutual disrespect. Program managers do not appreciate being considered simple-minded hewers of wood and drawers of water who waste public money and would not know a chi square if they met one in their soup. And evaluators do not like being thought of as heartless number crunchers who don't care about people and can't get a real job.

The trick is to keep dancing. Never mind that evaluation research is messy and program people can't seem to supply any data. Never mind that evaluators seem to have very strange notions about how behaviour change is achieved. Here's an example from an evaluation guide of what drives program managers wild. In describing a program effect the manual states, "Inputs to a drug education program might be three prevention workers, $25,000, a typewriter and a photocopier. The output might be 1,000 pamphlets about drugs and associated health risks. The effects of such a program might be that 50% of all students having received the information in this program have stopped using drugs." *Might*, indeed! Never mind that program evaluation takes so long that the results sometimes apply to a program that no longer exists. Never mind that in memoranda responding to evaluation recommendations, program managers have been known to make statements like, "Evaluators, pursuant to their role definitions, have a compulsive need to find sunsets and this is a case in which this compulsion has overwhelmed analytical capacity."

HEALTH PROMOTION REALITIES

The trick is to keep dancing, because these dynamics are further compounded by current realities in the health promotion field.

The contemporary conceptualization of health promotion does not seem to have been designed with evaluation in mind. The conceptualization I am referring to is reflected in the Ottawa Charter for Health Promotion as well as the Canadian document *Achieving Health for All: A Framework for Health Promotion*. In this conceptualization health promotion is defined as "the process of enabling people to increase control over, and to improve their health". This definition is both a blessing and a curse.

It's a joy to work in a field where the central integrative concept is enabling and which demands a participatory approach and the transfer of resources to those who do not have enough of them. We are surely on the side of the gods.

Health promotion can be somewhat less joyful in practice. Participatory planning and implementation of policy and programs requires good will and patience among many partners. National programs can require collaboration among 10 provinces and two territories as well as non-governmental organizations. The National Program to Reduce Tobacco Use has a steering group which involves 12 jurisdictions and eight national professional and voluntary organizations. Collaboration is hard-won and does not lend itself to precise, measurable objectives and systematic implementation and data collection. Instead, it lends itself to broad goals, compromise, and positive opportunism.

Health promotion also requires the understanding and support of politicians who tend to be more interested in results than in process. They speak continually of health promotion, but frequently mean narrowly defined lifestyle programs. This situation is not helped by the fact that health promotion is in a phase where many of its advocates seem to speak in tongues.

This situation creates a challenge not only for developers and implementers of health promotion but for evaluators as well. As Michel O'Neill said in a recent article in *Health Promotion*, "The health promotion ideology, in which public participation is fostered, thus conflicts with the ways scientific research and knowledge are currently built and disseminated." Furthermore, university people conducting health promotion research in government or service agencies are often not highly respected in the academic world, whatever their value.

In a sense, then, there is common ground between the evaluator and the evaluated where health promotion is concerned – both are suspect in traditional circles.

HEALTH PROMOTION PROGRAM EVALUATION

Last year an evaluation of the Health Promotion Directorate in the Department of Health and Welfare was completed. The evaluation was conducted in strict accordance with Treasury Board and Departmental policy and was something of a model. An evaluation framework was developed, data collected, a feasibility study undertaken and, finally, the evaluation was implemented. There was a literature review, a study of records, analysis of individual project evaluations, field visits, telephone and mail surveys, a key informant study, and an expert panel. On the surface, it was a model of protocol and decorum. Just below the surface, all the dynamics I described earlier were in play. In addition, the conceptualization of health promotion changed during the period under review and major new federal initiatives were introduced. *Achieving Health for All* began to influence the program in 1986, and the National Drug, Driving While Impaired, and AIDS strategies were launched.

The evaluation, nevertheless, has been useful. While underlining the problem of attributability, the program is seen, for example, to have contributed to change in smoking behaviour. And just as important, the Directorate is credited with having influenced the shape of health promotion in Canada. It also confirms the feeling we have had for some time in the Directorate that we need to pay more attention to strategic planning.

The point is that, through it all, we kept dancing.

NOTE
* edited transcript of talk

HEALTH PROMOTION/DISEASE PREVENTION: WHAT DO WE THINK WE KNOW?

Vivek Goel

Department of Preventive Medicine and Biostatistics, University of Toronto
Clinical Epidemiology Unit, Sunnybrook Health Sciences Centre

The methods available to evaluate health interventions have progressed in many ways in recent years. Such progress has included the development of new theoretical approaches, applications in diverse settings, and the use of the results of evaluations in policy development. Concepts such as the efficacy, effectiveness, and efficiency of health care interventions (Feeny, Guyatt, and Tugwell, 1986) are discussed in health care settings almost on a routine basis. Politicians, bureaucrats, and the public all frequently call for more "cost-effective" health care.

Concurrent with this surging interest in health care efficiency has been an increasing interest in health promotion and disease prevention (HP/DP). A common expectation is that widespread diffusion of HP/DP will reduce total health care expenditures. Several review committees in Ontario have called for increased expenditures on prevention as one means of achieving this objective (Evans, 1987; Spasoff, 1987).

Unfortunately, because of methodological and logistical reasons, as well as a lack of desire to evaluate many health care interventions critically and properly, we do not know as much about the evaluation of HP/DP as we would like to know. There have been some quite cogent arguments that have questioned whether prevention is more cost-effective than curative care (Russell, 1986; Russell, 1987).

Several aspects of HP/DP interventions themselves make them difficult to evaluate by bluntly applying the same methods that have been developed for evaluating diagnostic and curative interventions.

In the discussion that follows, it is important to keep in mind that the limitations described with respect to the evaluation of HP/DP can apply similarly to many other areas of health care evaluation.

This paper reviews some of the methodological issues involved in evaluating HP/DP. The first section describes an approach to considering different types and levels of health care interventions and looks at the implications of considering the differences between interventions in designing evaluation studies. The second section presents a very simplified model of the effects of different types of health care interventions. This model allows an appreciation of why the approach to the evaluation of HP/DP could be quite different from that for other health care interventions. The next section discusses several methodological issues of particular importance. The paper concludes with consideration of reasons some evaluations have been "successful" and the limitations inherent in using such evaluations to develop policy.

TYPES AND LEVELS OF HEALTH CARE INTERVENTIONS

In this paper, the *type* of health care intervention refers to the intervention's goal. Three broad classes of intervention can be described: health promotion, disease prevention, and treatment. Within each of these classes are various subdivisions. For example, prevention is often subdivided into primary, secondary, and tertiary preventions, and treatment may include curative, rehabilitative, and palliative interventions.

These subdivisions tend to become blurred when particular interventions are considered. For example, many primary disease prevention interventions can be implemented as health promotion manoeuvres, and many tertiary preventions may be considered rehabilitative treatments. Diagnostic interventions may be used for either prevention or treatment; mammography, for example, could be considered as either a screening (preventive) or diagnostic (treatment) intervention. In considering an evaluation of a particular intervention, one must therefore keep in mind what the 'target' type was for the intervention in that case.

In this discussion, the three types of interventions are distinguished as follows: Health promotion is defined as in the Ottawa Charter on Health Promotion (World Health Organization, 1986) and uses a positive definition of health. Health promotion maintains the health of individuals and communities and attempts to maximize their potential well-being. Disease prevention and treatment are based on more restrictive and classic definitions of health, which have been referred to as "negative" definitions, that is, "health" is the absence of disease. It follows that disease prevention aims to avoid or reduce the negative impact of illness prior to its occurrence. Treatment interventions, which include curative and rehabilitative interventions, aim to eliminate or reduce the impact of illness after its occurrence.

The distinction between health promotion and disease prevention is based on the definition of health. Although the distinction between negative and positive definitions is quite clear, there are many more subtle issues, for example, whether health should include economic well-being. Discussion of these components of health is beyond the scope of this paper (Stachtchenko and Jenicek, 1990). The key concern is that without a clear and complete definition of health, it is difficult to devise a good measure of health status. Since measurement of outcomes is obviously a crucial component of evaluation, what is to be measured must first be defined. If health is defined broadly, then many social programs, for example, housing, can be considered to fall into the realm of HP/DP. Evaluation of such programs in the context of other health programs thus becomes much more complex.

A further note of confusion is the usage of the term health promotion in the United States *Healthy Peoples* document (Healthy People, 1979). In this document, health promotion would seem to be used almost interchangeably with disease prevention, a confusion that has led to many evaluations of "health promotion" that are really evaluations of disease prevention.

In the last 25 years treatment interventions have begun to be evaluated rather extensively, comparatively speaking. Preventive services have also been critically examined, with the Canadian Task Force on the Periodic Health Examination leading the way (Spitzer, 1979). Similar work has been done in the United States by the Task Force on Preventive Health Services (Guide to Clinical Preventive Services, 1989). These groups have restricted themselves to interventions they consider to be clinical prevention interventions, i.e., those that can be carried out by a clinician. Some of these interventions could also be applied in the framework of health promotion. The results of such critical appraisals must be considered carefully when being applied in the context of health promotion. The appraisals were done for interventions as implemented in a clinician's practice; clearly, implementation in the setting of a health promotion program could be quite different. Another important question is whether the criteria and the hierarchy for evidence developed by these groups for appraising the literature on clinical preventive interventions can be readily applied to the evaluation of health promotion interventions.

In addition to the different *types* of interventions, the *level* of each intervention must be considered. Traditionally, health interventions have been applied to the individual and are often evaluated from the perspective of the individual. However, an intervention can also be applied in the context of the community (a community fluoridation or heart health program) or society (taxation to reduce alcohol consumption or legislation to restrict smoking) and therefore can also be considered from these perspectives.

A further level of health intervention, the global level, is becoming obvious. Many environmental interventions, such as those to reduce depletion of the ozone layer, will have an impact on human health. It is clear that evaluating interventions across all of these many levels can be difficult, since comparison of health outcomes is not easy, let alone finding means to define and measure them in these contexts.

When designing or appraising evaluations of health interventions, consideration of both the level and type of intervention is important, not only to assure selection of the appropriate methodology, but also to permit comparison across interventions.

A SIMPLIFIED MODEL OF THE IMPACT OF HEALTH INTERVENTIONS

Figure 1 illustrates a very simplified model of the manner in which the different types of health interventions may impact on health. Moving from left to right, the model shows the relationship between knowledge, attitudes, and behaviour on risk factors for disease, and the subsequent impact of these risk factors on disease occurrence. This model is based on the concept of the "web of causation, web of consequences" for disease etiology proposed by McMahon and Pugh (1970).

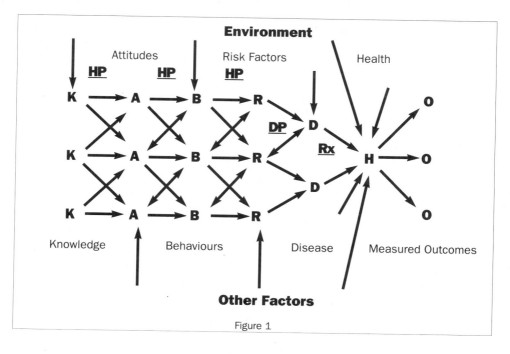

Figure 1

Many different facets of knowledge, attitudes, and behaviours can impact on several different risk factors. Similarly, different risk factors may impact on different diseases. This type of relationship is the basis for multiple risk factor interventions. Not shown is the fact that some behaviours (e.g., alcohol and trauma) may impact directly on disease. External factors (for example, social and environmental) can have an effect on these precursors to health as well as impact directly on health.

Illustrated on the right is the fact that health itself is not measured. Instead indicators, for example, mortality, hospitalization, or self-reported status, are usually measured using the "best" means currently available. The immediate result is that a certain error is already introduced as a result of problems with the measurement of these factors, as well as bias in the relationship between these factors and health (i.e, how well they actually relate to health).

Treatment oriented interventions – curative, rehabilitative, and palliative – operate at the right of this model. They take place after the occurrence of disease. Prevention is in the middle, trying to reduce or eliminate the impact of risk factors on disease. Health promotion takes place much earlier, trying to impact on knowledge, attitudes, and behaviours and to reduce the influence of external factors such as the environment or socio-economic determinants.

In considering the evaluation of an intervention, it becomes obvious that what is defined as the outcome of an intervention will influence the methodology and quality of the evaluation. An intervention that seeks to affect a factor in the model can be easily evaluated if only the area around the arrow following from that factor is considered. For example, an intervention that aims to affect attitudes could be evaluated by considering a change in attitudes following the intervention. However, to compare across interventions, we must be able to model the impact of the measured change on health, or those measures of health outcome that are currently available. Therefore, the evaluation must either directly consider the effect of the intervention on health or model it in some way. For example, the Stanford Five Cities Project measured changes in behaviour following a multiple risk factor intervention. A mathematical model was then used to estimate the impact on disease incidence and mortality (Farquhar et al, 1990).

Obviously, the further an intervention is from the health outcomes, the greater the uncertainty in considering its effects on those outcomes. In addition, understanding of the mechanisms through which many of these precursors impact on health, although perhaps more comprehensive than this simple model, is still quite limited.

Many of the external factors that impact on health are unknown or difficult to assess. Attempts to model the impact of changes in knowledge on health status can therefore become cumbersome and quite difficult. Clearly, the evaluation of the impact on health of a treatment intervention, by no means without problems of its own, can be quite rudimentary in comparison to that for health promotion interventions.

METHODOLOGICAL ISSUES

Many methodological concerns can arise in trying to evaluate HP/DP. Only a few of the most pertinent are considered here. These are grouped into three areas: study design considerations, measurement issues, and economic concerns.

STUDY DESIGN

In the evaluation of clinical interventions, the randomized controlled trial is considered to be the "gold standard" (Department of Clinical Epidemiology and Biostatistics, 1981). The Canadian Task Force on the Periodic Health Examination and the American Preventive Health Services Task Force both give the greatest weight to well designed studies that use such a methodology. Cohort and case-control studies receive less weight.

Non- or quasi- experimental designs and qualitative studies are usually not considered in such hierarchies of evidence or are given low weight. Yet in the case of many preventive interventions and most health promotion interventions, it is quite difficult to execute randomized trials. Reasons include the necessity of obtaining large enough sample sizes to gain adequate power to show effects on health outcomes, the need for long follow-up durations, problems with patient and provider compliance, and the presence of multiple confounders. Ethical problems in working with healthy individuals often preclude randomizing such individuals to receive unproven and potentially dangerous interventions, even if the absolute risks are quite small.

What is required is a basic reconsideration of the framework used for viewing study designs to evaluate health care interventions. The randomized controlled trial used for evaluating individual patient clinical interventions is not easily applied to other types or levels of interventions.

MEASUREMENT AND OUTCOME SELECTION

Measurement and outcome issues are another major methodological problem. Not only are current measures of health status poor proxies for actual health, they are often poor measures of even what they purport to be reporting. For example, the problems with the quality of mortality statistics are well known, yet they are considered amongst our most stable measures of health status.

A critical problem in comparing across different types of health interventions is obtaining a common unit of outcome. Although several measures are available to pool mortality and morbidity, e.g., disability-free days, quality adjusted life years, or healthy years equivalents, all have problems assigning relative weights to different outcomes. For example, averting a case of measles may have to be compared with treating a myocardial infarction. This comparison can have different results depending on the method used.

Although there are several general global measures available for determining health status (e.g., time trade-off or standard gamble), these global measures often do not have the specificity necessary to discriminate between similar health states. The effect of many health promotion interventions may be unmeasurable on such a global scale.

Problems with measurement relate not only to what is to be measured, but also to how it is measured. Clinical interventions have been traditionally evaluated in terms of their effect on relative risk, the proportional change in risk of disease after intervention. However, the impact of many HP/DP interventions may be quite small with respect to relative risk, but still be quite impressive in terms of absolute risk difference for the population as a whole. That is, even a small change in relative risk can have considerable impact on the total population when it is applied across a large group of individuals. Therefore, both relative and absolute risk must be considered in evaluating a health care intervention.

ECONOMICS

Economic evaluation has been proposed as a means to improve the allocation of scarce health resources and has been applied to all types of health interventions.

Since determination, or estimation, of the effectiveness of an intervention is a fundamental component of economic evaluation, all the problems discussed above, and many others not discussed, also apply in the case of economic evaluation. Furthermore, many problems arise in trying to compare economic evaluations of HP/DP with those of treatment interventions.

The fundamental components of an economic analysis are assessments of costs and outcomes. Assessing the costs of an intervention and its outcomes is never easy, and assessing the costs of a preventive intervention can be particularly troublesome. Since such interventions are applied across many individuals, assessing indirect costs is quite difficult. Health promotion interventions are often applied cooperatively with other agencies. For example, an exercise program may involve schools, parks, and retail stores. Assessing the costs incurred by other agencies can be very complicated.

A problem in assessing the value of outcomes is future productivity gains and health care costs. These should be included in an economic evaluation (Weinstein and Stason, 1977), but are often ignored in evaluations of clinical interventions because of the short time horizon being considered. However, they cannot be easily ignored in evaluation of HP/DP. Not only are they difficult to measure or estimate, but they can have a serious impact on the outcome of an analysis. For example, a program that prevents cardiac events in seniors should count as a cost the extra costs of medical care in the years of life that are added. Including such costs can reverse the results of the analysis. Determining which costs should be included is also important. For example, should only health care costs be considered, or should extra social support costs, such as pensions, also be included?

An even more fundamental problem is posed by discounting, the economic adjustment of future gains or losses to current terms to account for time preference. In general, individual and societal time preference favours the present over the future. Therefore, discounting will reduce the impact of interventions that require expenditure in the present but yield benefits in the future.

There is no economic doubt that future occurrences, both costs and consequences, need to be discounted to current dollars. However, what is the appropriate discount rate? The rate used can seriously impact on the results of the analysis. It then becomes crucial whether a lower societal time preference rate should be considered in the case of HP/DP to reflect the societal thrust towards these interventions. In other words, should we implicitly favour such interventions in economic analysis if they are what society wants?

There are no ready solutions to these and other problems. The approach recommended in performing such analyses is to state the assumptions explicitly and conduct extensive sensitivity analyses to estimate the effect of these assumptions.

CONCLUSIONS

It is not the intent of this paper to take a nihilistic attitude towards HP/DP. Indeed, if anything, further development of such interventions is strongly supported. However, it is clear that all health care interventions must be rigorously and constructively evaluated.

Although it is possible to show in limited controlled circumstances that many interventions are indeed efficacious, it is often far more difficult to show that they can be effective in practice. However, even this effectiveness can be demonstrated for most interventions if evaluations use appropriate methodology and precautions.

Far more difficult is the final stage, which uses the evidence from evaluations to set public policy and make recommendations for individuals. A crucial step is the comparison of the effects of different interventions. To be able to allocate resources across different programs rationally, one must be able to compare those programs using a common unit of outcome.

The United States Preventive Services Task Force explicitly ignored issues of efficiency and concentrated only on evaluating effectiveness, because of the limitations of economic evaluation of disease prevention (Russell, 1990).

In assessing the evidence for HP/DP and treatment interventions in terms of a common outcome, one must bear in mind the proximity of treatment interventions to outcomes. In many instances, this will result in greater uncertainty in the estimates obtained for the effects of HP/DP interventions. This uncertainty can lead to inconsistent results when the same intervention is appraised by different investigators. The current controversy with regards to screening for cholesterol is one example.

In considering those HP/DP interventions that are often cited as having been successfully evaluated, such as neonatal screening for phenylketonuria and some childhood immunization programs, one notes that they were found to save costs and result in benefits. However, there are some preventive interventions that, when evaluated in economic terms, do not save costs. These include screening for colorectal, cervical, and breast cancer; detection and treatment of hypertension; and counselling for physical activity. In many of these cases the cost-effectiveness results are not as reasonable as those for treatment interventions.

In part, the results might be unreasonable because of the assumptions used (because of missing information) and the application of economic analysis methodology that may be controversial, e.g., use of a high discount rate or consideration of indirect costs that are otherwise ignored by other analysts. However, the results may actually be unreasonable, and if society is willing to accept the underlying tenets of economic evaluation, then those interventions should not be funded. Distinguishing between cases in which the results are really unreasonable and those in which they are so because of the reasons outlined above is the difficult terrain that must be traversed by those who hope to use such analyses to assist in the determination of public policy.

REFERENCES

Department of Clinical Epidemiology and Biostatistics, McMaster University: How to read clinical journals: to distinguish useful from useless or even harmful therapy. *Canadian Medical Association Journal* 124:1156-1162, 1981.

Evans J (chairman): *Toward a Shared Direction for Health in Ontario.* Report of the Health Review Panel. Toronto: Ontario Ministry of Health, 1987.

Farquhar JW, Fortmann SP, Flora JA, Taylor CB, et al: Effects of communitywide education on cardiovascular disease risk factors. The Stanford Five-City Project. *Journal of the American Medical Association* 264:359-365, 1990.

Feeny D, Guyatt G, Tugwell P: *Health Care Technology: Effectiveness, Efficiency and Public Policy.* Montreal: Institute for Research on Public Policy, 1986.

Guide to Clinical Preventive Services: An Assessment of the Effectiveness of 161 Interventions. Report of the United States Preventive Services Task Force. Baltimore: Williams and Wilkins, 1989.

Healthy People: The Surgeon General's Report on Health Promotion and Disease Prevention. U.S. Government Printing Office, DHEW-(PHS) Publication No. 79-55071, 1979.

McMahon B, Pugh T: *Epidemiologic Principles and Methods.* Boston: Little Brown and Co., 1970.

Russell LB: The cost-effectiveness of preventive services: some examples. In Goldbloom RB, Lawrence RS: *Preventing Disease: Beyond the Rhetoric.* New York: Springer-Verlag, 1990.

Russell LB: *Evaluating Preventive Care.* Washington: The Brookings Institute, 1987.

Russell LB: *Is Prevention Better Than Cure?* Washington: The Brookings Institute, 1986.

Spasoff RA (chairman): *Health for All Ontario.* Report of the Panel on Health Goals for Ontario. Toronto: Ontario Ministry of Health, 1987.

Spitzer WO (chairman): Report of the Task Force on the Periodic Health Examination. *Canadian Medical Association Journal* 121:1193-1254, 1979.

Stachtchenko S, Jenicek M: Conceptual differences between prevention and health promotion: research implications for community health programs. *Canadian Journal of Public Health* 81:53-59, 1990.

Weinstein MC, Stason WB: Foundations of economic evaluation for health and medical practices. *New England Journal of Medicine* 296:716-721, 1977.

World Health Organization: *Ottawa Charter for Health Promotion.* Ottawa, 1986.

CHOLESTEROL SCREENING: THE COSTS AND BENEFITS OF VARIOUS PROGRAMS

Michael M. Rachlis
Toronto, Ontario

INTRODUCTION

It has been observed for some time that persons with high levels of blood cholesterol are at increased risk for the development of coronary heart disease (CHD) (Toronto Working Group on Cholesterol Policy, 1990). In the last six years, experimental evidence has been presented that the pharmacologic reduction of blood cholesterol can prevent or postpone the development of CHD in middle-aged men (Lipid Research Clinics Program, 1984; Frick et al, 1987). Men with very high levels of cholesterol in their blood (e.g., above 7.75 mmol/l or 300 mg/dl)[1] have approximately three times the risk of developing CHD of those with total cholesterol levels below 5.0 mmol/l.

Several authors have suggested that mass epidemics of CHD can occur only when mean cholesterol levels of the population reach a certain threshold (Rose, 1989). CHD is very uncommon in populations with adult mean cholesterol levels below 4.5 mmol/l, but becomes very common in populations with mean cholesterol levels above 5.5 mmol/l (Blackburn, 1989).

The extra risk associated with hypercholesterolemia is much less for men than for women. There are some indications that specific cholesterol fractions are better than total cholesterol at predicting an individual's future risk of CHD. Unfortunately, these fractions are much less reliably measured, at least outside specialized research laboratories, than total cholesterol (Toronto Working Group on Cholesterol Policy, 1990).

Cholesterol levels are related to the consumption of saturated fats, other fats, and certain other nutrients (e.g., soluble vegetable fibre). Approximately one in 500 persons has specific genetic abnormalities which predispose them to high cholesterol levels. There is some evidence that a high ratio of saturated to polyunsaturated fats (high S/P ratio) in the diet leads to higher levels of blood cholesterol, higher S/P ratios in fatty tissues, and higher S/P ratios in cell membranes (Riemersma et al, 1986; Fordyce et al, 1983).

This paper reviews the studies that have evaluated the efficiency of the treatment of hypercholesterolemia, compares their results to those of studies of other interventions to prevent or treat CHD, and draws some conclusions for decision-makers.

METHODS

A Medline computer search was conducted to find all articles indexed by cholesterol and economics from January 1980 until March 1990. Various workers in the field were consulted, and references in published papers were traced. Altogether, 10 reports were found which examined the cost-effectiveness of the treatment of hypercholesterolemia.

Articles were selected for this review if they met the following criteria:

1. Results were included for middle-aged men;
2. Results were expressed as costs per life year saved;
3. Results were presented with discounting; and
4. Clear evidence was presented for the efficacy of the program being evaluated.

The articles were further evaluated for their validity using criteria from a textbook of economic evaluation (Drummond, Stoddart, and Torrance, 1987). Six reports met these criteria

(Kinosian and Eisenberg, 1988; Oster and Epstein, 1987; Taylor et al, 1988; Weinstein and Stason, 1985; Hjalte et al, 1989; Martens et al, 1990).

The results were inflated to 1989 levels using the United States medical care index for July (U.S. Bureau of Labor Statistics, 1989)[2]. They were then converted to Canadian dollars using the exchange rate for July 1989.

RESULTS
EFFECTIVENESS

Five of these studies (Oster and Epstein, 1987; Taylor et al, 1988; Weinstein and Stason, 1985; Hjalte et al, 1989; Martens et al, 1990) use some modification of the multivariable equations developed by the Framingham Study to estimate the risk of CHD in treated and untreated persons (Kannel and Gordon, 1977). The Framingham Study, a follow-up study of CHD and risk factors in Framingham, Massachusetts, is the longest-running prospective study of risk factors for the development of CHD. However, these mathematical equations do not apply equally well to all populations. For example, researchers in Texas found that the equations developed by the Framingham study overestimated the true CHD experience for Mexican-Americans (Mitchell et al, 1990). In addition, the mix of risk factors is not exactly the same for young people and older people (Benfante et al, 1989).

Kinosian and Eisenberg (1988) use the results of the Lipid Research Clinics experimental study of cholestyramine (Lipid Research Clinics Program, 1984) for an estimate of effectiveness. Five of the studies investigate cholestyramine (Kinosian and Eisenberg, 1988; Oster and Epstein, 1987; Taylor et al, 1988; Weinstein and Stason, 1985; Martens et al, 1990), while two investigate simvastatin, a drug from a new class of cholesterol lowering agents (Weinstein and Stason, 1985; Hjalte et al, 1989)[3]. Taylor investigated the efficiency of intensive dietary counselling based on the results of the Multiple Risk Factor Intervention Trial (MRFIT) (Multiple Risk Factor Intervention Trial Research Group, 1982). Kinosian cited a substantial body of evidence on the hypocholesterolemic effects of oat bran and then assumed that oat bran would have the same effectiveness as for cholestyramine.

There is experimental evidence that cholestyramine reduces CHD mortality (Lipid Research Clinics Program, 1984). There is no such evidence, as yet, for intensive dietary therapy, oat bran, or simvastatin.

There is also no evidence as yet that the treatment of hypercholesterolemia reduces overall mortality. In fact, a meta-analysis of over 20 randomized trials of cholesterol reduction (drug and diet) has shown a statistically significant elevation of non-CHD mortality (MacMahon and Peto, 1988). The studies of cost-effectiveness assume that the reduction in overall mortality is equal to the reduction in CHD mortality. This is almost certainly an optimistic assumption.

COSTS

Various authors have discussed the advantages and disadvantages of different cost-effectiveness ratios (Drummond, Stoddart, and Torrance, 1987; Russell, 1986). In particular, the inclusion or exclusion of indirect costs is a point of debate for economic analysts. However, as is seen later in this analysis, few studies look at indirect costs.

These studies do not consider all costs inherent in their programs. Researchers at McGill University have calculated that the costs of physician and laboratory services alone in the first year of a Canada-wide screening program would be approximately $500 million (Grover et al,

1990). There would be an increase of approximately 300 visits to each primary care physician in the first year of the operation of the program. It is not clear whether physicians would add these patient visits to their workload or decrease visits for other conditions, with no net increase in physician billings to provincial Medicare plans. There would certainly need to be major investments in laboratory capability and quality assurance (Toronto Working Group on Cholesterol Policy, 1990).

Each of these studies uses a discount rate of 5%.

TIME HORIZON

The studies adopt somewhat different time horizons. Kinosian examines only the first seven years of the program (Kinosian and Eisenberg, 1988). It is not clear what the horizon is for Weinstein's paper (Weinstein and Stason, 1985). The others use time horizons of at least 15 years.

CONCLUSIONS

Table 1 shows the results of the studies for middle-aged men with high levels of cholesterol (all above 6.85 mmol/l or 265 mg/dl).

Table 1

RESULTS OF THE COST-EFFECTIVENESS OF PRIMARY PREVENTION OF CHD – STUDIES INVESTIGATING THERAPY FOR HYPERCHOLESTEROLEMIA

Study	Age	Serum Cholesterol (mmol/)	Other Risk Factors	Cost per life year saved (1989 CAN $)
Kinosian				
Cholestyramine	45-50	> 6.85	Avg. U.S. profile	A. $ 190,000 (packets)
				93,000 (bulk)
				B. 170,000 (packets)
Oat bran	45-50	> 6.85	Avg. U.S.	15,000 - 28,000
Oster	45-49	7.50	Avg. U.S.	140,000
Taylor				
Cholestyramine	40	7.75	low	400,000
	40	7.75	high	46,000
Intensive diet	40	7.75	low	150,000
	40	7.75	high	17,000
Weinstein				
Cholestyramine	45-50	> 6.85	Not stated •	210,000
Martens				
Cholestyramine	50	7.00	Framingham	250,000
		8.00	Framingham	180,000
Simvastatin	50	7.00	Framingham	57,000
		8.00	Framingham	36,000
Hjalte				
Simvastatin	52	7.00	Avg. Swedish	34,000
		8.00	Avg. Swedish	27,000

• Probably Avg. U.S. profile

Kinosian's figures are presented for drug sold in packets (the most expensive formulation) and in bulk (Kinosian and Eisenberg, 1988). The 'A' scenario excludes the indirect benefits of saved production costs, while the `B' scenario includes these benefits. The low risk category for Taylor's paper includes men whose cigarette smoking habit and diastolic blood pressure are at the 10th percentile and whose HDL cholesterol is at the 90th percentile of the age and sex-specific population distribution (Taylor et al, 1988). Taylor's high risk category includes men whose cigarette smoking habit and diastolic blood pressure are at the 90th percentile and whose HDL cholesterol is at the 10th percentile of the age and sex-specific population distribution.

These studies agree fairly well in their estimates for the efficiency of cholestyramine treatment. Treating men in their late forties who have serum cholesterol levels in the top 10% of the Canadian distribution and who have an otherwise average risk profile for CHD would cost between $100,000 and $200,000 for each additional year of life. As Taylor's paper shows, the program is much more efficient if it treats only persons with very high levels of cholesterol (> 7.75 mmol/L or 300 mg/dl), especially if they also have exceptionally high levels of other risk factors. The cost for every life saved if the program is applied to those with low levels of other risk factors is about 10 times greater than if applied to those with exceptionally high levels of those factors. Oster's work shows the same trend.

SENSITIVITY ANALYSIS

A review of the six studies above and of an additional study which had originally been excluded because it dealt with children (Berwick, Cretin, and Keeler, 1980) shows that the overall cost-effectiveness of programs to treat hypercholesterolemia varies considerably depending upon:

a. the cost of the intervention;
b. the absolute effectiveness of the intervention;
c. the group to whom the intervention is directed; and
d. the choice of discount rate.

The cost of the intervention is the key part of the cost-effectiveness calculation. Expensive interventions like drugs or intensive dietary counselling generate high costs. Conversely, inexpensive interventions like the oat bran in Kinosian's study lead to low costs for every life year saved.

Most studies of effectiveness highlight the *relative* effectiveness of a therapy. Using this index, an intervention that reduced mortality from 2 per 1,000 to 1 per 1,000 would appear as effective as one that reduced mortality from 2 per 100 to 1 per 100. However, the efficiency of the intervention depends upon the *absolute* effectiveness of the therapy. The first program cited above would be only 1/10 as efficient as the second. Because economic efficiency depends upon absolute rather than relative effectiveness, the most efficient interventions are those directed to individuals with the greatest risk of dying from CHD.

The most favourable cost-effectiveness ratios are for the treatment of middle-aged men with very high (> 7.75 mmol/L or 300 mg/dl) serum cholesterol levels and other CHD risk factors.

Discounting markedly reduces the efficiency of the preventive interventions whose benefits gradually accrue over time. Kinosian found that discounting at 5% reduces the overall cost-effectiveness of hypercholesterolemia treatment modalities by up to 50% compared with no discounting. The other studies show similar results.

From the review of these reports, the overall cost-effectiveness of CHD programs does *not* vary much if one changes assumptions about:

a. compliance;

b. the costs of treatment for *future* CHD events; or

c. indirect costs and benefits.

Most of the expenses are generated by the cost of treatment. Non-compliance does reduce the overall effectiveness of the program. However, if patients do not receive treatment, they do not generate costs. This conclusion would be modified, of course, for patients who purchase drugs on an ongoing basis but fail to comply.

Because the costs of treatment of CHD are generated in the future, they are discounted in the analysis. Similarly, since most of the events averted occur far in the future (> 10 years), they have little influence on the overall results. Kinosian found that increasing the costs of treatment of myocardial infarction by nearly 100% and the costs of bypass surgery by almost 200% changed the cost-effectiveness ratio for cholestyramine by only about 2% (Kinosian and Eisenberg, 1988). Unfortunately, the other authors did not vary this factor in their sensitivity analyses.

This analysis also applies for the additional costs of the program associated with the treatment of non-CHD illnesses occurring in men whose CHD has been averted. Kinosian found that these costs had very little impact on the overall results.

Only Kinosian investigated the impact of indirect costs (Kinosian and Eisenberg, 1988). Because of the low absolute risk difference between treated and untreated persons, relatively few of the men treated have an event averted. Furthermore, these costs and benefits occur in the future and must be discounted in any event. However, inclusion or exclusion of indirect benefits can have more impact on the overall results than varying compliance or the cost of treatment of CHD or other illnesses. Kinosian found that inclusion of the indirect benefits of non-fatal CHD events averted improved the cholestyramine cost-effectiveness ratio by 10 to 20%.

Inclusion of indirect benefits can have a more dramatic effect on the relative cost of more efficient interventions. Kinosian found a net cost saving for the use of oat bran with the use of a more liberal estimate for indirect benefits.

DISCUSSION
COMPARISON WITH OTHER INTERVENTIONS TO TREAT OR PREVENT CHD

A Medline search was conducted looking for articles indexed by coronary disease or hypertension and economics from January 1980 to March 1990. Various workers in the field were consulted, and references in published papers were traced. Altogether, six articles were found which met the criteria for selection (Goldman et al, 1988; Oster, Colditz, and Kelly, 1986; Cummings, Rubin, and Oster, 1989; Weinstein and Stason, 1982; Lee et al, 1988; Hatziandreu et al, 1988).

A complete review of these studies is beyond the scope of this paper, but a few notes will be made of their methods.

EFFECTIVENESS

The treatment of hypertension has been shown conclusively to reduce overall mortality, although it is more effective in preventing cerebrovascular disease (stroke) than CHD (MacMahon et al, 1990; Collins et al, 1990).

Lee's study of exercise testing pools data from randomized and non-experimental studies of bypass surgery (Lee et al, 1988). Over the years, non-randomized trials have systematically overestimated the effectiveness of surgery (Frye et al, 1987). Therefore, Lee's study likely overestimates the benefits from surgery and the screening strategy. For similar reasons, the Weinstein study of coronary artery bypass surgery also likely overestimates the effectiveness of surgery (Weinstein and Stason, 1982). The studies of smoking cessation (Oster, Colditz, and Kelly, 1986; Cummings, Rubin, and Oster, 1989) base their effectiveness of cessation on meta-analyses of various randomized controlled trials. However, the reductions in mortality are then based on large cohort studies of smoking and non-smoking populations carried out in the 1950s and 1960s. These studies could underestimate the effectiveness of smoking cessation if smokers who quit did so because of symptoms. However, for three possible reasons, these studies might overestimate the effectiveness of smoking cessation.

1. Smokers who quit might be expected to be healthier in any event. This is similar to the 'volunteer' effect seen in non-randomized studies.

2. There is some evidence that lighter smokers are more likely to quit than heavy smokers (The Task Force on Smoking and Health in Ontario, 1982). There is a gradient of risk for CHD depending upon the amount smoked. Therefore, one would not expect the 'average' benefit to pertain if those smokers quitting were at less than average risk for the smoking population.

3. These studies base their absolute risk-reduction on death rates in the 1950s and 1960s. However, the CHD death rates have fallen 30-40% in the past 30 years.

The study of beta-blockers after myocardial infarction is based on pooled data from randomized controlled trials (Goldman et al, 1988). The authors then make some assumptions which have the effect of underestimating the efficiency of this program.

Therefore, there is some concern about the validity of the effectiveness data used in all studies, but the ones of beta-blockers and smoking cessation are more firmly based.

The evaluations of programs involving bypass surgery (Weinstein and Stason, 1982; Lee et al, 1988) do not consider the costs inherent in bringing the patient to the operating table. The difference in the cost-effectiveness ratios between the studies of bypass surgery and the study of exercise testing to detect patients with operable CHD (Lee et al, 1988) is partly explained by these costs.

OTHER STUDIES OF PRIMARY PREVENTION OF CHD

The results of these studies are shown in Table 2. The smoking interventions are the most efficient and are based on fairly strong evidence. Exercise is in the middle range, but would probably appear to be more efficient if its other benefits (e.g., prevention of osteoporosis) were also included. The treatment of severe hypertension is fairly efficient and is supported by several randomized controlled trials of the effectiveness of treatment in lowering overall mortality. The treatment of mild hypertension is much less efficient and the evidence for effectiveness is far less convincing.

Table 2

RESULTS OF THE COST-EFFECTIVENESS OF PRIMARY PREVENTION OF CHD – STUDIES NOT INVESTIGATING THERAPY FOR HYPERCHOLESTEROLEMIA

Study	Age	Other Risk Factors	Cost per life year saved (1989 CAN dollars)	
Hatziandreu				
Jogging	35	Avg. U.S.	best est.	$ 45,000
			conservative est.	160,000
			liberal est.	21,000
Oster				
Nicotine gum as adjunct to MD advice on smoking cessation	50-54	Avg. U.S.	best est.	7,000
Cummings				
MD advice on smoking cessation	50-54	Avg. U.S.	best est.	1,200
			conservative est.	9,100
			liberal est.	720
Weinstein (1985)				
Moderate/severe hypertension DBP[diastolic blood pressure] ≥105 mmHg	55	Avg. U.S.		24,000
Mild/moderate hypertension DBP 95 - 104 mmHg	55	Avg. U.S.		47,000
Mild hypertension DBP 90 - 94 mmHg	55	Avg. U.S.		110,000

TREATMENT STUDIES

Table 3 summarizes the cost-effectiveness reports of treatment interventions against CHD. Beta-blocker drugs used after myocardial infarction are very efficient and supported by strong evidence for effectiveness. Bypass surgery for left main coronary artery obstruction is quite efficient, but this condition is present in only a small minority of patients who have surgery. Surgery markedly reduces the absolute and relative risk of death for these patients (Takaro et al, 1982; Chaitman et al, 1981). Surgery for other patterns of coronary artery obstruction has not been subjected to a proper economic evaluation, but would be much less efficient.

Table 3
COST-EFFECTIVENESS OF VARIOUS TREATMENT PROGRAMS FOR CHD

Study	Age	Other Risk Factors	Cost per life year saved (1989 CAN dollars)
Goldman			
Beta blockers after myocardial infarction	55	*high risk:*	
		best est.	$ 3,300
		conservative est.	4,500
		medium risk:	
		best est.	5,000
		conservative est.	8,200
		low risk:	
		best est.	18,000
		conservative est.	32,000
Weinstein (1982)			
Coronary bypass surgery (left main stem disease)	55	*Avg. U.S.: best est.*	9,000
Lee			
Exercise ECG to screen patients with mild stable angina for left main stem disease	50	*Avg. U.S.: best est.*	12,000

DO THE RESULTS OF AMERICAN STUDIES APPLY TO CANADA?

Almost all these studies are American. None is Canadian. Because one of the main determinants of the cost-effectiveness of a program is the cost of the intervention, efficiency will differ between the two countries to the extent of the difference in program costs. The costs of most drugs are similar between the two countries and depend upon method of purchase (bulk vs. small packets) more than other variables (Toronto Working Group on Cholesterol Policy, 1990). The cost of physician and dietitian services would be less in Canada.

The overall costs of the programs depend upon many variables which differ from country to country. For example, the number of yearly physician visits for the treatment of hypercholesterolemia varies from one to six. For similar reasons, there would likely be similar variations from region to region.

The costs of hospital care are greater in the United States, and therefore the true efficiency of hospital based programs (e.g., bypass surgery, exercise test screening) might be better in Canada. However, the other concerns about these programs still apply. For the preventive studies, inclusion of the cost of care averted or provided makes very little difference in the overall analysis.

It is likely that there would be some minor cost differences in translating these results to the Canadian setting, but the rank order of the programs would not be likely to change much.

A POPULATION APPROACH

During the past 20 years several communities have attempted to reduce the incidence of heart disease by using community interventions (largely education) to reduce risk factors. The best known of these have been conducted in Finland (Puska et al, 1983; Puska et al, 1985) and Northern California (Farquhar et al, 1990). Because of the nature of these interventions, they cannot be evaluated with the same rigour as drug therapy for hypercholesterolemia. However, a recent report from the Stanford project shows reductions in cholesterol levels and other risk factors compared to control communities (Farquhar et al, 1990). A recent review of tobacco control policies concludes that increased taxation is more effective than the educational strategies (Godfrey and Maynard, 1988).

Unfortunately, there are no economic evaluations of these strategies. However, Farquhar reports that the cost of the educational intervention for the Stanford project was only $4 (U.S.) per adult (Farquhar et al, 1990). Farquhar estimates that the project resulted in a 2% decrease in cholesterol levels and a 16% decrease in risk for CHD. It appears that these types of interventions would be far more efficient than any of the other programs described above, if the evidence for their effectiveness is confirmed. The Stanford project will continue to report results over the next decade, and reports from two other large American projects will soon be available.

CONCLUSIONS

The studies of the efficiency of *treatment* of hypercholesterolemia are quite difficult to use for decision-making on cholesterol *screening* programs for a number of reasons. First, they do not incorporate all the preliminary costs of a program to test the cholesterol levels of the entire adult population. Second, it is difficult to estimate properly the costs of the follow-up of marginal cases. These costs include the deleterious effects of 'labelling' asymptomatic persons (Alderman and Lamport, 1990) with a 'disease' – hypercholesterolemia. Third, there is no evidence that the treatment of hypercholesterolemia lowers overall mortality. In fact, there is some evidence that the reduction in CHD mortality is matched by an elevation in non-CHD mortality. Fourth, while there is experimental evidence for cholestyramine's effectiveness in reducing CHD mortality, there is as yet none for the HMG CoA reductase inhibitors (simvastatin, lovastatin).

It is very likely that the treatment of men with very high levels of cholesterol (>7.75 mmol/L or 300 mg/dl) and other risk factors would reduce overall mortality and be competitive with other CHD programs. However, this cannot be said (at least at this time) of the treatment of men with lower cholesterol levels without other risk factors. These programs are almost certainly less efficient than other interventions to prevent or treat CHD.

The problems with screening programs for hypercholesterolemia have been well described (Rose, 1981). If the program casts its net widely to test and treat initially many persons at low absolute risk for CHD, the program becomes very inefficient. On the other hand, if the program confines itself to screening persons with high risk for CHD and treats only those with very high levels of cholesterol, it is much more efficient but averts few CHD deaths.

Researchers at McGill University have calculated that physician and laboratory services alone in the first year of a Canada-wide screening program would cost approximately $500 million (Grover et al, 1990). There would be an increase of approximately 300 visits to each primary care physician in the first year of the operation of the program. On the other hand, it would cost only approximately $120 million (per year) to replicate the Stanford program throughout Canada.

It must be admitted that there are a number of distributive questions regarding a population-wide strategy. For example, the tobacco industry has been set back by the reductions in smoking. The agriculture and food industry would be hard-pressed by sudden shifts away from foods with high levels of saturated fats. However, many economists and environmentalists would point out that the overall ecologic efficiency of food production would be enhanced if Canadians consumed fewer of their calories from animal fat. Furthermore, increasing exercise and reducing smoking and the consumption of animal fat would have positive impacts on many diseases other than coronary heart disease.

ACKNOWLEDGEMENT

This paper draws on the author's previous work for the Task Force on the Use of Medical Services (Toronto Working Group on Cholesterol Policy, 1990).

NOTES

1. $1 \text{ mmol}/l = 38.7 \text{ mg}/dl$ or $1 \text{ mg}/dl = 0.02586 \text{ mmol}/l$.

2. The medical care index includes all health care services and commodities, such as drugs. Because the programs described in the simulations incorporate services and drugs, it was decided to use the medical care index instead of the medical commodities index or the prescription drug index. In any event, the selection of index makes little difference to the results. The cost-effectiveness ratios would be only 3 to 5% greater if the prescription drug index had been used instead of the medical care index.

3. Simvastatin is an HMG CoA reductase inhibitor. A similar drug, lovastatin (Merck - Mevacor), has been marketed in Canada for two years.

REFERENCES

Alderman MH, Lamport B: Labelling of hypertensives: a review of the data. *Journal of Clinical Epidemiology* 43:195-200, 1990.

Benfante RJ, Reed DM, MacLean CJ, Yano K: Risk factors in middle age that predict early and late onset of coronary heart disease. *Journal of Clinical Epidemiology* 42:95-104, 1989.

Berwick DM, Cretin S, Keeler EB: *Cholesterol, Children, and Heart Disease: An Analysis of Alternatives.* New York: Oxford University Press, 1980.

Blackburn H: Trends and determinants of CHD mortality: changes in risk factors and their effects. *International Journal of Epidemiology* 18(3 suppl 1):S210-S215, 1989.

Chaitman BR, Fisher LD, Bourassa MG, et al: Effect of coronary bypass surgery on survival patterns in subsets of patients with left main coronary artery disease: report of the collaborative study in coronary artery surgery (CASS). *American Journal of Cardiology* 48:765-777, 1981.

Collins R, Peto R, MacMahon S, et al: Blood pressure, stroke, and coronary heart disease. Part 2. Short-term reductions in blood pressure: overview of randomised drug trials in their epidemiological context. *Lancet* 335:827-838, 1990.

Cummings SR, Rubin SM, Oster G: The cost-effectiveness of counseling smokers to quit. *Journal of the American Medical Association* 261:75-79, 1989.

Drummond MF, Stoddart GL, Torrance GW: *Methods for the Economic Evaluation of Health Care Programs.* Toronto: Oxford University Press, 1987.

Farquhar JW, Fortmann SP, Flora JA, et al: Effects of communitywide education on cardiovascular risk factors. *Journal of the American Medical Association* 264:359-365, 1990.

Fordyce MK, Christakis G, Kafatos A, Duncan R, Cassady J: Adipose tissue fatty acid composition of adolescents in a U.S.-Greece cross-cultural study of coronary heart disease risk factors. *Journal of Chronic Disease* 36:481-486, 1983.

Frick MH, Elo O, Haapa K, et al: Helsinki heart study: primary prevention trial with Gemfibrozil in middle-aged men with dyslipidemia. *New England Journal of Medicine* 317:1237-1245, 1987.

Frye RL, Fisher L, Schaff HV, Gersh BJ, Vliestra RE, Mock MB: Randomized trials in coronary artery bypass surgery. *Progress in Cardiovascular Diseases* 30:1-22, 1987.

Godfrey C, Maynard A: Economic aspects of tobacco use and taxation policy. *British Medical Journal* 297:339-343, 1988.

Goldman L, Sia STB, Cook EF, Rutherford JD, Weinstein MC: Costs and effectiveness of routine therapy with long-term beta-adrenergic antagonists after acute myocardial infarction. *New England Journal of Medicine* 319:152-157, 1988.

Grover SA, Coupal L, Fakhry R, Suissa S: Screening Canadians for hypercholesterolemia: an economic analysis. *Clinical Research* 38:323A, 1990.

Hatziandreu EI, Koplan JP, Weinstein MC, Caspersen CJ, Warner KE: A cost-effectiveness analysis of exercise as a health promotion activity. *American Journal of Public Health* 78:1417-1421, 1988.

Hjalte K, Lindgren B, Persson U, Olsson AG: The cost-effectiveness of a new cholesterol-reducing drug: The case of simvastatin. Paper presented to the European Health Economics Societies. Barcelona, September 21-23, 1989.

Kannel WB, Gordon T (eds): *The Framingham Study: An Epidemiological Investigation of Cardiovascular Disease.* U.S. Department of Health, Education, and Welfare publication (NIH) 74-610. Bethesda: Med Pub Hlth Serv, 1977.

Kinosian BP, Eisenberg JM: Cutting into cholesterol: cost-effective alternatives for treating hyper-cholesterolemia. *Journal of the American Medical Association* 259:2249-2254, 1988.

Lee TH, Fukui T, Weinstein MC, Tosteson ANA, Goldman L: Cost-effectiveness of screening strategies for left main coronary disease in patients with stable angina. *Medical Decision Making* 8:268-278, 1988.

Lipid Research Clinics Program: The Lipid Research Clinics coronary primary prevention trial results. 1. Reduction in incidence of coronary heart disease. *Journal of the American Medical Association* 251:351-364, 1984.

MacMahon S, Peto R: Randomized trials of cholesterol reduction in the context of observational epidemiology. Paper presented to the Canadian Consensus Conference on Cholesterol. Ottawa, March 9-11, 1988.

MacMahon S, Peto R, Cutler J, et al: Blood pressure, stroke, and coronary heart disease. Part 1. Prolonged differences in blood pressure: prospective observational studies corrected for the regression dilution bias. *Lancet* 335:765-774, 1990.

Martens LL, Rutten FFH, Erkelens DW, Ascoop CAPL: Clinical benefits and cost-effectiveness of lowering serum cholesterol levels: the case of simvastatin and cholestyramine in the Netherlands. *American Journal of Cardiology* 65:27F-32F, 1990.

Mitchell BD, Stern MP, Haffner SM, Hazuda HP, Patterson JK: Risk factors for cardiovascular mortality in Mexican Americans and non-Hispanic whites. *American Journal of Epidemiology* 131:423-433, 1990.

Multiple Risk Factor Intervention Trial Research Group. Multiple Risk Factor Intervention Trial: risk factor changes and mortality results. *Journal of the American Medical Association* 248:1465-1477, 1982.

Oster G, Colditz GA, Kelly NL: Cost effectiveness of nicotine gum as an adjunct to physician's advice against cigarette smoking. *Journal of the American Medical Association* 256:1315-1318, 1986.

Oster G, Epstein AM: Cost-effectiveness of antihyperlipidemic therapy in the prevention of coronary heart disease: the case of cholestyramine. *Journal of the American Medical Association* 258:2381-2387, 1987.

Puska P, Nissinen A, Tuomilehto J, et al: The community-based strategy to prevent coronary heart disease: conclusions from the ten years of the North Karelia Project. *Annual Review of Public Health* 6:1470-1493, 1985.

Puska P, Salonen J, Nissinen A, et al: Change in risk factors for coronary heart disease during 10 years of a community intervention programme (the North Karelia Project). *British Medical Journal* 287:1840-1844, 1983.

Riemersma RA, Wood DA, Butler S, et al: Linoleic acid content in adipose tissue and coronary heart disease. *British Medical Journal* 292:1423-1427, 1986.

Rose G: Causes of the trends and variations in CHD mortality in different countries. *International Journal of Epidemiology* 18(3 suppl 1):S174-S179, 1989.

Rose G: Strategy of prevention: Lessons from cardiovascular disease. *British Medical Journal* 282:1847-1851, 1981.

Russell LB: *Is Prevention Better than Cure?* Washington: The Brookings Institution, 1986.

Salonen JT: Did the North Karelia Project reduce coronary mortality? (letter). *Lancet* 2:269, 1987.

Takaro T, Peduzzi P, Detre K, et al: Survival in subgroups of patients with left main coronary artery disease: Veteran's Administration Cooperative Study of Surgery for Coronary Arterial Occlusive Disease. *Circulation* 66:14-22, 1982.

The Task Force on Smoking and Health in Ontario (chair, Dr. J.A. Best): *Smoking and Health in Ontario: A Need for Balance.* Toronto: Ontario Council of Health, 1982.

Taylor WC, et al. Cost-effectiveness of cholesterol reduction for the primary prevention of coronary heart disease in men. Cost-effectiveness background paper for the United States Preventive Services Task Force (USPSTF), February 1988.

Toronto Working Group on Cholesterol Policy (Naylor CD, Basinski A, Frank JW, Rachlis MM): Asymptomatic hyper-cholesterolemia: A clinical policy review. *Journal of Clinical Epidemiology* 43:1021-1121, 1990.

U.S. Bureau of Labor Statistics, personal communication, September 21, 1989.

Weinstein MC, Stason WB: Cost-effectiveness of coronary artery bypass surgery. *Circulation* 66 (suppl 3):56-66, 1982.

Weinstein MC, Stason WB: Cost-effectiveness of interventions to prevent or treat coronary heart disease. *Annual Review of Public Health* 6:41-63, 1985.

DISCUSSION
Chair: C. David Naylor
Sunnybrook Health Science Centre/University of Toronto

C. David Naylor

I'm wondering. What about a societal perspective in these costing endeavours? Should we be applying that rather than a third party payer perspective, or some mix? And how would health promotion and disease prevention fare as compared to therapeutic endeavours, if we were to follow a strict societal perspective? What is going to happen to all these evaluations of health promotion if we include all the broad social ramifications?

Vivek Goel (Sunnybrook Health Science Centre/University of Toronto)

It's a hard question to get at. I think, sort of continuing on from Michael [Rachlis]'s point, one of the important issues that we have to get at is, are we doing these evaluations to allocate resources between treatment and prevention, to get a little bit more than that 4% or whatever, 2%, across the entire country that goes to prevention and health promotion, or are we doing the evaluations to find out which interventions themselves are working, so with that 2% we can maximize our dollars? And, in the latter case, I don't think it makes any difference what the external ramifications are – you are really looking within the focus of the program. You can use intermediate outcomes to decide how best to spend that money. But when it comes to trying to convince the policy makers and the public, who elect the policy makers, we hope, how to allocate those dollars, I think you've got to include all of the consequences of any program. And whether it's heart surgery and all the consequences of people waiting on lists and the negative effects that impact on the health care system when people die waiting on those waiting lists, or it's tobacco farmers out of work, those effects have to be included. All types of evaluations have to include a societal perspective, if you're going to be making societal decisions.

Michael Rachlis (Toronto)

I'll have to tell a Meech Lake joke about human health resource planning, if someone doesn't ask me. I just want to make a very important point that I did not make in my presentation, which is that the review of two dozen experimental studies that have looked at reducing cholesterol have found, of course, that there is a statistically significant, and very clinically significant, reduction in fatal and non fatal coronary heart disease events. However, there has been found to be a statistically significant elevation of noncoronary heart disease deaths. So that there is really no difference in the overall mortality in these studies. There isn't one cause of death that is statistically significantly elevated in the treatment group, but cancer and trauma deaths approach statistical significance. This is a finding that is just completely dismissed by the National Cholesterol Education Program in the United States, which is out to test everybody's cholesterol in supermarkets, but it is a finding that has certainly distressed those of us who worked on the report for the Task Force on Utilization of Medical Services and distresses some other people. And the studies that I've presented, in fact, assume that the reduction in mortality for coronary heart disease events is equivalent to an overall mortality drop. And so that's yet another reason that in the studies I've just shown, even though the numbers still seem too high, they should even be higher when we look at the cost-effectiveness ratio.

C. David Naylor

In the interests of stimulating some discussion from the audience, I'll pick on Dr. Battista a little bit here. The Canadian Task Force on the Periodic Health Examination has a set of rules of evidence to which Vivek made passing mention, and that many of us – I will speak for myself here – that some of us feel may be a little inappropriate in terms of the weighting of quantitative evidence and the difficulties in evaluating community health promotion endeavours and disease preventive endeavours in the strict random-ized trial framework. Should the Canadian Task Force be rethinking some of its recom-mendations and its hierarchy of evidence and taking more of a broad based view of looking at other sources of evidence? Or are you happy with staying with the gold stan-dard, given what we've heard today and from other sources?

Renaldo Battista (Montreal General Hospital)

That's a very tricky question. I think that, insofar as the Task Force was looking at clin-ical preventive care, the rules of evidence it was using were really serving its purpose very well. I think the problem right now is that we've reached the point where clearly we need to look at community health interventions, and certainly as we move into the area of health promotion, which is certainly much more complex, I think that some of these rules of evidence will not hold. And certainly this is the time for a total rethinking of the ways we approach evidence, especially when we look at these very complex interventions that were described. So I think that there's a lot of space for innovative work in development of new methodologies.

Vivek Goel

Can I make a point there? I think something to keep in mind, though, is that the focus of the Task Force is on the clinical evaluation of an asymptomatic patient in a doctor's office, and perhaps what we need is a similar type of body to review evidence on health promotion, to make recommendations for public health agencies or hospitals that might want to expand their borders to get into [such activities]. In the same sense that the Task Force has had an impact on how clinicians, we hope, practice, we would have some sort of authoritative review of the existing evidence.

C. David Naylor

I think the only thing I'd say is that if you don't integrate the two, you get yourself into trouble, because the ambit of clinical preventive services may well end up being much broader than it needs to be. If you had a very effective community health promotion strat-egy, some of what clinicians do would no longer be necessary. And certainly we made those tradeoffs in the cholesterol policy formulation that was produced as background in Ontario. I'm not at all sure we made them correctly. But those considerations – the bal-ance point between a community health promotion strategy and individual clinical pre-ventive care – were taken into account. And I worry about two solitudes – one being clinical preventive medicine and the other being health promotion at a community level – and I really think those two task forces had better be very closely knitted together in what they do.

Steve Elson (Niagara District Health Council)

I was surprised that nobody mentioned the Ontario Health Status Survey, which is currently being implemented in Ontario, partly because with the 60,000 interviews that are going to be done as part of that survey, it really does for the first time provide us with an opportunity to assess what the health status of the province of Ontario is, from a very broad and societal perspective. And with the prospect of repeating that survey at a later date, it really gives us the opportunity to assess what kind of changes can take place and be mobilized and stimulated within communities in the areas of health promotion and disease prevention, as has been discussed this afternoon. And as a person working in a District Health Council, I am very excited and I hope optimistic, and not unduly so, about the impact that kind of a survey can have on some of the rigour and some of the impact of health promotion within local areas. I guess the other comment that I would like to make, and it's been touched on – mainly, I think, it's a policy issue – is for local communities who are trying to implement a lot of the results, or trying to keep up with the kind of results that have been discussed this afternoon in the area of health promotion and disease prevention. We are hampered by the current policies of issuing – basically – time limited grants that allow communities to become excited and stimulated in the areas of undertaking health promotion, but with the exception of public health, which is, at least in the province of Ontario, restricted to funding arrangements between the province and local government, there is very little opportunity for sustained funding of health promotion initiatives within our communities. And certainly I know within our area and others, that's really hurting the development of health promotion.

Michael Rachlis

That's of course because governments don't care about the health of their people. They really don't, except if they're at war.

Vivek Goel

Or it gets into the newspaper.

Lavada Pinder (Health and Welfare Canada)

I couldn't agree more. I think the gains that have been made in health promotion and disease prevention are actually quite remarkable, given the fact that there's no infrastructure. The health promotion field is in its infancy. There are very few resources. There isn't enough exchange. Given this, I think that the gains have been very great. We do not have a system for health. We have a health care, or sickness care, system which is very well maintained, and what we must begin to think about is a system for health, and then our questions will have a chance of being answered.

Alex Berland (Vancouver General Hospital)

I'm not a health economist, and I guess my comments will be more an anecdotal caveat that I would like to toss out. Vivek's slide of the suntanner, of course, was filmed in Vancouver. And though you might not appreciate the effect of the sunshine we've had out there this summer, we've all appreciated it a great deal. And it reminded me of a discussion I had with a dermatologist friend not too long ago. I had mentioned something to him about sunscreen and he said, "Yes, but you know, we can go much too far in that direction." He cited a situation in Australia where, of course, they have a very high incidence of skin cancer and subsequent melanoma, and they mounted a very effective health promotion campaign involving a film of a young man who was dying of melanoma going around to beaches and talking with suntanners about how he had contracted the disease. The consequence of this very effective campaign was a tremendous interest in the problem and lineups of people going to dermatologists' offices worried about every little mole on their body. Tremendous expenditures on mole removal. And we have in Vancouver a Mole Patrol which goes around beaches. To some extent, it reminds me of Dr. Wright's comments this morning about needs and demands. And in this instance we have a situation where the public demand, incited by perhaps a particular group of specialists' interest in generating the demand, resulted in a greatly disproportionate amount of interest in a preventive measure which probably wasn't justified for the relatively small number of melanomas which develop each year. I don't know whether it's possible to predict in advance to what extent people will overreact – will eat too much oat bran, will worry too much about moles, will perhaps develop high blood pressure worrying about their high blood pressure – but it seems to me that it is an important concern that we need to recognize.

Vivek Goel

Just related to that, and to the earlier comment about the health status survey, in the United States the C.D.C. [Centers for Disease Control] runs a behavioural risk factor surveillance system. Every month they do a survey across, I think, 40 or 30 of the states, and they get a sense of what people's attitudes towards smoking and alcohol and a variety of other behaviours are, on a regular basis. And they are able to plot these out just as they do with communicable disease rates. And an interesting graph is women's attitudes towards mammography. And they plotted along, and there's a little spike when the American Cancer Society had a screening program, and then there's a massive spike, I think it was March of 1987, when Nancy Reagan had her lump diagnosed. It was a three-fold increase in the proportion of women that had had a mammogram the previous month. People react to what's in the news and what they perceive as being important. And ill-mounted programs, or early educational interventions, or noninterventions, like the oat bran, can lead to false expectations. And when information comes out that they are negative, it can lead to a lot of disappointment with the health care system. The oat bran, as you said, was everywhere. Kellogg's had a massive program in conjunction with the American Cancer Society; they were running TV programs – ads. They supported a national hot line for information on oat bran and cancer. And later on, I don't know whether the American Heart Association got involved as well. In this past year, the American Heart Association got into a controversy with its endorsement of particular products, where manufacturers were paying to be able to use the American Heart Association logo on their product. Health promotion is one of those things that at least the food industry sees as a marketing tool. And we've got to be careful that the results of preliminary evaluations don't get used as marketing tools, because those are going to lead to false expectations.

C. David Naylor

I'm not sure that you're entirely fair to oat bran, because number 1, even if the net effect is simply to fill the stomach and serve as a substitute for other foods, that's not exactly terrible. Number 2, you're basing the critique on a single crossover study with about 20 patients that happened to get into the *New England Journal,* whereas there's a whole boatload of other studies in other places that don't all support the notion that it has no hypolipidemic effects. So, as someone who never ever got on the bandwagon but continues to feel guilty as I look at the cereal boxes, I think there's still some life in oat bran.

Ronald Baigrie (Sunnybrook Health Science Centre)

This question has been nagging at me for years, and I'm glad to have the opportunity to ask this panel. It's probably a very naive question, but let me ask it anyway. Could we change the title of this panel to "What Gains Can We Expect from Health Promotion and Disease Delay, or 'Whither Oat Bran?'". In other words, what epidemiologic data is there to suggest that you're preventing, as opposed to delaying the inevitable by a period of time that hasn't yet been studied?

C. David Naylor

That's an excellent question, and I think I'll toss it over to the panel.

Michael Rachlis

I think that the evidence is very strong that the unofficial community heart health program that's been going on in North America for the last 25 years has had very beneficial effects not only on heart disease, but overall mortality. What I'm talking about is that over the last 25 years coronary heart disease death rates have fallen about 40% in Canada. And in fact, just looking between 1979 and 1987, particularly for young men, men in their forties and fifties, just in those eight years coronary heart disease death rates have fallen 35-45%, in only eight years. And this is almost totally because of fewer incident sudden deaths, associated, it seems, with lower cholesterol levels, certainly with lower rates of smoking, and not only are they not dying of coronary heart disease until later, but they're not dying of other things right away either, because the reduction in coronary heart disease mortality is one of the major reasons there have been extensions in life expectancy for middle aged people, and particularly for middle aged men. So yes, I guess the iron law of epidemiology might be that everybody dies sometime, but I think that it's pretty conclusive, at least in that area, that you're going to have a longer life and a healthier life if you don't die of coronary heart disease in your fifties. It doesn't apply to everything.

Raisa Deber (University of Toronto)

As the person who has to apologize for the much maligned session title, I think it's very appropriate that Dr. Baigrie has gone to a Keynesian metaphor which is, "In the long run, we are all dead."

Ronald Baigrie

If I am right, Mr. Chairman, it costs a lot more money to be alive with cardiac disease today than it does to be dead with cardiac disease today.

C. David Naylor

The only thing I would say is that I think there is some truth in Ron Baigrie's observation. I think there has been a compression of incidence. I think that there is a lot of controversy about the actual change in incidence and new MIs in various age brackets. There may be a drop in the younger group, but it's not clear to me that it is really falling in the older group. And I think that there has been some squeezing up of the burden of morbidity from coronary disease. The change in life expectancy is small. The change in overall mortality is small. And I think that we are getting something of a compression of morbidity, which is the Fries hypothesis. Now if you look at the medicalization of the elderly, which I know Morris Barer and colleagues have talked about, and you go out on the wards and you listen to residents who say, "He's a great 78 year old", or, "He's a great 88 year old", you have this whole sense of a difference in expectations, and where it all ends I don't know. I just have this vision of a society of 90 year olds who are on life support machines and getting bypass procedures. So, at some point, the music has to be faced.

Jane Sisk (Office of Technology Assessment, U.S. Congress)

I just wanted to make an observation about some of the scoffing at the cereal companies and everybody else who was getting on the oat bran band wagon. I've been in sessions where policy makers are trying fervently to figure out ways to get the commercial sector to find it in their economic self interest to engage in promotional activities that, as a side effect, will promote health or prevent disease. Here was a situation where there was a commercial interest in promoting a product that might have had some health benefit. I've been in situations where people are talking about trying to figure out ways to have profit-making organizations engage in activities – advertising or whatever – promoting their products in ways that will promote our health. For example, condoms, condom sales – or vaccine use in developing or developed countries. So I just wanted to make that point, that here was a situation where it was potentially a win-win situation, except people probably went overboard. But that's ultimately what we'd like to have happen, I think, as people concerned about the public's health and having an economic bent, that there be situations where it's win-win – everybody benefits.

C. David Naylor

I think those are very appropriate comments. I think I'd like to raise one caveat, though. And that is that the disutility of dietary change, for individuals who, particularly starting in their thirties or forties, let alone in their sixties, are faced with some injunction to change their diet, consume more fibre, drop their saturated fat intake, and so on, is such that if you consider even a rapid discount, decline in the disutility over three or four years, and you think about how many people have to change their diet to avert a certain number of coronary events, that promoting community-wide dietary change, promoting the consumption of some of these foodstuffs, actually may carry some penalties in terms of giving up bacon and eggs or whatever horrible things people are happy consuming. I often think we don't take into account the disutility of behavioural change in health promotion or disease prevention, which must always be factored into account, in fairness.

SOUTH
OF
THE
BORDER

U.S. INFLUENCES ON CANADA: CAN WE PREVENT THE SPREAD OF KURU?*

Robert G. Evans
Centre for Health Services and Policy Research
University of British Columbia

The title for today's session was selected, by me, several months ago at a time when it seemed like something suitably recherché and puzzling, the sort of thing that people would look at and say, "What on earth is that about?" Since it was selected, a number of things have happened which have suggested that the whole topic of kuru has become a great deal more important than certainly I would ever have expected at that time. I had no basis on which to expect anything, I just pulled it out of the air and thought that would really be something neat. But, as it happens – I was going to suggest that perhaps this is a case of Nature imitating Art, but I am not sure that this isn't just Nature imitating Bob – there have been some quite important developments in the news on this topic. "Kuru" – it's a name for a slow-acting disease called spongiform encephalopathy – brain rot. There are a number of versions of this. The mittel-European name for it is Creutzfeldt-Jakob syndrome. It turns up as scrapie among sheep. It turns up in Britain as bovine spongiform encephalopathy. If you say that quickly a number of times, you get to be able to do it reasonably reliably. BSE. Mad cow disease. It is now, of course, universally claimed by all the experts in this field in Britain that it doesn't spread to people, and you know what that means. Fifteen thousand cows have recently met their deaths in Britain as a result of this disease. Scrapie is spreading in North America among sheep. Should we worry about this? In the August 1990 *Scientific American* there is a long and rather chilling column on Oravske kuru. In two villages in a remote part of Slovakia where people deal with a lot of sheep, rates of infection from this illness are some hundreds of times the normal worldwide background rate. Very interesting. What is it? Is it a virus? Maybe, not clear. Still in debate. It seems – some people have done experiments on it – it seems to be able to survive temperatures up to 300 odd degrees Celsius – barely survive, as the article said. It's uniformly fatal, kills you within about seven months. Some kind of spongy protein is laid down in the brain; it basically is brain rot.

So why am I telling you this? Well, because you ought to get something interesting and new out of any of these meetings – after all, if this isn't basically fun, why are we doing it? That's one reason. Another reason is that about 10 years ago I was mooching through the back of the *New England Journal of Medicine,* avoiding reading what I was supposed to read, and I ran across a letter by some physicians in California to their colleagues saying, "Gee guys, we have noticed recently quite a lot of cases of Kaposi's sarcoma, and we're noticing them among young males, and we think this is unusual epidemiologically and we'd like to know whether anybody else out there is seeing something similar and whether anybody's got any thoughts about this." Well, at the time I had never heard of Kaposi's sarcoma. I still have no real idea what it is, but I've heard about it a lot more since. And that was obviously the very beginning of something really rather large and nasty. I do not know, nor does anybody else, whether this spongiform encephalopathy is the beginning of something rather large and nasty or whether it's just a rather awkward and rather terrible misfortune that will affect only a small group of people and a lot of sheep. But I just thought you might be interested to know that there is another one out there and exactly how it gets transmitted and all that stuff, and exactly what it is, is still really rather obscure.

However, that still leaves you wondering why I am telling you this. Kuru itself is a name that comes from New Guinea. It is the same, or appears to be the same, disease or family of diseases, and you get it by eating the brains of your dead enemies. So we're here talking about the communication of ideas from the United States to Canada – brain rot.

Now cast your minds back, so to speak, to yesterday's session with Martin Barkin, where a lot of very interesting things were said – most of them by Martin, as usual. He, among other things, detected a shift in the Canadian consensus over health insurance, what traditionally has been interpreted as Canada's special attachment to, and special definition by, its healthcare system. He felt that consensus might be breaking down and shifting. And he made this point in the context of a greatly increased concern for the competitive position of Canada in a multi-polar trading world. And you will have heard that rhetoric in a number of quarters, the notion that we are no longer able, if we ever were, to hide ourselves behind trade and other barriers and to rely upon our natural resource endowment, but that we are already in the position of being much more intensively competitive with the rest of the world. And in that context we may find ourselves not able, or not willing, any longer to maintain this kind of social consensus. Now that was not made as a firm prediction, but just something that we want to think about. But what is really intriguing about that is that, if true, it comes at a time when exactly the reverse situation is developing in the United States, where grave concerns about the international competitiveness of the U.S. economy are surfacing – have surfaced – coincident with concerns about the extraordinary cost of their healthcare system. And you get it particularly from Chrysler and Ford and some others of the Rust Belt industries, the notion that their extraordinarily high cost healthcare system is one of the factors – not necessarily the only one – but one of the factors which is making it very difficult for Americans to compete in world markets.

So we do have this extraordinary situation – at least it seems extraordinary to me – of Canadians starting to worry that we can't afford, in this new world, a universal social program which our neighbours to the south regard as something that they would like to get because it's so much cheaper than the alternative that they have. That's a rather convoluted way of saying, "Why on earth do we think that we want to abandon the cheaper form in order to take on the more expensive form, in order to make ourselves more competitive? Why do we want to make the thing worse?" So the argument about abandoning universality, bringing back and increasing the role of the private sector, all that kind of stuff, is really weird when you look at it from the south side of the border. However, what's that got to do with kuru? An American might quite reasonably respond – John [Iglehart] may respond, but I'll get there first – that it's got nothing to do with the transmission of ideas, that it's got to do with Canadians being ignorant and stupid. And that's something that they can manage at home without any help from their neighbours. If Canadians insist on not doing their homework, why should we get mad at the Americans? Well, it's an excuse at least, but it is not intellectually very sound.

Second point – in addition to failing to do our homework and understanding what the alternatives are – the second point is, I think, one of setting. We are in Canada a smeared line of small colonies along the northern American border. And so there is an extraordinarily high level of information generation that comes from the south that we pick up regularly on our televisions and newspapers and magazines and everywhere else. As soon as we begin to think about problems in our own system and think about alternatives, the alternatives that naturally intrude on our consciousness immediately are the alternatives that are presented in the United States. And because we're embedded in that broader culture we see ourselves as always different, with reference to the United States as normalcy (if you can imagine such a thing). So that a part of our problem is that any search for alternatives or any thinking about what else one might do, immediately one winds up looking at American examples because they're sitting there in front of you, they're in the same language, they are very highly promoted – the United States is an information-rich economy. But there again, that's a problem of geographic setting for which we can hardly blame the Americans; it just so happens that we're here and they're there. And that doesn't fit within the rubric of kuru, but it is something that you want to keep in mind as a problem in trying to think about how our healthcare system stacks up, how it might be better managed, and so on and so forth – that the context and setting makes life difficult for us.

Now when we start talking about the transmission of ideas, though, there I think we do find stuff coming north, and I would suggest that that falls into two categories, and I'll mention examples of them as we go along. The first I've called just 'general background noise'. Being immersed in U.S. culture and communications, we just pick up a lot from them of their attitudes and their ways of viewing the world which have nothing to do with them actually trying to do anything deliberate, but they are transmitted to us. They come north. We don't pick them up by going south, they just are sent north to us. And that's in the nature of the beast.

The second one, though, I think is the more interesting pattern, and that is what I would say is a very recently stepped-up campaign of attention in the United States to Canada, which I think is having some direct effects up here. And that's the one I want to put a little more emphasis on. Back in the early 1970s, going through until about 1974, the United States was heavily involved in studying national health insurance programs and was particularly interested in Canada, because of course we had just developed one although we didn't have much operating data yet. And there were then a number of conferences and studies and so on of health insurance which looked at Canada. Then about the mid 70s that dropped completely off the agenda. National health insurance in the States was no longer anything that anybody was interested in. There were other things that they were going to do. And between about 1974 and about 1988 it was a dead issue. That was a good time for comparative research, because it meant that researchers could plug along in their ivory towers using each country as a base-line against which to compare the results from the other, to ask "what if" questions or questions about counter-factuals. "Supposing we had not done what we did, but we did what those other guys did, what would the outcomes maybe have been?" So we can measure the impact of our own policies in an environment which is strictly academic. Nobody is worrying too much about policy implications. Now since 1988, there has been an explosion of interest in Canada in the United States. I think it's waning a bit at the moment but it's hard to tell, because there's so much goes on down there that it's hard to know what the averages are. But again, starting in the fall of 1988, suddenly I think the dissatisfaction with their own system crystallized, and a lot of that dissatisfaction was rhetorically associated with the inadequacy of coverage – the 37 million or 40 million or 30 million or however many people there are who don't have insurance coverage in the United States. But secondarily it was related to the problem of uncompensated care, which was making life very difficult for a lot of the big city hospitals. Perhaps even more important, there was the growing realization that a lot of the private sector corporations in the United States might be technically bankrupt, because if they were required to carry on their books the actuarial value of the commitments which they had made to their workers and retired workers for health insurance, that actuarial value might very well exceed the shareholders' net worth. And there is an ugly technical term for firms whose balance sheets have that characteristic. Furthermore, the FASB (Federal Accounting Standards Board) was making a lot of noises about requiring firms to report those unfunded liabilities, which would, as I say, bring into the open this rather distressing situation. Under the circumstances, it was not terribly surprising that a lot of American corporations decided that it would be a whale of a good idea if they could get a public insurance system which would cause those liabilities to be moved onto somebody else's books.

So, arising out of the combination of inadequate coverage, escalating cost, relatively high levels of public dissatisfaction, you suddenly got the rediscovery of Canada. Gosh! Up there, there is universal coverage, there is relative – relative to the U.S. – cost control. There seems to be a high level of public satisfaction. We're getting into a free-trade agreement, why don't we trade systems?

Well, the American intellectual immune system kicked into action immediately. You know an immune system's primary function is to distinguish between self and non-self. It is to detect antigens displayed on the surface of cells and recognize antigens as non-self and destroy those cells and mop up the agent involved. I am not going to get into a lecture on immune system function for at least two very good reasons. One has to do with the level of your understanding, and the other has to do with mine. But the point is that the immune system response occurred and is occurring on quite a substantial scale, and it's coming from the people that you might expect. It's coming from the vendors of care in the United States – the American Medical Association has been quite prominent in launching publicity campaigns trashing the Canadian system. The Health Insurance Association of America is equally prominent, with a somewhat different spin, in criticizing the Canadian system. And in an interesting way that you want to keep your eye on, some members of the economic intellectual community in the United States have in a more subtle way been carrying out quite deep-rooted criticisms of the way things are done in Canada. The problem is that our perceptions of our own system become heavily influenced by the perceptions of it which are generated in the United States, simply because that's true of everything in Canada – that any negative campaign in the United States is going to wind up coming across the border and undermining, influencing, affecting, getting into the background and even into the foreground of the way Canadians think about their own system. And the problem I think is that most people most of the time – well it's not a problem, actually, it's a good thing – most of the people most of the time don't have any direct personal experience with the healthcare system. And that's great. That's the last thing that anybody in his right mind would want is a lot of direct personal experience with the healthcare system. But it means that most of the population is then relying on faith, past experience, experience of friends, but also I think more than in many other fields vulnerable to distortions of perception as a result of claims and counter-claims made in the media. So the transmission of ideas affects the climate within which people are able to try to make health policy within Canada. Another way of looking at it is that the components of the American immune system pass across the border. I was going to say pass across the blood-brain barrier, but we would be a little obscure as to which is on which side of the fence.

Now why that violent immune response? Two reasons, I think. One – remembering that this is also an economics conference – one has to do with the notion of quasi-rents. And I think these are quite important for people to keep in mind, particularly our non-economics colleagues. A rent, in economics, is a technical term which refers to the payments made to a provider of a good or service over and above the amount necessary to keep that person in the market. We're coming back actually to Peter Ruderman's comment yesterday about physician payment. A quasi-rent is a payment to somebody for a fixed piece of capital equipment that is over and above what is needed to keep that capital in place, but not necessarily above what was necessary to get it committed in the first place. In another words, if you've already got people to make commitments, then they don't have to be paid as much to continue those commitments after the fact. So anybody who has invested in physical or human capital is earning quasi-rents on that capital over and above the marginal cost, but maybe – maybe not – over and above the full long run cost. What we have in the U.S., what we have in every healthcare system, is a lot of providers of care who have a lot invested in the existing system. We have in the U.S. a huge insurance industry, ditto, people who have acquired skills, capabilities, at expense to themselves and are earning a return on those. We have intellectual capital. We have economists who have invested in a particular way of viewing the world and have made a quite substantial personal investment in that, and they earn a return on that investment by virtue of potential buyers' willingness to accept their interpretation of events as especially privileged or enlightened. If you change the rules of the game dramatically, as by changing the American healthcare system to become Canadian, you wipe out a lot of quasi-rents. You destroy a lot of human capital. Overnight, the insurance industry becomes pure waste motion. It ceases to be highly skilled, highly paid clever individuals doing clever things and becomes a bunch of guys generally adding to the cost of healthcare by shuffling bits of paper around. Pure waste motion. Much of the payment to providers – more ambiguous – but generally American providers perceive reimbursement rates being lower in Canada. The intellectual interpreters of the system – all those who have made a heavy investment in envisioning healthcare systems in market and competitive terms – suddenly find their intellectual apparatus at a severe discount because nobody in the rest of the world looks at things that way. And when your intellectual apparatus is discounted, so are your fees, or so are your prospects for employment. So we do have a lot of quasi-rental streams in the U.S. tied up in maintaining this view of the world. In addition to that, there are ideological roots which feed these quasi-rental streams, because of course the U.S., more than any other country, is embedded in this notion of individualism, in this notion that goes back into the U.S. constitution. So let me sum up by quickly listing some of the things which I think come north as a result of that. One is – we've already mentioned it – "universality being more costly". We know it isn't, but a large proportion of our population still thinks it is. Surprisingly, educated and informed people who know very little about healthcare think that we are paying more because it's universal. Background to that is the distinction between government and private. "When the government does things they're done badly, when the private sector does them they're done well." Again, a surprising proportion of Canadians routinely pick that up and think it applies in healthcare as well, the notion that you can control costs on the demand side rather than on the supply side, that this whole deductibles and coinsurance – the D and C approach to cost control – will somehow work. Again, the American results there are conclusive. It doesn't work. And we know it doesn't work. And we know that our own approaches sort of do work. But you go out there in the regular community among the public, among particularly the business community – who ought to know better and never talk to their American colleagues about what's really going on – their first reaction is, "Gee, we ought to bring back some charges to patients, that would fix things up." Some of my colleagues and I have referred to these as zombies, ideas that are intellectually dead but keep walking around doing damage. And they do so for good sound economic reasons.

Perhaps the most difficult, the most troublesome thing of all, we constantly see ourselves, as the Americans do, in some kind of polar relation to the United States, either the cheap and nasty Canadian system in contrast to the American richly endowed and effective – that's sort of the AMA line – or alternatively, the lean and virtuous Canadian system in contrast to the American bloated and evil, which again some of the promoters of public health insurance in the United States would say. But the point is that either of those views, whether or not distorted, involves a polarity. And I guess this is my final message that I think we need to get out of. It involves a polarity between us and the U.S., when the U.S. is an extraordinary outlier on the world scale. We are not just a lot cheaper and a lot more universal than the U.S. We are relatively expensive but kind of in the top of the pack compared to the Europeans. And if we do a lot more comparing ourselves with the European systems, I think we'll learn a great deal more from it. But what I want to leave with you is partly that – that we need to see ourselves in a world picture and much less focusing on the projection of us that comes north of the border – but also, how the devil do we communicate this much more complex view to the people out in the rest of the Canadian community whose views, as Martin pointed out right at the beginning of his talk, really in the end are the critical ones?

NOTE
* edited transcript of talk

CANADIAN INFLUENCES ON THE U.S.:
IMMUNE SYSTEM RESPONSES?*
Discussant: John Iglehart
Health Affairs

It is always a pleasure to follow Bob Evans on the rostrum; he was really quite easy on us this morning. I do have a couple of announcements. First I wanted to thank all the Canadians who have spent time with me and helped me along over the last five years in my various pursuits of the Canadian system. It's really been a pleasure, and they have all been helpful and particularly generous with the most important resource we all have – time. Secondly, I just want to say a word about *Health Affairs*, the journal I have edited for the last decade in the U.S. It's a health policy journal. It's peer reviewed. I am trying to put more information in it on the Canadian system and would welcome submissions to it in the future.

I'd like to start out by quoting one of my favourite economists about health systems and how they relate one to another. He is a Canadian. In fact, he is Bob Evans. And I quoted him in one of my 1986 pieces in the *New England Journal,* because I thought he was particularly on point. Bob said at the time, and he was writing in an American journal, "Nations do not borrow other nations' institutions. The Canadian system may be 'better' than the American. I believe it is, though that is a very complex question, and as I have just pointed out, my views, like yours" – meaning Americans' – "are contaminated by my origins. Even if it is better, I am not trying to sell it to you. You cannot have it. It would not 'fit' because you do not see the world, or the individual, or the state, as we do.... The point is that by examining others' experience you can extend your range of perceptions of what is possible." I think that really is the point upon which all examinations of systems of other countries really should be pursued. I think it is clear to all of us that healthcare systems in any country, certainly in the industrialized world, reflect the cultural beliefs and the political priorities and the medical imperatives of the country in which they evolve. Healthcare spending in the entire industrialized world, including Canada, has year by year outstripped the growth of economies. In this era – 1975 to 1987 – West Germany really has the best record in terms of measuring the growth of its health spending against the growth of its national income, and the U.S. and Japan rank the worst. But a snapshot of the western countries at this time or really at any time shows that they are all struggling with that never ending question – challenge – of matching insatiable demands against limited resources. I think Bob made a valid point, and that is that the grass always seems greener in the other country. So it is not unusual that Canada looks longingly on occasion at the U.S. and some of the things we do in terms of research and development, and all the money we spend, and the U.S. looks at Canada, and West Germany looks at England, and so forth and so on. The looking always seems to be that those programs that are essentially public long for some of those private resources, and those systems that are permanently private such as the U.S. often are asking the question, "How can we tap those public treasuries a little more heavily than we are at the moment?" If you look across Europe at the moment, you see that all of the countries, in one form or another, are either debating or enacting reforms. The Netherlands is implementing recommendations of a recent commission to change the structure of the financing and delivery – at the margin – of its health service system. West Germany is implementing its 1988 reform law that introduces new controls on drug expenditures and higher user fees. Sweden is in the middle of a review of its system. The British parliament in July enacted major reforms, resisted by the medical profession, that will influence the directions of the National Health Service in the future. And Canada obviously has a wide variety of activities under way, some of which Doug Angus referred to yesterday in his remarks.

In the U.S., what's going on? It seems, I am sure, to anybody, to an outsider and even to an insider, that the U.S. is paralyzed in terms of trying to move off the dime and address directly and seriously the problems that it confronts. I think yesterday Rashi Fein made a very perceptive point about the kinds of issues we talk about in the U.S. and the fact that the questions we must address are really quite fundamental in terms of the future shape of our system - dealing with not only structure and organization, but things as basic as values. Essentially, the U.S. system is a system in trouble. You look at public opinion surveys conducted over the last year and they indicate that more than 70% of Americans favour some form of national healthcare program. The kicker there, though, is that this support for a plan financed by the government dwindles when the fundamental question about financing and who pays the bill comes up.

One of the first things that I think the U.S. must deal with more effectively than it has to date are the values upon which we base a healthcare system. It is those basic questions that still remain unanswered in our system – often addressed, but unanswered – things like, "Is it important that the U.S. healthcare system preserve freedom of choice in terms of the consumer going to the doctor? Should he or she be able to go to any physician at any time?" That is an unanswered question in our system, particularly for those millions who are uninsured. Another value question that's unanswered at this point is, "Is it more important to keep taxes down than it is to make sure that everyone has health insurance?" The U.S. devotes the lowest proportion of its GDP in the western world to taxes, yet the thing you hear more about, particularly from the politicians in the last decade through today, is taxes – "We must lower our taxes" – even as our budget deficit increases. Another value that has not been addressed, or at least has not been answered, is, "Should tax dollars, as in Canada, be used for basic health insurance for people who are not covered by other plans and can't afford to buy insurance policies?" You find in the United States that the game that is being played and has been for some years is cost shifting – making the other guy foot the bill. That obviously is not a viable long term strategy.

In the few minutes I have remaining I wanted to talk directly about what Americans have learned from the Canadian system in this pursuit – this examination that has been going on over the last five years. I think it is fair to say that many Americans, particularly Americans that you might put in the opinion moulding or opinion forming set, are fascinated by Canada's commitment to universality. I think the campaigns that have been going on – the self-interested campaigns that were sponsored by, say, the American Medical Association or the commercial health insurance lobby in the U.S. – really have not stuck. In fact, if you look at the A.M.A. campaign and just see what's happened to it in recent months, it is fair to say that they really have quietly withdrawn it because it wasn't based on fact, it was based on ideology.

So what have we learned? We have learned that in North America, systems that blend mostly public finance with private medical practice can and do work, and there is a living example, obviously, here in Canada. We've learned that the control of health expenditure through strengthening the hands of public funders as opposed to imposing higher costs on consumers is an approach that's broadly acceptable to the public. In the U.S., you must remember that about 26% of the expenditures are out-of-pocket – directly from consumers. We have learned that universal access appeals to all Americans of all economic strata, and the American media are particularly struck by Canada's achievement in this regard. There is an upcoming documentary on public television in December that Walter Cronkite is narrating that very effectively makes this point. Where Americans obviously come up short in deciding how their system should be shaped is the financing, who should pay the bill, and how it should be configured – private versus public.

My time is about up. Let me just finish by saying that the very presence of Canada's health insurance system has increased the pressure on the U.S. to remedy the flaws in its healthcare system. And I would like to quote from George Bush's health policy advisor – at least up until several months ago – Bill Roper, who has now moved on to be the director of the Centers for Disease Control. I quoted Bill late last year in an article in the *New England Journal* in relation to all this activity that was going on in Canada and he said, "As an individual trained in medicine, but who has worked since 1982 in several capacities for the federal government, I am not sure where this unprecedented level of activity is heading, but it is unusual in my experience. At the most basic political level, Canada's achievement says to us, 'Our neighbours to the north have accomplished several important health policy goals. Why can't we?'" In other words, Canada is challenging America's 'can do' spirit. That does not mean we will follow Canada's approach, but the attention that we are paying it certainly is accelerating the American debate. I will conclude by saying that it's my sense that the U.S., for all the problems it has, is going to muddle through for a few more years before it directly addresses them, and I think the event that will bring it about is that some aggregate number of chief executive officers from the Fortune 500 companies will go marching up Pennsylvania Avenue one day and knocking on the White House door and telling whoever is the occupant at that point, "We can't take it any more, and we need a national health program of some shape and form." And that's when it will happen.

NOTE
* edited transcript of talk

DISCUSSION
Chair: Greg Stoddart
McMaster University

Michael Rachlis (Toronto)

This question is particularly for John [Iglehart], I guess. I've been impressed, talking to Americans over the last year, that there seems – even by intelligent people – there seems to be this immediate upset at the idea that a worker would have deducted from his paycheque increased taxes that would go to government to pay for universal health insurance, instead of the deduction that now goes to an insurance company. So even if the dollar figures were exactly the same but the money was taken off the cheque to go to government instead of to an insurance company, that could result in the loss of an election for a politician that advocated it. Are people in the United States so upset at the idea of paying extra taxes that they would not take universal health insurance just because their deductions would go to taxes instead of to an insurance company? Is that a major problem?

John Iglehart *(Health Affairs)*

Time is short, Michael, so I'll say "Yes".

Larry Wiser (Manitoba Ministry of Health)

I don't know whether, Bob, you caught Saturday Report on the CBC, but they interviewed the Premier of British Columbia, who is once again behaving like the Premier of British California, and he is on again about user fees to cut down what he perceives as unneeded, unwarranted visits to the physician. And it looks like you've got some homework waiting for you when you get back to British California, Bob, and I can hardly wait for that.

Robert Evans (University of British Columbia)

I'm not sure there was a question there. I think the answer, though, is you don't spend your time on things that are likely to be unproductive. I think that why the Canada Health Act is so important is that it protects us, to some degree, against those zombies. The one country in the world that makes heavy reliance on user fees is the most expensive country in the world and that's the United States. And while I agree with John Iglehart – how could one disagree – that every country in the developed world is struggling with the same set of problems, I do believe that the United States represents a very distinct outlier in terms of both the combination of measures that it has taken and the relative lack of success of those measures. And prominent among those are the kinds of demand-side controls that the Premier of British Whatever is, once again, advocating. But I don't think there is any use in arguing with folks like that.

William Tholl (Canadian Medical Association)

John, a question to you. There's been a number of visiting delegations going in and out of Ottawa over the last six months, a lot of action in Washington, but there's also a lot of action at the gubernatorial level in terms of different states taking different initiatives, some of which are very closely modelled on the Canadian system. What's your sense as to whether there is a consensus emerging, particularly at the gubernatorial level? That's point 1. Point 2 – Is there likely to be a bottom-up versus a top-down development of alternative ways of financing the American health care system?

John Iglehart

There is a lot of activity at the state level, but I don't look for an initiative at that level that over the future will be important in terms of shaping the system that the U.S. finally ends up with. I think one of the real obstacles there is that big business, which drives a lot of U.S. public policy, does not want to have to deal with 50 different health systems, and when you see more than a handful of states going down that road, then you'll see reactions from big business that will retard those kinds of initiatives. So I think you'll see, as you have already seen in several states – Massachusetts and Hawaii and maybe one or two others – some activity that's leading to universality, but in terms of a national trend, I certainly don't look for that.

Participant

Just one question for Bob. Aside from the effect on the Canadian public, it seems to me that there is a lot of energy being spent by folks like the ones in this room, by researchers, by people in the civil service, doing Canada-U.S. comparisons, responding to the kinds of things that are being put out in the press. Is there anything constructive, Bob, that you think can come – on the Canadian side – from attention to these ideas, the zombies and so on?

Robert Evans

Sure, in the sense of constructive that can come from it. I think one of the ironies that was implicit in John's remarks, though, was that he was suggesting that the most constructive results of the comparisons will come from the Americans learning from the Canadian experience. And I guess one way of reading my remarks would be a more pessimistic view that maybe we won't learn from our own experience. And that's consistent with the previous comment/question about cycling back to ruddy user fees. I think one of the things that can come was well illustrated by Mike Rachlis' book, and that's only the latest in a long series of things, that by examining the U.S. experience we can get a much broader view of what is possible. In patterns of medical care, the examples of control of hospital utilization that the Americans present are extremely important ones, have been recognized as such all over Europe as well as in Canada, and I think those are the things that we can learn from. What troubles me is that it is the people like the people in this room who do learn from them, and that there's very little that happens in terms of communicating that information to the general public, and that's why I think Mike Rachlis' book is important, because it empowers the politicians. It doesn't help if they know the right answers, if they're constrained by a public that thinks what they really want is more medical care.

Brian Copley (British Columbia Ministry of Health)

Both speakers mentioned Europe and looking at European experience. I was wondering if you could both comment, from your different perspectives – i.e., Canadian and U.S. – on the developments in Europe and whether there are some things there that we should be looking at very closely.

John Iglehart

I will limit my remarks to Germany, since that's the system I'm looking at at the moment, and I would say yes, indeed there are. The one thing that has fascinated me most about Germany in relation to physician fees is the way they have absolutely bound the relationship between volume and fees for the ambulatory care physician so that the pot of resources available for ambulatory fees is essentially fixed and physicians draw on it. Basically, they can provide as many services as they like, but as services increase the fees are proportionately reduced, because the total pie is fixed. So there is no direct control – or as in the U.S., voluntary exhortations – for the physicians to behave in a cost-effective manner. In Germany, it's strictly a mechanical act that takes place. You provide more services, then your per unit fee is reduced. And I think it's really rather an ingenious way of doing it.

Robert Evans

Yes, I would agree with that. Technically, it's not difficult to devise a way of doing the same thing within the Canadian system, but politically it's much more difficult because you'd run into the sense both from providers and from users and payers, "Why should we bother doing that?" I think the way in which the German financing system is structured makes it very clear to powerful groups in the society why this is a good idea. But I would underscore that there is no technical difficulty at all in building that kind of apparatus directly into the Canadian system.

What I would draw from some of the European experience is that every country in Europe – well, I'm not sure I would know every country, but virtually all – have at some time during the late 1970s or early 80s found some way of limiting the rate of growth of health expenditures. John emphasized sort of that the glass is half full, in that everybody is wrestling with the same problems, and that over some time period health expenditures have been expanding as a percentage of GDP or GNP. Nevertheless, if you look at each country individually, you find a period of rapid growth followed by a period of flattening, and in Germany it begins in 1975-76. In Canada it begins in 1971 and then we get the break in the early 1980s and then a reestablishment in 1982-3-4 and through to the present. In Sweden, and in Denmark as well, you actually get a substantial reduction in health care expenditures as a share of GDP. What I'm getting at is that while there are very different structures in each of those countries, some combination of political will and universal coverage, or almost universal coverage, enables you to put a cap on expenditures. Not perfectly, not without a lot of controversy, and in somewhat different ways, but everywhere but the U.S. it has been done in recent years. Whether those caps will stick and hang on, and what effects they have, are all, I think, matters for much more serious study.

One of the things also, though, I think – going in the other direction that one can draw from the European experience – is the way in which the old issues, just like our zombies, don't seem to go away. And so the struggle continues, partly in terms of old language, partly in terms of new language, and you get things like the British White Paper, which is partly fed by old ideologies, partly motivated by much more recent American (among others) thinking, which is really quite interesting, but if you ask the people involved who are going to turn their system upside down, or at least claim they are (they won't in the end because it is going to be much less of a revolution than initially planned), "How will you know whether you've won or not at the end of that overturning?", the answer is that they don't really know. There seems to be a lot of enthusiasm for reform, without nearly as careful thinking through as to how you'd evaluate the reform afterwards. And that seems to me to be a very general problem.

YANKEE INFLUENCES: PLAYING IN THE BUSH LEAGUES?

MANAGED CARE: WHAT IS IT, AND CAN IT BE APPLIED TO CANADA?*

Marianne Lamb
Raisa B. Deber
Department of Health Administration
University of Toronto

What is managed care? Increasing attention is being paid to what, if any, lessons can be learned from the alphabet soup of (largely American) organizations with such names as HMOs, PPOs, and IPAs, as well as from the new Canadian experiments with CHOs or OSIS.

This talk is based on a literature review and case study of the proposed Comprehensive Health Organization at The Toronto Hospital (Lamb et al, 1991). We will focus on the concept of managed care and offer suggestions on how it might be applied in the Canadian context.

It is clear from the literature that managed care means different things to different people. The term can be used as an umbrella one that covers both managed care approaches and managed care systems. A managed care approach involves application of a management policy or procedure that affects either the financing or delivery of a service to achieve a specific goal. For example, implementation of a case management system can be described as a managed care approach aimed at coordinating care or reducing length of stay in hospital.

The idea of a managed care system is that for a predetermined amount of money, a specific and comprehensive *range* of services (rather than *number* of services) will be provided as required and the delivery of these services will be organized, monitored, and controlled so as to meet established health care delivery goals. A managed care system thus combines the financing and delivery of comprehensive health care services for a defined group of individuals.

In other words, there are degrees of managed care, ranging from a few managed care approaches to highly structured managed care systems. The concept of managed care is therefore not confined to alternative delivery systems, although it is most frequently, if not always, more fully developed within such systems. This paper focuses primarily on managed care systems.

THE GOALS OF MANAGED CARE

The goals of a managed care system can be multiple and overlapping. The two most frequently mentioned are *cost containment,* either for the system as whole or for a single institution, and *quality of care,* which can include continuity of care, coordination of care, technical quality of care, prevention of illness and promotion of health, and a multidisciplinary team approach. Although these two general goals are not mutually exclusive, it is interesting to note that much of the literature in which the term managed care is used focuses on cost containment; in contrast, the literature on case management often has a quality of care focus.

THE ELEMENTS OF MANAGED CARE

All managed care approaches contain, either singly or in combination, three elements: formal agreements, risk assumption, and utilization management.

FORMAL AGREEMENTS

We consider formal agreements to include contract or salaried employment agreements between organizations and providers, risk contracts between two organizations, and agreements between consumers and health care delivery organizations. Formal agreements provide financial predictability, accountability, and the ability to plan, and establish a framework within which health care goals can be realized. In contrast, the traditional fee-for-service system is more open-ended in terms of services, costs, and practice behaviour.

Formal agreements are found within all systems of health care, but the specificity of an agreement and the extent to which it covers all parties indicate the extent to which health care is managed within that system. In a managed care system, the network of agreements constitutes vertical integration so that comprehensive services can be provided.

RISK ASSUMPTION

Medical care costs money. Who will pay for that care? The usual possibilities are patients, providers, and third party insurers.

Medical insurance systems are built on the assumption that the costs will be predictable and that fixed pre-payments can therefore be used to cover them. If the cost estimate proves incorrect, however, who will assume the financial risk to pay for the added care?

In the traditional fee-for-service system, most of that risk is assumed by the payers and insurers of health care, or by the patient (through deductibles and co-payments). A key feature of managed care is an assumption of risk by those who *deliver* health care. Patients are liable only for their pre-set fee, although some managed care systems also use deductibles, co-payments, and/or service limitation to shift at least a portion of the risk to clients. Risks may also be shifted to providers (e.g., through capitation arrangements or bonus arrangements). However, in the final analysis, the financial risk for additional care rests with the managed care system itself.

The challenge in risk sharing is to assume risk only to the degree to which it can be offset through management of care. The assumption of financial risk is presumed to encourage an organization to be as efficient as possible in meeting the goals of health care. Managed care systems therefore have the incentive, and perhaps the legitimacy, to monitor utilization and implement management strategies to identify and eliminate any utilization found to be inappropriate. Where such monitoring and control cannot take place, risk can be reduced by off-loading it to direct care providers who then have an incentive and the means to influence utilization.

UTILIZATION MANAGEMENT

Utilization is managed in order to achieve the goals of health care, meet the responsibilities set out in agreements, and minimize financial risks. The management strategies may be aimed at influencing the behaviour of either users or direct providers of the service.

Mechanisms to influence the use of services include incentives, deterrents, the organization of care delivery, rules or guidelines, and "softer" methods such as feedback and education.

One approach is case management, whereby the care of and utilization of services by an individual client are overseen and coordinated by one person. Another approach is the "gatekeeper" role of the primary physician, whereby a consumer's access to care is limited to a single point of entry and the gatekeeper authorizes all services. Other authorization procedures include preadmission certification before hospitalization and mandatory second opinions prior to surgery.

Both consumers and providers may be influenced to modify the utilization of services through the "softer" methods of information feedback, education, and incentives. HMOs frequently give physicians statistical reports on performance and utilization that allow comparisons with peers. One plan gives new mothers who are discharged within two days following a normal delivery a check for $75.00 and a home visit by a pediatric nurse practitioner.

MANAGED CARE: APPLICATIONS TO CANADA

How might an alternative care model that incorporates the concept of managed care be implemented in the Canadian health care system? Applications to Canada will be discussed in terms of the three elements of managed care outlined.

FORMAL AGREEMENTS

A managed care system involves agreements between payers and organizations, organizations and providers, and organizations and users.

Government-organization

Within Canada's universal system of health care, provincial governments are the payers, so agreements between government and organizations will have to address a number of issues.

1) Capital funding: In the past, governments, with the exception of Quebec, have been reluctant to invest in new organizational models.

2) Range of services: Existing formal agreements with regard to health care in Canada are those spelled out in federal and provincial health care legislation. Such legislation sets out the services for which citizens are eligible - essentially medical care and hospital care, with some variation in additional services from province to province. What is less clear is what additional services could be offered and how they could be financed. There is some uncertainty as to whether the government as payer could agree to benefits that go beyond those available to residents of the province who do not have access to the alternative model. If the government agrees to permit new organizations to manage their own finances and services, it is possible that savings generated by an organization could be used to enhance services to include dental or vision care or other uninsured services.

3) Rate setting: Currently, provincial governments pay for most medical care on a fee-for-service basis, although there is some experience with capitation payments. A major concern with managed care models is that they may enroll healthier individuals and yet be paid at rates more suitable for populations that have greater needs for health care.

A variety of risk adjustments to premiums based on age, sex, disease condition, and previous utilization have been suggested as ways to counter the effects of biased selection.

4) Marketing: For new organizations to become viable, they must be able to inform the public about their services and about the advantages of enrolling. Both tradition and the organizations responsible for the regulation of professions in Canada inhibit advertising of health care services, although this traditional stance is now in the process of change.

5) Professional regulation: To allow cost-effective use of multidisciplinary teams, professional regulations may require modification, particularly as they relate to scope of practice and supervision issues.

Organization-consumer

1) Lock-in: Agreements binding users to the new organization might be open to legal challenge; enrolled patients are not really "captive" and they can engage in out-of-plan use without financial penalty. Either policy changes will be required that permit lock-in of enrollees for a specified length of time, or alternative models will have to make extra efforts to maintain voluntary enrollment and minimize out-of-plan use.

2) Attractions: Not only is advertising restricted, but the advantages of enrolling are unclear. What would the new organization offer that is different from or better than what is currently available to individuals (universal, comprehensive, first-dollar coverage with free choice of provider)? Unless the provincial government allows the funds saved through efficiency to be used for the development of added benefits, attraction to the alternative model may have to be based on non-price benefits such as improvements in coordination of care, convenience, or other factors.

3) Out-of-plan use: In theory, there are two kinds of out-of-plan use in a managed care system: care that would otherwise have been provided within the managed care setting, and care that the gatekeepers would have decided was unnecessary. The cost implications vary accordingly; if the services can be provided less expensively in another setting, managed care systems might even benefit from encouraging selective out-of-plan use of necessary services. In contrast, out-of-plan use of unnecessary services is a pure add-on. In Canada, the balance between these two types of out-of-plan use can be crucial to the fiscal health of the organization.

Organization-provider

1) Reimbursement system: If formal agreements provide for an attractive income, some family practitioners may find the resulting freedom from volume-driven practice appealing, particularly if they wish to work with a multidisciplinary team. However, the issue of attracting physicians (especially specialists) may be a difficult one for new managed care organizations.

2) Professional autonomy: Although resistance to alternative payment mechanisms has diminished over the years, there remains potential for conflict between the physician's role as patient advocate and his/her responsibility to assist in cost reduction. Some physicians are uneasy and concerned about the growth of managed care, particularly about management by nonphysicians and how that might "interfere" with clinical judgment.

RISK ASSUMPTION

In the Canadian system of health care, almost all of the risk is assumed by governments who pay for insured health care. There is continuing reluctance to adopt policies whereby consumers would assume financial risk with regard to insured services.

Managed care systems offer the government the opportunity to off-load some risk to an organization. Rather than the government's trying to manage care directly, the incentive to manage is transferred to a health delivery organization. In turn, the organization may establish risk contracts with providers that encourage them to manage care or incorporate providers into the organization which itself implements utilization controls.

Although features of a managed care system may attract primary care physicians, the attractions for specialists are not as great. A new organization is not likely to provide much employment for specialists and there is apt to be greater difficulty in finding a range of specialists willing to assume risk through capitated contract arrangements. A health care delivery organization would have to be quite large before market share provided it with enough leverage to negotiate agreements with specialists.

UTILIZATION MANAGEMENT

In theory, managed care systems may have an incentive to under-service. The relative emphasis on the goals of quality and cost containment is key.

If utilization management means improving continuity of care – e.g., use of case managers – it is likely to be supported by clinicians. In contrast, if the goal is cost containment – with the incentive to deny potentially useful care – it is likely to meet deserved opposition from both providers and the general public.

Health care personnel in Canada have limited experience with the use of utilization control measures although there are some examples, such as Vi-care in Victoria, British Columbia. There may be considerable opposition to utilization review, restrictions on referrals or use of diagnostic facilities, or any other organizational measures perceived to erode the autonomy of the physician or interfere with clinical decisions. Nonetheless, it is recognized that such measures can improve quality (as well as efficiency) of care, and the trend towards instituting them in many hospitals is likely to continue.

Providers are more likely to accept control mechanisms if they are participating in management decisions and if the control mechanisms are viewed as justified and credible. More sophisticated information systems will be necessary to facilitate decision-making and monitor quality of care. Some managed care organizations have been able to accommodate both management and clinical perspectives, and this seems to be a necessary ingredient for organizations to succeed. There will be a need for more sophisticated communication systems.

In sum, alternative models that begin to implement utilization management will have to ensure that health care professionals have input into decision-making. Communication with all providers associated with the organization will have to convey the rationale for the management so that the approaches are not perceived as intrusions on clinical care decisions. Quality assurance mechanisms will be needed to ensure that utilization management does not adversely affect quality of care.

CONCLUSION

Applications of managed care systems to Canada will have to take specific features of Canadian health care into consideration. In particular, attention will have to be given to how to attract and retain patients and how to ensure that health professionals participate in management decisions. Incentives rather than deterrents, as well as managed care approaches that focus on quality of care rather than only cost containment, will be necessary.

NOTE

* edited transcript of talk by Marianne Lamb

ACKNOWLEDGEMENTS

We thank NHRDP for funding this study through the Healthcare in Transition competition (6606-4009-HT) and are grateful to the many individuals at The Toronto Hospital who cooperated in the research and to our co-investigators C. David Naylor and J.E.F. Hastings. A more detailed report of the study and an annotated bibliography on managed care are given in:
Lamb M, Deber RB, Naylor CD, Hastings JEF: *Managed Care in Canada: The Toronto Hospital's Proposed Comprehensive Health Organization*. Ottawa: Canadian Hospital Association, 1991.

THE AMERICAN EXPERIENCE WITH A PROSPECTIVE PAYMENT SYSTEM: SOME LESSONS FOR CANADA

Lee Soderstrom
Department of Economics
McGill University

Since late 1983 the United States has used its Prospective Payment System (PPS) to reimburse hospitals for inpatient services provided to Medicare patients. PPS is best known through its Diagnostic Related Groups (DRGs) patient classification system. Many American health planners seem pleased with PPS, which has reduced health costs for people 65 and over.

This review of the American experience with PPS was undertaken to determine whether a PPS-type system would improve the performance of Canadian hospitals. A Canadian version seems possible. Technically it is feasible, though it would apply to all patients, not just to patients 65 and over, as in the U.S. It is also consistent with the principles underlying our public financing programs.

A PPS-type reimbursement system provides hospitals with financial incentives to control their costs. This is the principal attraction of such a system for health planners. However, the financial incentives are more complicated than most analyses of PPS suggest. The U.S. experience also indicates that there is much more to such a system.

The next section of this paper describes the key elements of PPS. The financial incentives are then clarified. The third section summarizes the available evidence regarding the utilization, cost, and health effects of PPS. Finally, the fourth section considers the impact of a PPS-type system on a variety of problems currently affecting Canada's hospitals. A key conclusion is that each province should establish an advisory council on hospital services patterned after the Americans' Prospective Payment Advisory Commission.

PPS: THREE KEY ELEMENTS

Only a simplified view of the three key elements of PPS is presented here. Russell (1989) and Vladeck (1984) provide more detailed descriptions. PPS was introduced October 1, 1983, the start of Medicare's 1984 fiscal year. It covers only the operating costs for inpatient hospital services for Medicare beneficiaries, essentially Americans 65+. PPS does not cover services in psychiatric, rehabilitation, or long-term care hospitals, or services provided in psychiatric or rehabilitation units in acute care hospitals. Nor does PPS pay the capital cost of new hospital equipment or the salaries of interns and residents.

ELEMENT #1: PAYMENT FORMULA

For reimbursement purposes patients are grouped according to their health conditions, using the DRG classification system. Given the patient's age, the principal diagnosis and surgical procedure (if any), and any secondary diagnoses and/or procedures, the patient is assigned to one of the 477 DRGs. Each DRG includes health problems that are clinically similar and whose case management costs are supposed to be similar (Fetter et al, 1980; Vladeck, 1984). Associated with each DRG is a "Relative Weight", which indicates the average cost of treating patients in the DRG relative to the average cost of treating all Medicare patients (Coffey and Goldfarb, 1986; Cotterill et al, 1986; Lave, 1985).

To determine the payment to a hospital for a patient, the Relative Weight for the patient's DRG is multiplied by the hospital's "Standardized Payment", a fixed amount of money applicable to all the hospital's Medicare cases, whatever their DRG. One can think of the Relative Weights and the Standardized Payment as being fixed at the start of each fiscal year and the same Weights and Payment as applying to hospitals across the U.S. Thus, for each Medicare case a hospital receives a predetermined amount of money, the amount depending on the patient's health problem[1]. Then, if the hospital's costs for a case exceed the PPS payment, the hospital itself must make up the deficit. If its costs are less than the payment, the hospital may keep the surplus.

Although this description of the payment formula is adequate for this review of PPS, the actual formula is more complicated. The Standardized Payment is not the same for all hospitals. It is higher for urban than for rural hospitals, and for hospitals in high wage areas than for those in low wage areas. In addition, there are three special adjustments. Extra "Outlier Payments" are made for a limited number of cases with unusually long hospital stays or high costs. Hospitals serving a relatively large proportion of low income patients receive an extra "Disproportionate Share Adjustment". Finally, "Indirect Teaching Payments" provide extra payments to teaching hospitals, which have higher (case-mix adjusted) costs than nonteaching hospitals.

ELEMENT #2: DETERMINATION OF THE STANDARDIZED PAYMENT

The Standardized Payment is determined politically. The law that established PPS stipulated that the Standardized Payment for 1984fy had to equal an estimate of the national average cost per case for Medicare patients in 1983 plus a prescribed growth factor. Subsequently, periodic increases – called "Update Factors" – have been approved by Congress and the administration. Given that PPS was introduced to reduce Medicare hospital cost increases, the Update Factors have been small, ranging between 0.2% in 1986fy and 4.72% in 1990fy (Russell, 1989).

This Update Factor is not determined by cost increases. There is no formula linking it either to cost increases expected during the forthcoming year or to increases actually realized during the preceding several years. Therefore, the Standardized Payment is not the average cost of treating Medicare patients; it is simply the payment the government is willing to make for the average patient.

While deliberating about the next Update Factor, Congress takes advice from many sources. One is the Health Care Financing Administration (HCFA), the federal agency responsible for administering the Medicare program. Another important source of information has been the Prospective Payment Assessment Commission (ProPAC), which provides advice to both the Congress and the Secretary of Health and Human Services on PPS-related matters. The Commission itself is composed of part-time commissioners who are experts in health economics, hospital finance, or health care.

Each year ProPAC recommends a specific numerical value for the next year's Update Factor. When preparing its recommendation, it draws on the work of its small staff as well as contract and other outside researchers. In its recommendation, ProPAC makes provision for cost increases expected in the next year because of increases in the prices of hospitals' labour and nonlabour inputs. It also makes provision for the change in the Standardized Payment it believes warranted by changes in hospital productivity, advances in technology, real changes in the severity of patients' health problems, quality of care, and long-term cost effectiveness of hospital services (ProPAC, 1990a).

ELEMENT #3: UTILIZATION REVIEW

The third element of PPS is utilization review, primarily by Peer Review Organizations (PROs). When PPS was established, there was concern that the financial incentives would result in unnecessary admissions, premature discharges, excessive transfers to other hospitals, and undesirable curtailing of services. Consequently PROs were established and mandated to monitor utilization. Most are sponsored by state medical societies and are responsible for utilization review for an entire state. They operate under contract to HCFA.

Since the beginning of PPS, the PROs have focused on reducing admissions. They review a sample of discharge records to determine the need for the admissions and encourage hospitals to develop lower cost ambulatory services to replace inpatient care. They also review all readmissions, inter-hospital transfers, and cases involving Outlier Payments. In addition, the PROs check for inaccuracies in hospitals' diagnostic coding. More recently, HCFA has required them to review a sample of cases each year for indications of poor quality care.

ProPAC is also involved in utilization review, though it has only an advisory role. It maintains an ongoing review of the impact of PPS on the utilization of services by Medicare beneficiaries, on the quality of care provided them, and on hospitals' financial situation. Each year its staff and contract researchers prepare analyses of particular issues, and the results are published in its discussion paper series. It also publishes a comprehensive annual evaluation of PPS (ProPAC, 1990b).

MACRO AND MICRO FINANCIAL INCENTIVES OF PPS

PPS, a form of case-based reimbursement, creates both macro and micro financial incentives for a hospital. Although no distinction is made between them in most discussions of PPS, treating these two types of incentives separately facilitates understanding the American hospitals' reactions to PPS and the impact of a PPS-type system in Canada[2].

The macro incentive encourages hospitals to curtail their costs. It stems from two features of PPS. First, the hospital must fund any Medicare deficit and can retain any Medicare surplus. Second, a hospital's total PPS revenues are largely beyond its control. Given its case-mix and admissions[3], a hospital's total PPS revenue is determined by its Standardized Payment, which is set in Washington. The higher this payment, the higher the hospital's payments for each case, and in turn the higher its PPS revenue.

If a hospital's total cost for treating Medicare inpatients exceeds its total PPS revenue, the hospital must either eliminate the deficit or finance it from other sources of revenue. The hospital's ability and desire to subsidize Medicare services are limited, so if the anticipated deficit is "large", the hospital must reduce it. To do this, the hospital must curtail its Medicare costs; its PPS revenues are fixed. Costs must be curtailed wherever possible, by producing specific services more efficiently, reducing the clinical services provided patients, and discharging patients sooner. The deficit will be reduced by cutbacks affecting patients in any DRG, not just those in DRGs for which the hospital's costs per case exceed its PPS payments. One less dollar spent on any Medicare patient will reduce the Medicare deficit. Moreover, the steps taken to curtail Medicare costs can also reduce non-Medicare costs; a policy encouraging shorter hospital stays can affect Medicare and non-Medicare patients alike.

On the other hand, if the hospital's PPS revenues exceed its Medicare costs, it can retain the surplus. This too provides the hospital with an incentive to curtail its costs. PPS revenues being fixed, it can increase its surplus only by reducing its costs, again wherever possible. However, the threat of a Medicare deficit may spur greater cost constraint than the possibility of gaining a surplus. The financial stability of the hospital is in greater danger, and an inefficient hospital has more scope for cutbacks than an efficient one.

The micro incentives result from having predetermined case-based payments. A hospital can compare the PPS payment for a DRG with its costs for Medicare patients in that DRG. This may affect the hospital's admission decisions. If it earns a surplus on patients in a DRG, the hospital would gain financially by admitting more of them. If the hospital loses money, it would gain financially by not admitting patients in that DRG. Of course, admission decisions reflect more than financial considerations, so the hospital may admit patients on whom it loses money.

The micro incentives may also affect services provided patients. In theory, a hospital's decisions about the services it provides patients in a particular DRG should not depend directly on whether it makes or loses money on them. A hospital gains financially from cutbacks for any DRG[4].

As a practical matter, however, when searching for ways to reduce costs, a hospital may identify the DRGs for which it is losing money and then make a special effort to curtail services provided patients in such DRGs.

According to this analysis, evidence that PPS reduced hospital costs does not demonstrate that case-based payment was the active ingredient. The cost reduction may be caused by the macro incentive, which does not require such payments. It requires only that total revenues be predetermined, and this is possible with other reimbursement plans, including Canada's negotiated budget system. Case-based payments are required only for the micro incentives. To show that such payments are important, evidence is required that admission or case management decisions for patients in specific DRGs were influenced by the difference between the PPS payment for the DRGs and hospitals' costs of treating these patients.

This analysis also implies that the importance of the macro and micro incentives depends on the size of the Standardized Payment. The smaller this payment, the smaller will be the hospital's PPS revenue and the larger any Medicare deficit. Therefore, the smaller the Standardized Payment, the larger the number of hospitals threatened with large deficits unless they reduce their costs. Similarly, the smaller this payment, the smaller the PPS payment for any particular DRG relative to the hospital's costs, and the greater the hospital's financial incentive to avoid admitting patients in that DRG and to curtail services for them. Thus, the determination of the Standardized Payment is an important element of a PPS-type system.

THE EFFECTS OF PPS

The rapidly growing literature on the effects of PPS is informative, though evaluating PPS has proved difficult. Given the information available, most analyses involve a comparison of the values of some performance indicators for the PPS period with their values for the pre-PPS period. But the differences observed may not be caused just by PPS. In the mid-1980s other changes were being made in the structure of the Medicare program (e.g., TEFRA cost-constraints in 1983fy and expanded home care benefits in 1981). There were major technological changes (e.g., ambulatory lens extractions). Some state governments were taking steps to reduce the hospital costs of their Medicaid programs, and employers were taking steps to reduce their health insurance costs.

Many of the studies rely on data for the first years of PPS. But these were transition years. Hospitals were learning about the revenue constraints of PPS and introducing better information systems to make better cost calculations. Utilization review was new, and structural details of the program were also changing[5].

UTILIZATION EFFECTS

PPS is associated with a significant reduction in the use of inpatient hospital services. There is considerable evidence of reduced admissions (Feder et al, 1987; ProPAC 1990a; Russell, 1989); reduced lengths of stay (DesHarnais et al, 1987a, 1987b; Feder et al, 1987; Fitzgerald et al, 1987, 1988; Morrisey et al, 1988; ProPAC, 1990a; Smith and Pickard, 1986; Weinberger et al, 1988); and fewer services per case (DesHarnais et al, 1987; Fitzgerald et al, 1986, 1988; Long et al, 1987; Sloan et al, 1988; Weinberger et al, 1988). The admissions rate for people 65+ rose 4.8% per year between 1978 and 1983, fell -2.9% per year during the first 3 years of PPS, and then rose again 1.2% per year between 1987 and 1989 (ProPAC, 1990b). There does not appear to have been a significant jump in hospital readmissions following the introduction of PPS (Russell, 1989). However, interhospital transfers have increased (ProPAC, 1990b; Russell, 1989). Over half the decline is caused by the shift of lens extraction from an inpatient to an outpatient procedure (Russell, 1989; Schramm and Gabel, 1988).

There are several reasons for this admissions decline. In part, as the shift in location of lens extractions suggests, it is the result of new knowledge whose application would have occurred without PPS, though the macro incentive of PPS may have hastened its diffusion. In addition, PPS's utilization review has been important (Russell, 1989); the PROs have been active and their main task has been to reduce admissions.

Lengths of stay also apparently declined, though this effect is more difficult to see than the decrease in admissions. Hospital stays for people 65+ fell in 1984 and 1985. But they fell throughout the 1970s and early 1980s. Since 1985 the average length of stay has increased slightly (Newhouse and Byrne, 1988; ProPAC, 1990b). It is reasonable, however, that there was an effect. The decline in 1984 was far larger than in any preceding year. Survey data also indicate that hospital administrators were encouraging physicians to discharge their patients earlier (Russell, 1989).

The decline in inpatient hospital services has been accompanied by an increase in the use of other health services. Greater use is now made of hospital outpatient services (ProPAC, 1990b; Weinberger et al, 1988). Hospitals have considerable incentive under PPS to do this. Greater use of these services is one way to reduce inpatient costs. Hospitals also receive cost-based reimbursement from Medicare for most outpatient services, which are outside the domain of PPS. If an outpatient test is done prior to an admission, the hospital can receive reimbursement for the outpatient test plus the PPS payment for the admission.

In addition, more patients are now discharged to home care programs (DesHarnais et al, 1987b; Morrisey et al, 1988; ProPAC, 1990b; Russell, 1989) and to skilled nursing facilities (DesHarnais et al, 1987a; Fitzgerald et al 1987, 1988; Morrisey et al, 1988; Sager et al, 1987, 1989). Although not all researchers agree, it appears that the proportion of the patients discharged to nursing homes who are seriously ill has increased (Lyles, 1986; Russell, 1989; Sager et al, 1989).

There has also been a change in the composition of physician services. The decline in these services for hospital inpatients has been offset by an increase in physician services for hospital outpatients. The fraction of total Medicare payments going to physicians for office visits and other services, however, remained unchanged between 1982 and 1986 (Fisher, 1987, 1988). Holahan et al (1990) found that PPS resulted in a small increase in Medicare spending on physician services. The apparent substantial decline in inpatient hospital services has therefore not resulted in any decrease in total payments to physicians.

Several aspects of the utilization effects have been of particular concern. Given the financial incentives, there has been concern that severely ill people who require relatively costly care may now have trouble gaining access to hospital services. The existing empirical evidence does not indicate whether this has in fact occurred.

Another concern relates to rural hospitals, many of which have been pressed financially by PPS. For example, in 1988, when urban hospitals had PPS operating costs 2.6% less than their PPS revenue, rural hospitals had PPS costs 2.3% higher than their PPS revenue. The probability of a rural hospital's closing has also been much higher (ProPAC, 1990b).

Consequently, there has been considerable concern that access to hospital services has become more difficult for Medicare beneficiaries in rural areas. Initial research, however, suggests that this has not happened (ProPAC, 1990b).

COST OF HOSPITAL SERVICES

The cost effects – a central issue in discussions of PPS – can be viewed on different levels. The effect on hospital costs indicates the impact of PPS on hospital behavior. The effect on Medicare program costs indicates the impact on government spending. The impact on total health costs indicates the effect on social costs. Available evidence suggests that at least Medicare program costs and social costs have been reduced by PPS.

When PPS was first introduced, it apparently did slow hospital cost increases (Feder et al, 1987; Hadley and Swartz, 1989; Hadley et al, 1989; Sheingold, 1989; Zwanziger and Melnick, 1988). There is evidence of such PPS effects even after controlling for other sources of pressure on hospitals to control their costs (Hadley and Swartz, 1989; Zwanziger and Melnick, 1988). For example, Feder et al (1987) compare a sample of hospitals covered by PPS in 1984fy with a sample not covered that year[6]. Between 1982fy and 1984fy the PPS hospitals had·a smaller change in admissions (-0.4% vs. 3.4%) and a smaller increase in inpatient costs per Medicare patient (7.6% vs. 18.5%). Moreover, the increase in Medicare outpatient costs was slightly lower for the PPS hospitals, implying that the smaller increase in inpatient costs for those hospitals was not offset by a larger increase in their outpatient costs.

However, these cost analyses relate only to the initial PPS effect. ProPAC (1990b) reports that the increase in the cost per Medicare case was substantially lower in the first year than in subsequent years[7]. In 1984fy it increased only 2.1%, while in the next four years the annual rate of increase was 10.0%. During the first five years of PPS, this cost per case increased 8.4% per year. At the same time, prices of hospital inputs increased 4.1% per year, so hospital costs per Medicare case increased about 4.3% per year in real terms. If – as ProPAC has assumed – real case severity increased 1.5% annually, then real costs per case (severity adjusted) still increased 2.8% per year during the first five years of PPS. ProPAC's data do not indicate whether this is lower than the real rate of increase in pre-PPS years. But from a Canadian perspective 2.8% does not represent much hospital cost constraint! It would be a large increase in Canada. It also seems large because hospital costs in the U.S. were already high relative to those in Canada (Evans, 1988; Newhouse et al, 1988).

These cost increases are understandable, because hospitals were actually under little financial pressure to curtail spending during the first five years of PPS. In 1984fy PPS payments per Medicare case were 18.9% higher than they had been the previous year (ProPAC, 1990b). Costs per case being only 2.1% higher, hospitals' PPS operating margins increased substantially. While Medicare operating costs were 9.8% less than PPS payments in 1983fy, they were 14.5% less in 1984fy. In the second year, costs per case increased 10.4% and PPS payments per case 10.3%, so PPS operating margins remained high. But these margins were much higher than PPS planners had intended them to be, so the government approved only small Update Factors for the following years (Russell, 1989; Sheingold, 1989). The effect of these small Update Factors was partially offset by other program changes and "DRG creep".

Nevertheless, the average PPS payment per case increased 4.6% per year between 1985fy and 1988fy, while average cost per case increased 9.8% annually. Thus, by 1988fy the aggregate PPS operating margin had fallen to only 2.6%, and ProPAC estimates this margin will be negative in 1990 (ProPAC, 1990b). Moreover, in 1988fy Medicare costs exceeded PPS revenues at 51.2% of the hospitals, up considerably from 18.3% of the hospitals in 1984fy.

The idea that hospitals' willingness to reduce their costs is directly tied to their operating margins has been corroborated by several researchers using data for large samples of hospitals (Feder et al, 1987; Hadley et al, 1989; Sheingold, 1989). They have found a significant negative relation between the size of hospitals' deficits and the size of their cost increases. During each of the first several years of PPS, hospitals with large negative PPS margins in the preceding year had the smallest cost increases. Hospitals with large positive margins had the largest cost increases.

Here is evidence that hospitals do respond to the macro incentive of PPS. But evidence regarding the importance of the micro incentives has not yet appeared. Although most discussions of the financial incentives of PPS focus on the effects of having predetermined case-based payments, the impact of such payments on hospital costs has not yet been determined.

Although these studies indicate that individual hospitals have curtailed their costs when squeezed by PPS, the aggregate data for the first five years show little sign of constraint. Apparently most hospitals were able to sustain significant nominal and real cost increases because of their sizable operating margins. This indicates the importance of the size of the Standardized Payments. Initially the PPS payments were large relative to costs. But by limiting the increases in Standardized Payments in subsequent years, the government has been able to squeeze more and more hospitals' operating margins. Hospitals are now under much more financial pressure to curtail their costs than when PPS started. This increased pressure has little to do with fixed, case-based payments, however. It is the consequence of small increases in the Standardized Payments, resulting in small increases in government funding for hospital services. As Vladeck (1988) observes,

> Hospital administrators have increasingly come to understand that the most important aspect of any payment system is not its unit of payment (e.g., days or DRG) or its formulas, but the amount of money it contains. Although the mechanics of the system have not materially changed, PPS was far more popular in the hospital community in 1984 and 1985, when it was paying too much, than it has been since, as the real level of payments has declined.

Russell (1989) argues that PPS has significantly reduced the rate of increase in the federal government's Medicare costs for inpatient services. She reports that the Trustees of the Hospital Insurance Trust Fund have substantially reduced their estimate of program costs for 1990 after reviewing the first year's experience with PPS. However, her evidence is based on changes in expected program costs in 1990, not changes in actual costs, and the reliability of the Trustee's program cost projections is unclear. Nevertheless, her conclusion seems reasonable. As late as early 1984 the Trustees could not have anticipated the decline in admissions in 1984 and 1985, or the small increases in the Standardized Payments in the late 1980s. Note, however, that the limited growth in program costs has not been matched by limited growth in hospital costs per case. Medicare spending has been curtailed in part by reducing admissions, but largely by eliminating hospitals' Medicare surpluses.

Russell also argues that the reduction in Medicare spending on inpatient services has not been offset by increased spending on other services. This suggests that social spending on health services for people 65+ has been reduced by PPS. According to her analysis, the increase in Medicare spending for hospital outpatient services, physician services, etc. was much smaller than the decrease in spending for inpatient hospital services. Russell also reports that the increase in user charges paid by Medicare beneficiaries was not significant. However, her data apparently relate only to user charges for Medicare covered services; data on total user charges for nursing home services, most of which are not covered by Medicare, are not available. Finally, she finds little evidence of cost-shifting to other users of hospital services. In fact, both Russell and Sloan et al (1988) suggest that PPS has reduced hospitals' non-Medicare costs; this is the expected effect of the macro incentive.

HEALTH EFFECTS

The available evidence presents mixed signals regarding the health effects of PPS. For some aggregate measures, there is no evidence indicating negative effects. There was no apparent rise in the incidence of selected acute conditions, restricted-activity days, or bed-disability days among the population 65+ between 1982 and 1987 (ProPAC, 1989b). Data on the utilization of hospital services by various socio-demographic groups and for selected health conditions do not suggest widespread access problems (ProPAC, 1989b, 1990b). Mortality rates seem unaffected (Russell, 1989). Lindberg et al (1989) report increased mortality in the Minneapolis area, but the increases they describe started at least one year before PPS.

Nevertheless, there has been concern that important medical services have been sacrificed to shorten hospital stays and that nursing home and home care services are imperfect substitutes for hospital services eliminated. There is concern about the availability of nursing home and home care services, the financial problems confronting their potential users, and the quality of care provided (Institute of Medicine, 1986; Sager et al, 1989; Vladeck, 1988). For example, while Medicare finances hospital services, it provides very little coverage for nursing home care. Most patients must pay their nursing home costs from their own pockets, impoverish themselves to qualify for Medicaid coverage, or forego nursing home services.

The results of two related studies by Fitzgerald et al (1987, 1988) give credence to these concerns. These researchers compared PPS and pre-PPS cohorts of hip fracture patients. The PPS patients had shorter hospital stays, received less physiotherapy while hospitalized, and had a much higher probability of being discharged to a nursing home. They were also less ambulatory when discharged. Most importantly, the proportion of PPS patients who remained bed-ridden in a nursing home six or 12 months after their hospital discharge was dramatically higher.

Weinberger et al (1988) compared small pre-PPS and PPS cohorts of noninsulin-dependent diabetes patients hospitalized for glycemic control. They too found that the post-PPS patients had shorter hospital stays and less access to various inpatient services, including training in proper dietary practices – training which is an important element of glycemic control. During the year following hospital discharge, the PPS patients had significantly more outpatient visits and poorer glycemic control.

These results relate to case management practices for only two health conditions at three Indiana hospitals. It remains to be seen whether researchers elsewhere will find similar results using data for other hospitals and other health conditions. Nevertheless, these are troubling results. These are the only published case studies, and they all indicate negative health effects. The picture of hospital behavior is also disturbing. The hospitals involved, apparently seeking to reduce their Medicare costs, reduced important services. These are not marginal services like an extra day of bed rest or the infamous sixth stool guaiac of Neuhauser and Lewicki (1975). Moreover, they did not assure that the patients received appropriate substitutes elsewhere. Fortunately, such behavior is not an inevitable consequence of PPS. If changes in hospital case management practices are properly planned, such negative effects need not occur; adequate physiotherapy services and dietary training could have been arranged.

SOME IMPLICATIONS FOR CANADA

It is technically feasible for the provinces to replace their current negotiated budget system (NBS) with a PPS-type system (PPS*). There would be differences between the American and Canadian versions. PPS* would apply to all admissions. However, the many chronic care patients in the acute care hospitals would probably be excluded from PPS*.

Whether the DRG classification system or some other one were used, it should be based on Canadian data. The American DRGs and their relative weights reflect American hospital utilization patterns, and Canadian patterns are different from them (Newhouse et al, 1988; Anderson et al, 1989). However, though each province would operate its own PPS*, it is not clear whether there is sufficient inter-provincial variation in hospital use that each province would need its own distinct classification system. If that were necessary, the cost of PPS* would be greatly increased.

There could also be increased use of outpatient hospital services, nursing home services, home care programs, etc. The supply of these services would need to be increased. Who would do that? Who would pay for them? Outpatient hospital services are publicly financed, but not all home care programs are.

PPS* is technically feasible and compatible with the principles that underlie our public programs. But would it improve the performance of a province's health system? Would any favorable effects justify the substantial costs for organizing and operating such a reimbursement process? To facilitate discussion of these questions, the impact of PPS* on some current problems with NBS is discussed.

PROVINCIAL FUNDING FOR HOSPITAL SERVICES

A key current problem is determining total provincial spending for hospital services. Certainly there continues to be much debate each year over the adequacy of provincial spending. Undoubtedly some of the ruckus stems from political maneuvering (Evans et al, 1989). But this does not necessarily imply that provincial spending is appropriate. PPS* would not necessarily change this situation. Provincial spending with PPS* would continue to be determined politically. The provincial governments would set their Standardized Payments[8]. The level of funding would continue to depend on what these governments thought was appropriate, given such considerations as their fiscal positions, their nonhospital spending priorities, the prices of hospital inputs, patient case-mix, and their perceptions of hospital productivity and the social value of new services.

Possibly, provincial governments might make different spending decisions with PPS*. If PPS* included an agency like ProPAC, its recommendations could result in different decisions. Governments, providers, and the public would have better information with which to assess the need for additional spending. Of course, Canadian ProPACs could be introduced independently of the other parts of PPS*. If they were the source of any positive effects of PPS*, their benefits could be obtained simply by adding these advisory commissions to the present provincial health systems.

In addition, if the financial incentives of PPS* did improve hospital efficiency, governments might make different decisions. For example, if Quebec hospital efficiency were improved, the Quebec government might be more receptive to hospital requests for additional funding. It would be harder for it to argue that the hospitals should make better use of available resources, and it might believe that an additional $50 million would yield greater social benefits in such circumstances than it would at present.

However, there is nothing about PPS* which assures how governments would react if hospital efficiency improved. If Quebec hospitals improved their efficiency, the government might capture that "extra" savings by approving an Update Factor well below the average rate of increase in hospital input prices. And when the hospitals requested more funding for new services, the government might continue to argue that it could not afford more hospital services.

PPS* would open up new opportunities to circumvent provincial spending constraints. Although government would set the Standardized Payments, public spending would also depend on hospital case-mix and admissions. Given a fixed Standardized Payment, a hospital could generate more revenue by describing its patients differently, resulting in their being classified in DRGs with higher relative weights. This "DRG creep" has occurred in the U.S., though it has not been a major problem (Hsia et al, 1988; ProPAC, 1990b; Sheingold, 1986; Simborg, 1981; Steinwald and Dummit, 1989)[9]. In addition, it is financially attractive to admit more patients whose PPS* payments exceed the hospital's added costs.

However, hospitals' ability to engage in such practices requires government acquiescence. A government can compensate for DRG creep by granting smaller annual Update Factors. It can limit both DRG creep and extra admissions with utilization review. The Americans have done both. Thus, the evolution of public spending on hospital services would remain in the political domain with PPS*.

HOSPITAL EFFICIENCY

A standard argument for PPS* is that it would provide hospitals with a financial incentive to improve their efficiency. Although the American evidence suggests that a PPS-type system can lower costs, this experience also indicates that even this result is not automatic. It requires that government squeeze hospitals by constraining their Standardized Payments. The provincial governments, of course, long ago realized that they could constrain hospital costs by squeezing hospital budgets. Moreover, even if PPS has improved American hospitals' efficiency, it is questionable whether the incentives of PPS* would generally improve our hospitals' efficiency.

One reason is that the introduction of PPS represented a much greater change in financial incentives for American hospitals than would the introduction of PPS* for Canadian hospitals. PPS replaced cost-based reimbursement, which provided little incentive to be concerned about either productivity or ineffective services. PPS* would replace NBS, which already provides a financial incentive to be efficient. Indeed, the incentives of NBS are very similar to the macro incentive of PPS*. Both confront hospitals with fixed revenues, and both require them to fund any deficits and allow them to retain any surpluses. Thus to the extent that government budgetary constraints and the macro incentive are the active ingredients in PPS, PPS* would change very little.

However, the micro incentives of PPS* do not exist with NBS, though the importance of these micro incentives in the U.S. is still unclear. PPS* would provide a greater financial incentive to admit some patients. If the PPS* payment for a particular health condition exceeded the hospital's treatment costs for such patients, the hospital would gain financially by admitting more of these patients. With NBS, however, there is no such gain; more admissions only increase costs, there being no revenue increase[10]. But the desirability of encouraging hospitals to admit more patients is questionable. Canadian admissions are apparently not systematically lower than those in the U.S. (Anderson et al, 1989). Utilization review was made an integral part of PPS because it was feared that the financial incentives otherwise would result in excessive admissions.

Both PPS* and NBS provide a financial reward for keeping patients' hospital stays short, though the force of this incentive is greater with the former. With either scheme an additional day increases costs, but not revenues. With NBS, however, a hospital has some incentive to allow patients to stay an extra day or two to avoid some costly new admissions. The cost of the work-up and treatment for a new admission with a four-day length of stay often exceeds the cost of keeping four post-treatment patients in the hospital an extra day. With PPS*, the incentive to do this is reduced; as long as the new admission added more to a hospital's revenues than to its costs, the hospital would gain financially by discharging the four convalescing patients one day earlier in order to facilitate that new admission.

This difference between PPS* and NBS is important because lengths of stay in Canadian hospitals are relatively long, at least by American standards (Anderson et al, 1989; Newhouse et al, 1988). PPS* could affect health costs if it lowered hospital stays significantly. However, predicting its effect on stays is difficult. It depends, in part, on the reason for these long stays. If they result largely from the financial incentives of NBS, PPS* could reduce hospital stays. If they result from long-stay chronic care patients, the effect of PPS* could be limited, because such patients would probably be exempted from PPS*. In addition, the effect of PPS* on hospital stays for chronic and nonchronic care patients depends on the availability of alternatives for hospital services. The reduction of hospital stays in the U.S. has been facilitated by an increase in access to nursing home and home care programs. It is not clear, however, that current providers of these services in Canada could handle many more patients. Moreover, transferring patients to nursing homes and home care programs might yield little savings in overall health care costs (Hochstein, 1984; Soderstrom, 1987).

These financial incentives could also cause negative health effects. There would be a micro incentive to avoid admissions that added more to costs than to revenue; a hospital could lose money on severely ill patients with above average treatment costs. The macro incentive to reduce lengths of stay and inpatient services per case could also harm patients' health.

The limited American evidence gives some credence to at least the latter concern. But PPS* could have different health effects from PPS. The performance of the nursing home and home care sectors may be different in Canada; the negative effects found in the American case studies might be avoided through better planning. Moreover, as just noted, the change in financial incentives would be less dramatic here; PPS* would replace NBS, which already provides some incentive to avoid costly admissions and curtail services for admitted patients. Of course, Canada's budget constraints may have caused significant negative effects which have gone unrecognized because Canadian researchers have not looked for them[11]. On the other hand, the potential for problems is greater here, the Canadian average length of stay being so much longer.

There is a second reason a PPS-type system might improve the efficiency of American, but not Canadian, hospitals: the problems of American and Canadian hospitals are different. Canadian hospitals, which have been subject to budget constraints since the 1970s, already spend less per case than their American counterparts (Evans, 1988; Newhouse et al, 1988). Consequently, American hospitals have greater scope to reduce costs. Canadian hospitals should already be doing their laundry efficiently, and they should have made the easy cutbacks in hospital services.

Now the need is to curtail any service of low value (i.e., a service that is ineffective or for which the social value of the positive health effects is less than the cost of the service).

PPS* is not well-suited for this complicated problem because it provides the hospital with distracting information. Consider the decision to admit a patient. This person should be admitted if the social value of the hospital services exceeds the cost of providing them. The micro incentives of PPS* focus the hospital's attention on the difference between the PPS* payment for the patient's DRG and its cost for caring for this patient. But the PPS* payment is not a measure of the social value of the admission. It is an odd construct, obtained by multiplying a measure of the relative cost of treating people in the DRG and the hospital's Standardized Payment. The social value of the admission could be higher or lower than the PPS* payment. Suppose it is much lower than both this payment and the hospital's cost of treating the patient. In this case, the person should not be admitted. But if the PPS* payment exceeded the hospital's cost for the case, the hospital would have a financial incentive to admit the patient. PPS* would provide the hospital with an incorrect signal.

INTRODUCTION OF NEW TECHNOLOGY

Access to effective new technology has been a central topic in the debates over hospital funding in Canada. The use of inefficient technology has also been a central topic in debates over hospital efficiency. The central issue with respect to PPS* is its impact on the availability of additional public funding for the operating costs of new services. If the American model is followed, PPS* would not cover capital costs; hospitals would remain dependent on their provincial governments and private sources for capital funding.

Descriptively, there are two ways additional public funding for the operating costs of new services could be provided. Both require government action. First, the provincial government could set a higher Update Factor. This would provide hospitals with a general increase in funds. Second, a health condition for which a costly new technology had been developed could be reassigned to an existing DRG with a higher relative weight or to a new DRG created specially for it.

There has been much concern in the U.S. about that impact of PPS on the availability of new technology. Some critics have been concerned about its potential effects (Anderson and Steinberg, 1984; Bourque, 1984; Smits and Watson, 1984; Stern and Epstein, 1985). Others argue that PPS has already unduly restrained the diffusion of some new technologies (Kane and Manoukian, 1989; McCarthy, 1988). There have been some complaints that the Update Factors have been insufficient to cover the cost of new services. But most concern has focused on the willingness of government to reassign health conditions affected by new technologies to different DRGs or to create new ones for them.

Although its judgment is based on limited evidence, ProPAC (1989b, 1990b) has not expressed great concern that PPS has in fact adversely affected the diffusion of major new technologies. Indeed, its last two recommended Update Factors have included no allowance for additional operating costs for new technologies. ProPAC (1989a, 1990a) has argued that hospitals should be able to finance new, socially desirable services through productivity increases.

The Americans' concern is understandable. With cost-based reimbursement, the additional costs generated by a new service would be matched by additional Medicare payments. With PPS the situation is quite different. Consider the financial implications of providing a new service to patients who would be admitted whether or not the new service were available. If the health condition's PPS payment were not changed, providing the costly new service to these patients would mean additional costs uncompensated by higher revenues. The hospital would have to finance the costly new service by cutting back other services. This discourages use of the new technology[12]. PPS* would have less effect on the diffusion of new technology for two reasons. First, PPS* would not greatly change the role of government in financing new services. PPS has provided the U.S. government with a new financial tool with which to shape diffusion. But the provincial governments already have this tool. With PPS* additional funding could be provided either by a larger Update Factor or by assigning the health condition to a different DRG. With NBS, however, provincial governments do the comparable thing when they agree to increase hospitals' budgets to finance new services. If a province is now unwilling to increase global budgets to finance new services, it is not clear why with PPS* it would be any more willing to approve higher Update Factors or alter DRG assignments.

Second, PPS* would not greatly change the incentives confronting Canadian hospitals. Again, consider the case of a new service for patients whose admission would occur independently of the new service. With PPS* the hospital would have to absorb the cost of the new service, unless the government approved a higher PPS* payment. But this is exactly the situation with NBS; the hospital must absorb the cost of the new service, unless the government grants it a higher budget. Therefore, if the hospital is not willing to finance a new service from its global budget now, it should not be willing to finance the same service under PPS* without a DRG change[13].

INTER-HOSPITAL ALLOCATION OF FUNDS

PPS* might provide a more acceptable way to distribute available public funds among hospitals. In Quebec, for example, some hospitals complain that they do not receive their "fair share" of available public funds (DesRochers, 1988). Certainly with PPS* government bureaucrats would have much less discretion in allocating available funds. Every hospital's revenue would be determined by the same "objective criteria". One criterion would be its case-mix (i.e., the distribution of its patients among DRGs). In addition, as in the U.S., there could be higher payments for urban hospitals and teaching hospitals as well as extra payments for "outlier" cases.

However, the American experience warns that setting "objective" criteria acceptable to all hospitals is difficult. PPS* might reduce the grumbling, but it would not assure all hospitals "fair treatment". In the U.S. a frequent criticism of PPS is that the DRG patient classification system is too coarse. There is much variation in resource use among patients in specific DRGs because of variation in case severity (Berki et al, 1984; Horn et al, 1985a, 1985b, 1986; Hughes et al, 1989; McMahon and Newbold, 1986; Rhodes et al, 1986). Hospitals that treat a disproportionate share of the more severe cases having above average costs are penalized financially. Although alternative schemes have been proposed, neither HCFA nor ProPAC has found any of them to be clearly superior to the DRG scheme.

There is considerable agreement in the U.S. that urban and teaching hospitals should receive larger payments because they have higher costs (case-mix adjusted) than other hospitals. But PPS planners have had trouble deciding how much more the urban hospitals should be paid per case. This problem is compounded by the fact that special treatment for urban hospitals also affects rural hospitals, a significant fraction of which are having financial problems. Higher payments for urban hospitals mean lower payments for rural hospitals[14]. Consequently, there has been considerable controversy over the size of the extra payments for the urban hospitals.

Similarly, determining the appropriate size of the extra payments for indirect medical education costs has proved difficult. Teaching hospitals have apparently done very well financially under PPS (Guterman et al, 1990). In 1988fy when all hospitals had PPS operating costs that averaged 2.6% less than their PPS payments, the costs of the major teaching hospitals were 15.1% less than their PPS payments (ProPAC, 1990b). The size of this extra payment has already been reduced twice – and the size of the payments going to nonteaching hospitals correspondingly increased twice.

ADMINISTRATIVE BURDENS

With PPS* hospitals would no longer need to have their budgets approved by the provincial government each year. These budget negotiations require time and treasure for both the provincial government and the hospital. But the savings from eliminating them must be stacked against both the added cost to the hospital of preparing payment claims for each discharge and the added cost to the government of processing these claims. Resources would also have to be devoted to establishing and managing PPS*.

Other budget-related problems with which hospital managers now grapple would not be eliminated. PPS* would not necessarily eliminate year-end deficits, whose resolution could still involve negotiations with the provincial government[15]. Collective agreements with hospital workers and various provincial regulations would continue to exist. Moreover, utilization review would create new problems for hospital administrators.

INFORMATION ABOUT HOSPITAL PERFORMANCE

A striking feature of PPS is the small advisory commission ProPAC. As already indicated, it makes annual recommendations regarding both the size of the next year's Update Factor and possible modifications of other parts of PPS. Equally important, it prepares an annual review of the performance of PPS. It reviews hospital performance, the utilization of hospital and other services by Medicare beneficiaries, and the available evidence regarding quality of care. The reports and recommendations of this commission provide substantive, independent information for HCFA and Congress as well as for others involved in the continuing debates over PPS and Medicare. ProPAC's work appears to have had a positive impact on government decision-making.

No comparable commission exists in Canada; certainly there is no such commission in Quebec. Nor is the information and analysis comparable to that provided by ProPAC readily available from other sources here. This is unfortunate. Good information does not necessarily imply good decisions, but it can facilitate them. It is striking how little descriptive information and substantive analysis is now available to fertilize our health policy debates and decisions[16]. Often relevant data exist, but they are not analyzed and readily available publicly.

To deal with this information problem, each province should consider establishing an advisory commission comparable to ProPAC. Such commissions could be established without implementing any other part of a PPS-type system. As a first step, a detailed review should be made of the organization, role, and impact of ProPAC, to assess the usefulness of establishing such commissions here and to help determine their structure and functions.

A commission's membership and mandates could be analogous to those of ProPAC. Its descriptive information, analyses, and recommendations should focus on hospital financing and performance, the utilization of hospital services, and the quality of care being provided. It should have sufficient resources that it could maintain a small staff of researchers and commission some outside research. It would make regular public reports, addressed to the provincial health minister. However, a number of design questions remain: Should the focus of the commission be limited to hospital services? Would it be sufficient for it to report every two or three years? What access should the commission have to information collected by government on hospital operations, people's use of services, etc.?

Given the history of our health policy debates and the financial pressures now on governments, it is probably wise that the information be reviewed and presented by an independent agency – at least an agency as independent as any agency appointed by government can be. These commissions should not be forums for providers, either. ProPAC is composed of thoughtful people who are experts in health economics, hospital finance, and health care. The work of these provincial commissions would complement the work of the technology assessment councils now taking root in Canada, as well as the work of regional health councils such as those now being contemplated in Quebec.

Although such commissions could improve public decision-making, a provincial government might be reluctant to establish one, fearing that the commission would create political problems for it. Undoubtedly, the commission's reports and recommendations would occasionally be critical of some government policies. But, as ProPAC's record indicates, a commission could also provide support for government policies. Sometimes opposition from providers makes it difficult for governments to implement good policies. The work of the advisory commission could be an effective antidote for providers' opposition in such situations. Moreover, the commission could be a source of new ideas for governments.

DISCUSSION

Three themes emerge from this review of the American experience with PPS. First, PPS has altered the performance of the American health system, and the explanation for this involves more than the incentive effects of case-based reimbursement. Federal spending on the Medicare Program and apparently the social cost of health services for people 65+ have been reduced. However, it is not clear that PPS has yet caused a significant reduction in hospital operating costs per Medicare patient. There is also troubling evidence that hospital cutbacks have had negative health effects.

Canadian health planners seem attracted to a PPS-type system largely because of the financial incentives associated with case-based reimbursement. But the American evidence does not indicate how important these incentives have been. PPS involves both macro and micro incentives. Only the latter require case-based payments, and little evidence is yet available on the significance of their micro incentive effects. It is important that Canadians realize this. Although PPS has reduced costs, health planners should not jump to the conclusion that this is the result of case-based payments. The evidence points to three other explanations: the macro incentive, government determination of the Standardized Payments, and utilization review. But Canada's negotiated budget system already provides incentives comparable to PPS's macro incentive. The provincial governments already have the power to determine hospital spending. And utilization review could be introduced into our present system; case-based reimbursement is not a prerequisite for it.

Nevertheless, case-based reimbursement built around DRGs is very important in the U.S. Its role is similar to that of the old Trojan Horse. It facilitates having a potentially effective hospital cost control system that does not require the federal or state governments to become involved in approving each hospital's budget. The Canadian experience indicates that hospital costs can be controlled using negotiated budgets. But such detailed government involvement in hospital affairs remains politically unacceptable in the U.S. Although it is probably more costly to administer, case-based reimbursement built around DRGs averts the need for negotiated budgets; each hospital's revenues are determined mechanically by a formula. Thus, it provides the government with a politically acceptable tool with which it can control hospital spending. Although the literature has been focused on DRGs and case-based reimbursement, the active element of PPS is government determination of the Standardized Payments.

The second theme is that the efficiency effects of a PPS-type system on the provincial health systems are uncertain. Certainly, any effects here would be different from those in the U.S. PPS was a much more dramatic change in reimbursement institutions in the U.S.

than a comparable plan would be here. Indeed, it is very striking that the introduction of such a plan would not appreciably change key aspects of our health system which shape its performance. The provincial governments would continue to control spending on hospital services, and it is not clear that governments would make decisions greatly different from those they now make. There would not be a substantial change in the financial incentives confronting hospitals. And the reimbursement process would still create headaches for hospital managers, though their current problems with budget negotiations would be replaced by problems involving utilization review and the proper classification of patients in order to be paid for services rendered.

Nevertheless, a PPS-type system would mean change. Utilization review would be needed to avoid unnecessary admissions. Such a system might also reduce hospital lengths of stay. The size of any reduction would depend on the reasons for the long stays and on the availability of adequate replacements for some inpatient hospital services. The available American evidence warns, however, that such reductions can cause some negative health effects if they are not properly managed.

The final theme is that every province should seriously consider establishing an advisory commission on hospital services, patterned after ProPAC. From a Canadian perspective, this little advisory commission is one of the most interesting aspects of PPS. It certainly provides more information on a regular basis about the performance of PPS than is currently available on the performance of our provincial hospital sectors.

Whether our negotiated budget system is retained or replaced with a PPS-type system, government will continue to have a major role in our provincial health systems. That is to say, the performance of the provincial systems will be shaped through political processes. However, the lack of information about the performance of our health systems is a major problem for health policy development in Canada. The creation of provincial advisory commissions on hospital services would help overcome this problem.

NOTES

1. For each admission the patient must also pay a government determined deductible, $592 in 1990fy. Therefore, the total amount of money a hospital receives for each Medicare case is slightly larger than the PPS payment. But this amount is predetermined by the government.

2. Although a formal model of hospital behavior is not presented here, one has in mind non-profit, preference-maximizing hospitals, which for decision-making purposes group patients according to their health conditions. The hospitals' preferences depend positively on the number of patients in each group admitted and on the perceived quality of care provided patients in each group. The form of the hospitals' budget constraints depends on the reimbursement process used. Hospitals also face capacity constraints because their beds are limited.

3. A hospital could increase its revenues by changing its case mix or increasing its admissions of patients whose treatment costs would be less than their PPS payments. But there are limits on the extent to which a hospital can reclassify its cases, and admissions are controlled by utilization review. Moreover, even if the hospital did alter its case-mix and admissions, it would still have an incentive to behave as described in the text.

4. Decisions about quality of care reflect the way the hospital values the amenities and clinical services it provides patients. If a hospital reduced the quality of care for one DRG, it could provide more services to another DRG. When considering whether to do this, the hospital compares the value to itself of the services not provided patients in the first DRG to the value of providing additional services to patients in the second DRG.

5. Now the Standardized Payments are based on national hospital cost data. But as part of the process of phasing-in PPS, each hospital's Standardized Payment was initially based on a weighted average of the hospital's own average cost per Medicare patient, the regional average cost, and the national aver-

age cost. Between 1983fy and 1989fy the weights for the hospital's own cost and the regional average were periodically reduced and the weight for the national average increased.

6. Not all hospitals were covered by PPS when it started. Hospitals were first covered at the start of their next fiscal year following September 30, 1983. Thus, hospitals whose fiscal year began July 1, 1983, did not enter the program until July 1, 1984, at the beginning of their 1985fy. These are the non-PPS hospitals used by Feder et al; they continued to be reimbursed by Medicare for their actual costs, subject to a TEFRA-imposed ceiling.

7. These cost data come from the cost reports hospitals file with HCFA indicating their operating costs for Medicare patients. The quality of these data apparently needs improvement, but the discussion here based on them is not sensitive to the particular numbers used.

8. When case-based reimbursement is discussed, it is often suggested that increases in the Standard Payment could be determined by increases in the average cost per case. This has not happened with PPS. There are several problems with such a mechanical formula. The necessary cost data only become available with some lag. Such a formula locks "DRG creep" into the payment base, and it limits new funding for new services. Perhaps most importantly, it is doubtful that any government would commit itself to budget increases in a major program over which it has no control.

9. Medicare's Case Mix Index increased 3.3% annually between 1984fy and 1988fy. Estimates of real changes in case severity range between 1.5% and 2.1% (ProPAC, 1990a), so creep was between 1.2% and 1.8% per year.

10. Two caveats: First, if admissions prove larger than expected, a hospital may be able to renegotiate its global budget. Second, more admissions in the current fiscal year may result in larger budgets in the next fiscal year.

11. Within five years of the introduction of PPS three informative case studies of the quality of care effects of PPS had been published. But 15 years after the introduction of provincial constraints on hospital budgets in Canada no comparable Canadian studies have been published. Many Canadian health planners – myself included – have supported the provincial constraints, arguing that hospital costs could be reduced by eliminating ineffective services. But, as the three American case studies indicate, there is no guarantee that when Canadian hospitals have taken steps to curtail costs they have eliminated only ineffective services. If, in fact, they have done that, it should be documented. If they have eliminated some important services, that too is important to document.

12. PPS has a similar effect on the diffusion of a new service targeted to people who would not be admitted unless the service were available for them. With cost-based reimbursement, funding for the additional operating costs of the service would be assured. Not so with PPS. Unless the PPS payment covered the operating costs of the service, the hospital would have less incentive to introduce it. The effect of this disincentive is inversely related to the ratio of the PPS payment to the hospital's incremental cost of treating these patients.

13. However, in the case of a new service for patients who would not be admitted unless the service were available, PPS* might make a difference. With NBS, their admission would result in no revenue increase unless the government granted a budget increase. With PPS*, their admission would increase hospital revenues even if the government did not increase the size of the payment. Thus, PPS* would provide an incentive to introduce new technologies that result in new admissions. However, if governments continue to require hospitals to obtain provincial approval before adding new services that increase admissions, this incentive would be checked.

14. Larger payments for urban hospitals are based on data indicating that the average cost per case in urban hospitals is higher than that in rural hospitals, after adjusting for wage and case-mix differences. Mathematically, given the average cost of all Medicare patients, the higher the average cost estimate for urban hospitals, the lower must be the estimate for the rural hospitals. Intuitively, the Standardized Payment for each type of hospital is proportional to its estimated average cost per case. Thus, the higher the estimated average cost for urban hospitals, the higher their Standardized Payment, and the lower the Standardized Payment for rural hospitals.

15. This could be a bigger problem in Canada than in the U.S. PPS covers only Medicare beneficiaries, so Medicare losses can be offset by surpluses for non-Medicare patients. With PPS* Canadian hospitals would not have a comparable safety valve.

16. For example, it is very striking to compare the information relating to the provision and utilization of hospital services in one of ProPAC's annual evaluations (1990b) and that in the recent works of Quebec's Rochon Commission (Quebec, 1988). Although the Commission's central area of inquiry was the adequacy of provincial funding for hospital services, it provided surprisingly little information about and analysis of the performance of Quebec's hospitals. ProPAC provides far more information useful for policy discussions.

REFERENCES

Anderson GM, Newhouse JP, Roos LL: Hospital care for elderly patients with diseases of the circulatory system: a comparison of hospital use in the United States and Canada. *New England Journal of Medicine* 321(21)1443-1448, 1989.

Anderson G, Steinberg E: To buy or not to buy: technology acquisition under prospective payment. *New England Journal of Medicine* 311(3):182-185, 1984.

Berki SE, Ashcraft MLF, Newbrander WC: Length-of-stay variations within ICDA-8 Diagnosis-Related Groups. *Medical Care* 22:126-142, 1984.

Bourque DP: Technology acquisition under prospective payment. *New England Journal of Medicine* 311:1189-1190, 1984.

Carroll N, Erwin WG: Patient shifting as a response to Medicare prospective payment. *Medical Care* 25(12):1161-1167, 1987.

Coffey R, Goldfarb MG: DRG's and disease staging for reimbursing Medicare patients. *Medical Care* 24(9):814-829, 1986.

Cotterrill P, Bobula J, Connerton R: Comparison of alternative relative weights for Diagnostic Related Groups. *Health Care Financing Review* 37-52, Spring 1986.

DesHarnais SI, Chesney JD, Flemming ST: The impact of the Prospective Payment System on hospital utilization and the quality of care: trends and regional variations in the first two years, 1987b. Paper presented at the October 1987 meeting of the American Public Health Association. (Cited in Russell 1989).

DesHarnais S, Kobrinski E, et al: The early effects of the Prospective Payment System on inpatient utilization and the quality of care. *Inquiry* 24:7-16, 1987a.

DesRochers G: Financement et budgetisation des hôpitaux, Synthèse critique 30, Commission d'Enquête sur les Services de Santé et les Services sociaux, *Les Publications du Québec,* Québec, 1988.

Evans RG: Split vision: interpreting cross-border differences in health spending. *Health Affairs* 7(5):17-24, 1988.

Evans RG, Lomas J, Barer M, et al: Controlling health expenditures – the Canadian reality. *New England Journal of Medicine* 320(9):571-577, 1989.

Feder J, Hadley J, Zuckerman S: How did Medicare's Prospective Payment System affect hospitals. *New England Journal of Medicine* 317(14):867-873, 1987.

Fetter RB, Shin Y, Freeman JL, Averill RF, et al: Case mix definition by Diagnosis-related Groups. *Medical Care* 18(2: supp):1-53, 1980.

Fisher CR: Impact of the Prospective Payment System on physician charges under Medicare. *Health Care Financing Review* 8(4):101-103, 1987.

Fisher CR: Trends in Medicare enrollee use of physician and supplier services, 1983-86. *Health Care Financial Review* 10, Fall 1988.

Fitzgerald JF, Fagan LF, Tierney WM, Dittus RS: Changing patterns of hip fracture care before and after implementation of the Prospective Payment System. *Journal of the American Medical Association* 258(2):218-221, 1987.

Fitzgerald JF, Moore PS, Dittus RS: The care of elderly patients with hip fracture: changes since implementation of the Prospective Payment System. *New England Journal of Medicine* 319(21):1392-1397, 1988.

Guterman S, Altman SH, Young DA: Hospitals' financial performance in the first five years of PPS. *Health Affairs* 9(1):125-134, 1990.

Hadley J, Swartz K: The impacts on hospital costs between 1980 and 1984 of hospital rate regulation, competition and changes in health insurance coverage. *Inquiry* 26(1):35-47, 1989.

Hadley J, Zuckerman S, Feder J: Profits and fiscal pressure in the Prospective Payment System: their impacts on hospitals. *Inquiry* 26(3):354-365, 1989.

Hochstein A: A cost comparison in the treatment of long stay patients. *Canadian Public Policy* 10(2):177-184, 1984.

Holahan J, Dor A, Zuckerman S: Understanding the recent growth in Medicare physician expenditures. *Journal of the American Medical Association,* 263(12):1658-1661, 1990.

Horn SD et al: Misclassification problems in Diagnosis-related Groups: cystic fibrosis as an example. *New England Journal of Medicine* 314(8):484-487, 1986.

Horn SD et al: Interhospital differences in severity of illness: problems for prospective payment based on Diagnosis-related Groups (DRG's). *New England Journal of Medicine* 313(1):20-24, 1985a.

Horn SD, Sharkey PD, Chambers AF, Horn RA: Severity of illness within DRG's: impact of prospective payment. *American Journal of Public Health* 75:1195-1199, 1985b.

Hsia DC, Krushat WM, Fagan AB, Tebbutt JA, Kusserow RP: Accuracy of diagnostic coding for Medicare patients under the Prospective-Payment System. *New England Journal of Medicine* 318(6):352-355, 1988.

Hughes JS, Lichtenstein J, Magno J, Fetter RB: Improving DRGs: Use of procedure codes for assisted respiration to adjust for complexity of illness. *Medical Care* 27(7):750-757, 1989.

Institute of Medicine, Committee on Nursing Home Regulation: *Improving the Quality of Care in Nursing Homes.* Washington, D.C.: National Academy Press, 1986.

Kane NM, Manoukian PD: The effect of the Medicare Prospective Payment System on the adoption of new technology: the case of cochlar implants. *New England Journal of Medicine* 321(20):1378-1383, 1989.

Lave JR: Is compression occurring in the DRG rates? *Inquiry* 22(2):142-147, 1985.

Lindberg G, Lurie N, Bannick-Mohrland S, Sherman RE, Farseth PA: Health care cost containment measures and mortality in Hennepin County's Medicaid elderly and all elderly. *American Journal of Public Health* 79(11):1481-1485, 1989.

Long MJ, Chesney JD, Fleming ST: Were hospitals selective in their product and productivity changes? The top 50 DRGs after PPS. *Health Services Research* 24(5):615-641, 1989.

Long MJ, Chesney JD, et al: The effect of PPS on hospital product and productivity. *Medical Care* 25(6):528-538, 1987.

Lyles YM: Impact of Medicare Diagnosis-related Groups on nursing homes in the Portland, Oregon metropolitan area. *Journal of the American Geriatric Society* 34:573-578, 1986.

McCarthy CM: DRGs-five years later. *New England Journal of Medicine* 318(25):1683-1686, 1988.

McMahon L, Newbold R: Variation in resource use within Diagnosis-related Groups: the effect of severity of illness and physician practice. *Medical Care* 24(5):388-397, 1986.

Morrisey MA, Sloan FA, Valvona J: Medicare prospective payment and posthospital transfers to subacute care. *Medical Care* 26(7):685-698, 1988.

Neuhauser D, Lewicki AM: What do we gain from the sixth stool guaiac? *New England Journal of Medicine* 293(5):226-228, 1975.

Newhouse JP, Byrne DJ: Did Medicare's Prospective Payment System cause length of stay to fall? *Journal of Health Economics* 7(4):413-416, 1988.

Newhouse JP, Anderson G, Roos LL: Hospital spending in the United States and Canada: a comparison. *Health Affairs* 7(5):6-16, 1988.

Pettengill J, Vertrees L: Reliability and validity in hospital case mix measurement. *Health Care Financing Review* 4(2):101-128, 1982.

Prospective Payment Assessment Commission: *Report and Recommendations to the Secretary, U.S. Department of Health and Human Services.* Washington, D.C., 1989a, 118 p.

Prospective Payment Assessment Commission: *Medicare Prospective Payment and the American Health Care System: Report to Congress.* Washington, D.C., 1989b, 187 p.

Prospective Payment Assessment Commission: *Report and Recommendations to the Secretary, U.S. Department of Health and Human Services.* Washington, D.C., 1990a, 118 p.

Prospective Payment Assessment Commission: *Medicare Prospective Payment and the American Health Care System: Report to Congress.* Washington, D.C., 1990b, 119 p.

Quebec: *Rapport de la Commission d'Enquête sur les Services de Santé et les Services sociaux.* Québec: Les Publications du Québec, 1988, 803 p.

Rhodes RS et al: Factors affecting length of hospital stay for femoropoplited bypass: implications of the DRG's. *New England Journal of Medicine* 314(3):153-157, 1986.

Russell LB: *Medicare's New Hospital Payment System.* Washington, D.C.: The Brookings Institution, 1989, 114 p.

Sager M, Easterling DV, Kindig DA, Anderson OW: Changes in the location of death after passage of Medicare's Prospective Payment System. *New England Journal of Medicine* 320(7):433-439, 1989.

Sager MA, Leventhal EA, Easterling DV: The impact of Medicare's Prospective Payment System on Wisconsin nursing homes. *Journal of the American Medical Association* 257:1762-1766, 1987.

Schramm CJ, Gabel J: Prospective payment: some retrospective observations. *New England Journal of Medicine* 318(25):1681-1683, 1988.

Sheingold SH: Unintended results of Medicare's national prospective payment rates. *Health Affairs* 5(4):5-21, 1986.

Sheingold SH: The first three years of PPS: impact on Medicare costs. *Health Affairs* 8(3):191-204, 1989.

Simborg D: DRG creep: a new hospital-acquired disease. *New England Journal of Medicine* 304(26):1602-1604, 1981.

Sloan FA, Morrisey MA, Valvona J: Medicare prospective payment and the use of medical technologies in hospitals. *Medical Care* 26(9):837-853, 1988.

Smith DB, Pickard R: Evaluation of the impact of Medicare and Medicaid prospective payment on utilization of Philadelphia area hospitals. *Health Services Research* 21:529-546, 1986.

Smits HL, Watson RE: DRG's and the future of surgical practice. *New England Journal of Medicine* 311(25):1612-1614, 1984.

Soderstrom L: Family care. In: Soderstrom L: *Privatization: Adopt or Adapt?* Synthèse critique 36, Commission d'Enquête sur les Services de Santé et les Services sociaux. Quebéc: Les Publications du Québec, 1987, 237 p.

Steinwald B, Dummit LA: Hospital case-mix change: sicker patients or DRG creep? *Health Affairs* 8(2):35-47, 1989.

Stern RS, Epstein AM: Institutional response to prospective payment based on Diagnosis-related Groups: implications for cost, quality and access. *New England Journal of Medicine* 312(10):621-627, 1985.

Vladeck BC: Medicare hospital payment by Diagnosis-related Groups. *Annals of Internal Medicine* 100(4):576-591, 1984.

Vladeck BC: Hospital prospective payment and the quality of care. *New England Journal of Medicine* 319(21):1411-1413, 1988.

Weinberger M, Ault KA, Vinicor F: Prospective reimbursement and diabetes mellitus: impact upon glycemic control and utilization of health services. *Medical Care* 26(1):77-83, 1988.

Zwanziger J, Melnick GA: The effects of hospital competition and the Medicare PPS program on hospital cost behavior in California. *Journal of Health Economics* 7(4):301-320, 1988.

RIVERVIEW/FRASER VALLEY ASSERTIVE OUTREACH PROGRAM

John A. Higenbottam
Bruce Etches
Yvonne Shewfelt
Riverview Hospital
Port Coquitlam, British Columbia

Michael Alberti
Ministry of Health
Victoria, British Columbia

BACKGROUND

The past three decades have witnessed major reductions in the populations of psychiatric institutions throughout North America and other parts of the world. These reductions have been largely achieved through:

a) the development of effective neuroleptic medication;

b) the application of admission policies intended to reduce the population of large psychiatric hospitals;

c) the development of community residential and treatment capabilities;

d) the introduction of psychosocial rehabilitation programs (Anthony, Cohen, and Vitalo, 1978) to prepare patients for community living; and

e) the development of aftercare systems to provide necessary clinical support to patients after discharge from hospitals.

In British Columbia, these factors have resulted in a reduction of the adult population of Riverview, the provincial psychiatric hospital, from a peak of over 5,000 patients in the 1950s to its current level of 800.

In addition to reduced institutional populations, major changes have occurred in the characteristics of the patients who are admitted to hospitals such as Riverview. With most mentally ill people requiring hospitalization being treated in public hospital psychiatric units, virtually all the patients now admitted to Riverview are the chronically mentally ill with multiple previous admissions either to Riverview or other psychiatric units. Over 80% of Riverview patients have been committed under the Mental Health Act, and most present serious behavior management problems. Many of these patients are also highly deficient in the life skills necessary for successful living in the community.

Despite a reasonably good supply of community residential accommodations, a network of mental health centres, and community care teams for providing post discharge aftercare, the rehospitalization rate for the chronically mentally ill remains very high. Of patients being discharged from Riverview, approximately 40% are readmitted within a year. This high rehospitalization rate is consistent with those reported in American settings (Anthony, Cohen, and Vitalo, 1978) – rates which are associated with enormous personal, social, and economic costs.

As an example of the enormous costs of serious mental illness, many will be familiar with the case of Sylvia Frumkin (a pseudonym), which was documented in the *New Yorker* magazine (Moran, Freedman, and Sharfstein, 1984). This 32-year-old American woman became mentally ill at the age of 14 and in 18 years had multiple admissions to hospitals as well as sessions of outpatient treatment. The direct treatment costs alone were estimated at over $636,000 in 1983 dollars. The indirect costs in terms of lost productivity, social service support, and family burden would probably be at least as much.

A number of studies have shown that it is possible to reduce substantially the high rate of rehospitalization of the chronically mentally ill through an intensive type of community-based aftercare. This aftercare is often referred to as Assertive Case Management but is also known as Assertive Outreach or Assertive Community Treatment.

The pioneer work with such programs was done by Pasamanick, Scarpitti, and Dinitz (1967). However, the best known and most influential of these programs has been the Program of Assertive Community Treatment (PACT) implemented in Madison, Wisconsin (Stein and Test 1985; Test and Stein, 1980). The model program not only resulted in a significantly lower rehospitalization rate of approximately 25%, but also, when rehospitalization did become necessary, in much shorter hospital stays.

The success of the PACT program has led to the implementation of a large number of similar programs throughout North America and other parts of the western world. One of the programs based on PACT, which has itself attracted a great deal of attention, is the Bridge Program, established in Chicago in 1978. Follow-up studies on the Bridge Program have shown rehospitalization rates ranging from 14% (Dincin and Witheridge, 1982) to 35% (Setze and Bond, 1983). Furthermore, Dincin and Witheridge (1982) have reported an average of 34 days of rehospitalization for Bridge Program clients compared with 591 days for those from a control group.

In one study (Bond et al, 1987) clients receiving Assertive Outreach were compared with clients attending a drop-in centre for the chronically mentally ill. During a year's follow-up, Assertive Outreach clients had approximately 50% fewer episodes and days of state hospitalization as compared to clients attending the drop-in centre.

The Assertive Outreach model has now been implemented in a large number of North American and European settings and has actually become the dominant paradigm of aftercare for the seriously mentally ill. Although significant variability may be seen among assertive outreach programs, the following key elements characterize the approach and its contrasts with traditional forms of aftercare:

1. The program uses in vivo intervention where clients are visited in their homes, where they work, or where they take part in leisure social activities. This is perhaps the most critical contrast with traditional clinic-based aftercare.

2. Outreach staff must be committed to preventing unnecessary hospitalization by assisting clients in solving community living problems which could lead to breakdown.

3. The approach addresses the satisfaction of each major area of human need. In terms of a client's ability to live successfully in the community, the importance of personal and social living needs may be equal to or greater than medical and psychiatric treatment needs.

4. Outreach staff must accept ultimate responsibility for their client. Outreach staff are where the "buck stops" in terms of responsibility for client welfare.

5. Outreach staff must provide assertive, occasionally aggressive, advocacy for their clients to assist them in dealing with government and agency bureaucracy.

6. Rather than being reactive, outreach staff must anticipate and prevent crises in the lives of the clients.

7. Outreach staff must be accessible to clients when the inevitable crises occur.

8. A low staff-to-client ratio is necessary to provide the high degree of contact required for assertive outreach. Most successful programs employ ratios in the order of 1:10.

9. A total team approach is important; each outreach staff member works with each client assigned to the outreach service.

10. A long term and perhaps lifetime commitment must be made to clients to meet their needs as long as those needs exist. Additionally, staff must develop a great tolerance for difficult or intractable client behaviors.

PROGRAM DESCRIPTION

The success of American assertive outreach programs generated strong interest at Riverview Hospital in validating this approach, particularly since Riverview's rehospitalization rate within a year of discharge has historically exceeded 40%.

It was considered important to conduct a rigorously controlled clinical and economic evaluation to validate this approach in a Canadian setting. Research funding was sought from the National Health Research and Development Program (NHRDP), and the investigators were fortunate in obtaining a major grant to permit a two-year longitudinal study.

The Riverview/Fraser Valley Assertive Outreach program has now been implemented in the Surrey and New Westminster Mental Health Centre areas in the province of British Columbia. The program is staffed by five psychiatric nurses from Riverview who have been trained in assertive outreach technique.

Subjects for the study have been selected on the basis of clinical history as being at high risk for rehospitalization. Clients have a psychiatric diagnosis of Schizophrenia or Major Affective Disorder with multiple previous psychiatric hospitalizations and recent system use.

Sixty clients have been randomly assigned to the assertive outreach experimental condition and 60 clients to a control condition. Both groups of clients receive full mental health centre services, except that control clients do not receive the assertive outreach.

Subjects in both conditions are being followed up over a period of two years. The two groups will be compared in terms of rehospitalization rate, number of days of rehospitalization, psychiatric symptomatology, and quality of life. In addition, a comprehensive cost benefit analysis is being conducted.

COST BENEFIT ANALYSIS

This project builds on the work of Burton Weisbrod (1981), who pioneered the application of cost-benefit analysis to mental illness treatment programs. Weisbrod developed a framework which aimed at measuring all the resources used and all the outputs generated in the treatment of difficult cases of mental illness. He applied this framework to costs and benefits in a controlled (random assignment) experiment comparing hospital-based care at the Mendota Mental Health Institute, Dane County (Madison and surrounding area), Wisconsin, and community-based care implementing the Training in Community Living Program (TCLP) developed by Leonard Stein and Mary Ann Test (Stein and Test, 1985; Test and Stein, 1980).

The present project aims to measure all the costs and benefits in a controlled experiment comparing the care provided by Mental Health Centres and the care provided by the Riverview/Fraser Valley Assertive Outreach Program, in the settings of New Westminster and Surrey, to patients diagnosed as having severe chronic mental illness.

This group of patients can be characterized as "high cost" in terms of utilization of health care and social resources. This cost is largely the result of their frequent, recurring, relatively long term rehospitalization in a psychiatric or acute care facility, a process called "the revolving door syndrome". The pattern of use of acute care hospital days in British Columbia by patients with a primary diagnosis of schizophrenic psychosis or affective psychosis is shown in Table 1.

Table 1

TRENDS IN THE USE OF ACUTE CARE HOSPITALIZATION WHERE THE PRIMARY DIAGNOSIS IS A MENTAL DISORDER

British Columbia, 1987/88 and 1988/89

ICD9		1987/88			1988/89		
Code	Description	Days	Cases	Days/case	Days	Cases	Days/case
295	Schizophrenic psychoses	65,325	3,137	20.8	59,108	3,093	19.1
296	Affective psychoses	75,233	3,439	21.9	80,825	3,663	22.1
Sub-total (295 + 296)		140,558	6,576	21.4	139,933	6,756	20.7
Total Chap. V (mental disorders)		329,811	20,607	16.0	326,183	20,909	15.6
Total acute care		3,571,419	442,661	8.1	3,476,275	439,158	7.9
295 and 296 as a % of Total Chap. V (mental disorders)		42.6%	31.9%	133.8%	42.9%	32.3%	132.7%
295 and 296 as a % of total acute care		3.9%	1.5%	264.2%	4.0%	1.5%	262.0%

Even though hospitals in British Columbia are now funded on a global budget basis, per diem rates are calculated for some billing purposes, such as for patients who are not residents of the province. These can be used with the data on the number of days of hospitalization to begin to establish the order of magnitude of the situation. Acute care per diem (standard ward) rates in 1990/91 range from $355 to $700. Even if patients with a diagnosis of schizophrenic or affective psychosis do not fully use all the resources represented by those average values, the amount would still be in the order of several hundreds of dollars per patient day. When this is applied to 140,000 days per year, the amount is significant.

Furthermore, Corrado and Doherty (1989) have shown that for patients in British Columbia similar to those who will participate in this study, there are high social costs beyond hospitalization. These costs are the result of the involvement of many of the patients with the legal system, which can occur following inappropriate behavior. They are in the thousands of dollars per patient per year, and include such costs as police, court administration, crown counsel, legal services, corrections institutions, probation, and bail.

Following Weisbrod's framework, the project measures expenditures in the following key areas:

Assertive Outreach Program and Mental Health Centres
- Direct and indirect time each registered psychiatric nurse spends with or on behalf of each client and time spent on other activities as recorded in log books
- Capital and operating costs

Hospitals
- Inpatient and outpatient (including emergency room and psychiatric day care program) use of services (labour, maintenance, tests and procedures and medication)

Medical Services Plan
- Services billed by physicians and other practitioners, amount paid

Pharmacare Programs
- Medication provided and amount paid

Law Enforcement
- RCMP and local police force contacts with clients
- Court, jail, and probation time
- Medico/legal, including hospital morgue and coroner's office
- Investigation of the possibility of quantifying impacts on any victims of encounters with clients

Forensic Psychiatric Services
Social Services and Housing
- Time and payments

Other Agencies
- Time, funds, and goods provided by the Salvation Army, Community Services Agency, etc.

Maintenance Costs
Family Burden
- Attempts are being made to quantify family burden

Benefits are being measured in terms of outcomes as assessed by various psychological evaluations, comparisons of the number of suicides (these patients are a high risk group for suicide), participation in the labour force, and earnings from employment, as well as in terms of the difference in amount and type of expenditure for each treatment condition.

The analysis will also provide detailed information on the patterns of use of medical services by the patients. For example, it will be possible to measure the use of general practice and specialist physician services, the types of services provided, and the continuity of care as revealed by treatment by few or many of the same physicians over time, for both the control and experimental groups.

SUMMARY

The Riverview/Fraser Valley Assertive Outreach Program is an important demonstration project with national as well as provincial implications for mental health service planning. If the present trend towards replacing large institutions with community alternatives continues, it is important that effective aftercare programs be developed to support the significant proportion of seriously mentally ill people who are at high risk for rehospitalization. We now have many years of experience to demonstrate that in the absence of effective aftercare programs, most seriously ill people cannot live successfully or happily in the community. It is our hope that the Riverview/Fraser Valley Assertive Outreach Program will validate this approach as cost-beneficial, resulting in substantially reduced rehospitalization with an improved quality of life for clinically high risk individuals. Although it may never be possible or desirable to eliminate facilities such as Riverview completely, the continuing development of community residential and service alternatives together with effective aftercare approaches will permit substantial reductions in institutional populations. Furthermore, as the "revolving door syndrome" is controlled, it will be possible for institutions to develop new roles as smaller, highly specialized short term assessment, diagnostic, and treatment centres for the seriously mentally ill.

REFERENCES

Anthony WA, Cohen MR, Vitalo R: The measurement of rehabilitation outcome. *Schizophrenia Bulletin* 4:365-383, 1978.

Bond GR: An economic analysis of psychosocial rehabilitation. *Hospital and Community Psychiatry* 35:356-362, 1984.

Bond GR, Miller LD, Krumwied RD, Ward RS: Assertive Case Management in three CMHSs: a controlled study. *Hospital and Community Psychiatry* 39:411-418, 1988.

Bond GR, Witheridge TF, Dincin J, Wasmer D, Webb J, Degraaf-Kaser R: A controlled evaluation of the Thresholds Bridge Assertive Outreach Program. Paper presented at the annual meeting of the American Psychological Association, New York, New York, August 28, 1987.

Corrado RR, Doherty D: A cost measurement of a non-random sample of ten cases referred to the multiservice network. Unpublished manuscript, Simon Fraser University, 1989.

Dincin J, Witheridge TF: Psychiatric rehabilitation as a deterrent to recidivism. *Hospital and Community Psychiatry* 33:645-650, 1982.

Endicott J, Spitzer RL, Fleiss JL, Cohen J: The Global Assessment Scale. *Archives of General Psychiatry* 33:766-771, 1976.

Kay SR, Opler LA, Fiszbein A: Significance of positive and negative syndromes and chronic schizophrenia. *British Journal of Psychiatry* 149:439-448, 1986.

Moran RI, Freedman RI, Sharfstein SS: Economic Grandrounds: the journal of Sylvia Frumkin: a case study for policy makers. *Hospital and Community Psychiatry* 35:887-893, 1984.

Pasamanick B, Scarpitti FR, Dinitz S: *Schizophrenics and the Community.* New York: Appleton-Century-Crofts, 1967.

Schneider LC, Struening EL: SLOF: A behavioral rating skill for assessing the mentally ill. *Social Work Research and Abstracts* 19:9-21, 1983.

Setze PJ, Bond GR: Community "survival" after entrance into a psychosocial rehabilitation program. Unpublished manuscript, Thresholds, Chicago, 1983.

Stein LI, Test MA: The evolution of the Training in Community Living Model. In: Stein LI and Test MA (eds.): *New Directions for Mental Health Service: The Training in Community Living Model: A Decade of Experience,* No.25. San Francisco: Jossey-Bass, 1985.

Test MA, Stein LI: An alternative to mental hospital treatment. III. Social cost. *Archives of General Psychiatry* 37:392-412, 1980.

Weisbrod BA: Benefit cost analysis of a controlled experiment treating the mentally ill. *Journal of Human Resources,* 16:523-528, 1981.

DISCUSSION

Chair: Jackie Muldoon
Trent University

David Kelly (Alberta Health)

I have a question for Dr. Soderstrom. Does the U.S. DRG funding system permit hospitals to use their budgets to develop home care and other community outreach services in order to move patients out of acute care beds, and if so, have they actually done it?

Lee Soderstrom (McGill University)

Yes, hospitals can use any PPS-derived savings to finance home care or other outreach services. PPS encourages hospitals to find lower cost ways of managing their Medicare caseload. A hospital may believe it can reduce these costs by admitting a group of Medicare patients for a day or two and then discharging them to a home care program. If so, it is free to use any PPS savings to develop such programs. Hospitals have two financial reasons for doing this. First, it will minimize any PPS losses. Second, any Medicare surplus provides financial resources which hospitals can use for other projects. They are not even required to spend any PPS savings on new programs for Medicare patients.

There has been a dramatic shift in the 1980s from inpatient to outpatient care in the U.S. But it is unclear now to what extent this has been a response to the financial incentives of PPS, as opposed to a response to other developments (e.g., new technology). Moreover, as I indicate in my paper, it is unclear whether paying hospitals a fixed sum per case has much effect on their behaviour. The active financial element of PPS may be the amounts of the payments themselves. PPS may have its biggest effect on hospitals' behaviour when the amounts paid them are low relative to their costs, thereby threatening hospitals with financial losses unless they improve their efficiency and case management practices.

Charles Wright (Vancouver General Hospital)

In the general feeling that a move towards some form or other of managed care is a desirable objective, I see that a major problem in Canada is the history we're coming from of universal accessibility and freedom of access. And anything that is done is going to have serious political repercussions in this. We had a beautiful example in B.C. recently where a large number of beds were transferred from tertiary hospitals to the community, with the laudable objective of having medical care provided where the community required it, but absolutely no system, or the beginnings of any ideas, as to how to implement it because of the political repercussions if any restraints of that kind are put on the public.

Marianne Lamb (University of Toronto)

Yes, I think certainly there is the issue of things like choice of provider – in Canada, there is no indication that anybody wants to change that. The question of whether you can still attract people to a managed care system and keep them there, even without lock-in, I guess is an empirical one. How big a problem would it be? I wonder if it really would be that difficult, and if there would be a lot of out of plan use? I don't think so, if people are satisfied once they are enrolled. There is still the question of how you would attract them to enroll in the first place, though.

Pete Welch (Urban Institute, Washington D.C.)

I have a comment, not a question. It pertains to ProPAC, which again is the commission for the prospective payment system. And I agree that ProPAC has done a lot of very useful analyses. But I think you should keep in mind that ProPAC is an arm of the Congress. The analyses that it does do could just as well, at least in a technical sense, be done in the executive branch in the health financing administration. The reason the commission exists is because, in the 1980s, the American federal government has been divided, with the Republicans controlling one branch and the Democrats controlling at least part of another. So there have been real questions as to whether Congress can trust the executive branch. It may be much more difficult in a parliamentary system to get a commission that has the political support and security to do what you're proposing. This may be one of the few advantages of the American political system when it comes to health care.

Lee Soderstrom

Two reactions. Certainly, you're right. The political context of – institutionally – a ProPAC is very different from what it would be in the Canadian context. And I would never envisage ProPAC-type organizations reporting simply to Parliament. The important thing, and the key idea, is that you have a commission that has some responsibility to provide an annual or biannual review, drawing widely on available data, to inform not only governments but the population at large as to what in the world is going on in the Canadian health care system. And I think one of the things Americans may find most striking about the Canadian system, despite the fact that we all write about how important the role of government is in managing the system, is how very little information is available on the operation of the Canadian health care system. ProPAC provides more information in its annual report than was provided by the Rochon Commission in Quebec on the functioning of the hospital system or the health system in Quebec operating three years ago. And it's that information idea that I'm trying to get at, not the political setting.

Al Erlenbusch (Ontario Ministry of Health)

My question is for Professor Soderstrom. In your presentation you mentioned a couple of case studies which you said may be alarming in terms of potential negative impact of prospective payment on health outcome. Can you give us a little more information in terms of either diagnostic or patient characteristics that might be associated with those studies?

Lee Soderstrom

There were two studies relating to the management of hip fracture patients and one study dealing with the management of diabetes patients. And with the hip fracture ones, which were probably the better designed studies, basically what was found, not unexpectedly, was that patients in the hospitals were discharged sooner, they got less physiotherapy, they tended to go into skilled nursing home facilities, and then a year later a much much higher fraction were still in bed in skilled nursing home facilities.

HOSPITALS: CHANGING PRESCRIPTIONS

CHANGING PATTERNS OF GOVERNANCE FOR HOSPITALS: ISSUES AND MODELS

G. Ross Baker
Department of Health Administration
University of Toronto

Hospital governance has become an important and widely discussed issue in Canada as hospitals and their boards face accelerating pressures to provide a clear vision of their future role and their relationship to the broader health care system. Some measure of the import of this issue can be seen in the number of recent reports focused on governance questions (B.C. Health Association, 1988; Croll, 1988; Knudson, 1990; Sinclair, 1990; Trypuc, 1988; Wilson, 1990). The salience of governance issues not only in Canada, but also in Britain and the United States, underlines their fundamental importance in the changing structure of the health care system. This paper provides an overview of hospital governance issues in Canada and examines alternative models of governance in the United States and Great Britain. Despite the different social and political contexts for hospitals in these health care systems, there is some apparent convergence in broader policy goals as key actors in these three jurisdictions seek to develop more effective governance structures which balance the interests of individual hospitals and regional bodies.

DEFINING GOVERNANCE

The use of the term "governance" suffers from a confusion between governance responsibilities and governance structures. The responsibilities of governance include developing policy to ensure the survival and well-being of an organization or, in Kovner's view, "the making or not making of important decisions and the related distribution of authority and legitimacy to make decisions" (Kovner, 1990). The structures of governance refer to the roles and composition of boards of trustees and other groups charged with making policy in the organization. Governance in this sense is usually contrasted with management, which administers the operations of the organization. Effective governance requires both organizational strategies and structures.

In hospitals, the relationship between the responsibilities and structures of governance has been complicated by the complex overlap in the roles of boards of trustees, medical staff, and administration. In many hospitals, policy setting is carried out by all three groups rather than being solely the responsibility of the board. Similarly, management activities (the enactment of policy) are also often shared. Thus, unlike "corporate" models of governance, which view policy-making functions as the sole purview of boards of trustees, hospital governance responsibilities have traditionally been divided among several constituencies within the organization.

THE CHANGING ENVIRONMENT OF HOSPITAL BOARDS

There is a considerable literature which discusses the limited effectiveness of governing structures in hospitals and, in particular, the failure of boards of trustees to develop a strategic orientation or assume a policy-making role. (For example, see Delbecq and Gill, 1988; Griffith, 1988; Kovner, 1990; Shortell, 1989; Umbdenstock and Hageman, 1990).

In Canada, as in the United States, many hospital boards have served either as forums for reconciling medical staff and administrative views on hospital policy, or as passive recipients of decisions made elsewhere. Despite the legal accountability of boards of trustees envisioned in provincial legislation, few hospitals in Canada have had strong boards capable of discharging their governance responsibilities.

For much of the post-World War Two period the limited effectiveness of hospital boards had few serious consequences. In the context of rapidly growing resources for health care and a policy consensus which supported the expansion of hospital activities, weak hospital boards and disjointed governance responsibilities had little impact, since administrators, medical staffs, and boards shared similar goals. Where differences emerged, resources usually permitted pursuing multiple, and sometimes conflicting, goals.

The consequences of failing to align governance structures with governance responsibilities in hospitals and the need to develop effective governing boards have become more critical as hospitals have experienced greater environmental stresses. Pressures are mounting within hospitals as they attempt to meet severe demands while the growth in health expenditures is constrained. Although funding for hospitals has grown rapidly in the last 20 years, most provincial governments have signalled a determination to limit this growth. Hospitals will continue to face the demands of an aging population, the pressures to acquire new technologies, and the rising costs of hospital labor, but they will have to meet these challenges without substantial new resources. New program priorities will compete with old commitments for resources, and conflicts will develop as professional groups are asked to abandon traditional roles in favor of more cost-effective patterns of service delivery. Shortages in hospital funding will force hospital boards to deal with difficult financial decisions as well as to address a variety of other issues resulting from the need to rationalize operations.

Although funding pressures will require greater financial creativity from board members, most trustees are at least familiar with financial issues. An equally important issue, the growing board mandate for assuring quality of care, requires that trustees assume responsibilities which, to date, they have largely avoided. New accreditation requirements assign boards of trustees the responsibility for establishing review systems to monitor and improve care. Many medical-legal experts believe that the Canadian courts are moving toward the principle of vicarious liability, breaking down the traditional distinction between the physician's liability for medical care and the hospital's liability for the quality of hospital services. In the context of increasing public concern that health services attain the highest quality possible, hospital boards have found themselves with the responsibility of assuring that quality review systems are capable of assessing the care of physicians and other health professionals, and that appropriate mechanisms for improving deficiencies are in place (Prichard, 1990; Scott, 1983).

Hospitals also need more effective hospital governance as they address their changing roles in the broader health care system. These pressures require strategic responses which balance competing priorities. For example, hospitals are under pressure to shift health care services from institutional settings to ambulatory or community-based programs and to coordinate their services with a wide range of other providers more effectively. Such initiatives assume that ambulatory programs will be less expensive and that community-based care will help to maintain patients in their homes and prevent future use of expensive inpatient services (Ontario Premier's Council on Health Strategy, 1989). At the same time, however, hospitals have been criticized for failing to expand their services to meet greater demands for such specialty care as coronary artery bypass surgery. With these conflicting pressures, making strategic decisions which enable hospitals to use their resources most effectively requires clear vision and a sophisticated understanding of the increasingly complex health policy environment.

Hospital boards also face increasing pressure from their communities to provide health care services which meet the evolving character of those communities. Members of many ethnic communities wish to see hospitals alter care strategies to incorporate the alternative health care teachings and practices preferred by those groups. They also want hospitals to provide mechanisms for local groups to influence hospital decisions and make them more responsive to community views on health care needs.

Finally, boards are being compelled to monitor the effectiveness of hospital management. Traditionally, most boards have relied upon CEOs for their understanding of hospital performance, and the CEO has had considerable influence on board decisions, including the selection of new board members. Faced with the new pressures of accountability for financial performance and quality of care and with the need to develop a strategic vision which may significantly alter existing hospital roles, trustees are being advised to develop procedures for a regular, comprehensive evaluation of the CEO, and are holding CEOs responsible for hospital performance. CEO turnover has increased considerably in the last decade in the U.S. (American Hospital Association, 1988) and probably in Canada as well. Although turnover may reflect board ineffectiveness as much as poor CEO performance (Kovner, 1990), its increasing rate is creating greater expectations that boards establish fair evaluation processes and, when necessary, carefully manage the selection of a new executive. Some boards have found the transition to this new relationship with the CEO difficult.

POLICY ISSUES

Much of the policy discussion on governance deals with subsidiary rather than root questions. Several of the recent provincial hospital association reports have focused on the questions of "Who should the members of boards be?" and "How should they be selected?" Policy makers as well have focused on changing board composition to deal with broad organizational and health system problems and make hospitals more responsive to constituencies not traditionally represented on boards. Several years ago, Quebec legislation was altered to require increased representation by consumers and practitioners on hospital boards (Eakin, 1984). More recently, in Ontario, government regulatory changes have placed nurses on hospital board committees as a means of addressing the problems of job dissatisfaction, perceived powerlessness, and high turnover among hospital nursing staffs. The possibility that the Ontario government may initiate broad-ranging changes to board structure and roles in the redrafting of the *Public Hospitals Act* has led the Ontario Hospital Association to articulate its continuing support of voluntary hospital boards with membership largely composed of individuals elected from the local community (Ontario Hospital Association, 1989).

Although these issues of governance structure are important, they should follow such more fundamental considerations as roles and accountability. From this perspective, the key questions are: "What is the role of the board?" and "What is the relationship of the board to its internal constituencies and to the larger community?"

The traditional role of the board focused on attracting resources and maintaining the legitimacy of the hospital and its prestige in the community. Much of the management literature continues to highlight these external relationships and the so-called "boundary spanning" function (Morlock, Nathanson, and Alexander, 1988), but there appears to be no consensus on the appropriate division of responsibilities between boards and management. Umbdenstock (1983) suggests that the board has the responsibility for deciding on strategic direction and that management has the responsibility for implementing that direction. Others (e.g., Mintzberg, 1983) believe that the governing board should oversee and approve strategic direction, but that management should establish strategy.

The board's roles have important implications for its relationships with both internal and external constituencies. Relationships to community are obviously crucial, since this is one of the traditional roles of boards and such relationships are still important for raising funds and maintaining public support. Communities are becoming increasingly complex, however, and the traditional manner of choosing board members may no longer assure adequate representation. Hospitals must begin to develop alternative means to relate to their communities so the board is not seen as the only channel.

Board relationships with professionals also remains a significant issue. Considerable attention has been generated in both Ontario and Quebec by discussion about whether physicians and other professionals should be members of hospital boards. Relationships between hospitals and physicians have been in a state of flux for some years, particularly as administrators have developed physician manpower planning and utilization management strategies in an effort to improve their management of hospital expenditures. Some of the anxiety about the departure of physicians from boards is linked to status and power issues. However, for many hospitals the inadequacies of the medical staff organization as a management structure have reinforced the role of the board in managing medical staff issues. Organizational structures which integrate physicians into hospital management, or other innovative relationships between hospital organizations and physician groups, will be required if governing bodies are to become policy making forums.

Regionalization and the creation of regional boards have been important themes in many of the provincial reports issued in the last two years. New legislation in Quebec would give many of the responsibilities of existing hospital boards to regional councils. The proposals put forward in, among other provinces, Alberta and Nova Scotia, are less radical but would likely require a rebalancing of the relationships between individual facilities, regional bodies, and central government agencies. Although few groups oppose the goal of improving integration and coordination of health care services, there remains considerable dispute about the mechanisms for achieving this goal. A fundamental issue for hospital governance, therefore, lies in the division of responsibility between boards established for individual organizations and boards accountable for many organizations or for defined populations.

A related issue is the accountability of hospital governance to government and how that accountability is discharged. How will government deal with conflicts between the missions of individual institutions? What appeal will there be for individual hospitals that contest the allocations or strategic plans developed by regional bodies? To what extent should government have the authority to replace boards either temporarily or permanently? These questions require decisions about allocating accountability between different authorities in ways that serve the public interest.

These policy issues are important not only in Canada, but also in other jurisdictions. Two examples may be particularly useful: the multi-hospital system governance models in the U.S. and the developing self-governing hospital trusts model currently being discussed in the U.K. In looking at governance structures in these jurisdictions, it is important to note how they interact with regional bodies and other health providers, how they affect the roles of administrators and physicians and, perhaps most important, their impact on the effectiveness of health care organizations.

HOSPITAL GOVERNANCE IN THE U.S.

Kovner (1990) notes three different theoretical perspectives on the role of hospital boards which have been applied to hospital governance in the U.S. The first perspective sees the board as a "community steward" serving the local community and focusing on improving the health status of its residents (Seay and Sigmond, 1989). The second perspective builds on Shortell's (1989) vision of the hospital board as a strategic decision maker. In this view, board members need to develop skills as risk takers, strategic managers, and evaluators and to be experts in crucial policy areas such as marketing or vertical integration. The third view sees boards as rational advisors to management: board members improve decision-making processes and collaborate with managers and medical staff to develop better planning and financial processes. Although Kovner believes that these models are not necessarily mutually exclusive, their different perspectives suggest very distinctive accountability structures and relationships.

Variations in the perspectives on hospital roles stem in part from the considerable differences in structure and operations of U.S. hospitals depending on their ownership, teaching status, and affiliation in multi-hospital systems. Different forms of hospital governance have developed, for example: (1) independent non-profit community hospitals, (2) public non-profit urban hospital systems, (3) corporate (private) multi-hospital systems, (4) teaching hospital-university board structures, (5) religious hospital chains, and (6) government hospitals. Research studies indicate that even within these categories, the nature of hospital board structure, composition, and influence will vary systematically as a result of a number of hospital characteristics and external influences. Hospital boards must therefore balance the needs of particular types of institutions with local conditions and corporate status (Fennell and Alexander, 1989).

Given the increasing concentration of hospital ownership in for-profit multi-hospital corporations, and the considerable research focused on examining the structure of governance in these corporations, it is particularly worthwhile to examine how these organizations address governance issues. Governance is a crucial issue, since hospitals in multi-hospital organizations must be responsive to local needs but also participate in system goals and philosophy (Alexander and Schroer, 1985). These multi-hospital systems must decide how centralized or decentralized control should be over policy decisions. In a survey of 159 multi-hospital systems, Alexander and Morlock (1985) found six different types of relationships between the system-wide governance structure and the structures of the individual hospitals within the system:

- Both a system-wide board and separate local hospital governing boards (47%);
- A system-wide governing board only (27%);
- A system wide governing board with separate hospital advisory boards (14%);
- System-wide boards, regional boards, and individual hospital boards (4%); and
- System-wide and regional boards with no governing or advisory boards at the individual hospital level (2%).

A growing number of U.S. hospitals, particularly those in multi-hospital systems, have altered their boards so that their structure and operation resemble those of boards in private industry (Shortell, 1989; Delbecq and Gill, 1988). These "corporate" style boards are smaller than traditional hospital "philanthropic" style boards, are more likely to draw their members from business and professional backgrounds, and tend to focus more on effective decision-making and strategic planning. Shortell (1989) notes that the adoption of a corporate board model in hospitals has meant that many of the traditional community relations aspects of boards are being delegated to community advisory panels. These panels also serve as new locations for those board members who are not included in the smaller (and more business expertise-oriented) hospital boards.

Findings of a study by Alexander, Morlock, and Gifford (1988) show that boards in corporately restructured hospitals are more likely to conform to the corporate than to the philanthropic model. However, governance in these restructured hospitals has not moved completely to this model. Board size, in particular, has not been affected; however, if the number of board members was to be reduced by attrition, effects might not have been discernible at the time of the study. Alexander and his colleagues also speculate that a hybrid board form unique to hospitals may result from corporate restructuring. Hospital boards, for example, may require large numbers of members to continue to fulfil some of the traditional functions of philanthropic boards – constituency representation, public legitimacy, and linkage to key resources in the environment. These functions may remain important, regardless of the corporate form. This argument also explains why boards of corporately restructured hospitals are no more likely than boards of non-restructured hospitals to put limits on the numbers of terms members serve, since such turnover may defeat continuing board needs.

Changes in hospital relationships to corporate decision-making bodies have also had important consequences for the roles of CEOs and medical staff in hospital decision-making. Analysis of American Hospital Association data by Morlock, Alexander, and Hunter (1985) found that CEOs were more likely to have increased influence on decision-making in multi-hospital systems than in independent hospitals. At the same time, physicians were less likely to participate in governance activities in multi-hospital systems. Hospitals governed by boards accountable to higher authority were also more likely to monitor medical staff functions through non-physician board member participation on medical staff executive, quality assurance, and utilization committees.

In another study, which examined the locus of decision-making (at the corporate or local boards) for 15 decision-making areas, Alexander and Schroer (1985) found considerable variation in responsibilities for different decision-making areas. Corporate board power was retained in resource allocation and strategic planning decisions about assets, formation of new companies, and changes in the bylaws of system hospitals. Corporate boards also maintained significant control over the appointment of local board members and hospital CEOs. Local boards had their strongest influence on decisions related to budget formation, medical staff privileges, service changes at the hospital level, and other hospital strategic planning issues. These researchers also found that investor-based systems tended to be less centralized in their decision-making than other systems, particularly the secular not-for-profit ones. These latter systems, however, were more likely to be geographically concentrated, thus facilitating central control and coordination. Overall, older systems were less centralized than newer ones, suggesting that with time, decision-making responsibilities were increasingly delegated to local boards.

Attempts to investigate the impact of boards on other measures of effectiveness have yielded few significant findings. Kaufman et al (1979) found no linkage between measures of board size, composition, diversity, and influence on hospital efficiency or quality of care, although they did find that the more trustees knew about hospital operations, the less efficient the hospital was. Morlock (1979) studied the relationship of trustees' influence on hospital wide decisions and quality of care and found a positive correlation between quality of care and the board chairman's level of activity and influence, but suggested that this relationship was indirect and might be the result of tighter financial controls.

In general, the large number of endogenous and exogenous variables which are likely to impact on quality of care and financial performance make the impact of board characteristics on these measures difficult to assess. Indeed, Fennell and Alexander (1989) argue that, given the current status of outcome measures and the underdevelopment of research on effectiveness, attention to this issue is premature.

HOSPITAL GOVERNANCE IN GREAT BRITAIN

Changes proposed in the 1989 White Paper on the National Health Service, *Working for Patients* (U.K. Secretaries of State for Health, 1989b), do not augur for major administrative changes to the NHS, but focus instead on changing its managerial and professional cultures. Although details of the changes and the process of implementing the White Paper proposals are still being worked out, the original White Paper combines two major thrusts: first, it emphasizes the strengthening of managerial authority and challenging of medical autonomy, and second, it attempts to create internal competition between providers, giving patients greater choice in their selection of providers (Day and Klein, 1989; Robinson, 1989).

The reform does not alter the dominance of the Department of Health, but rather strengthens the line of managerial hierarchy running from central management of the NHS through the Regional and District Authorities. For hospitals, however, the major thrust of the reform is to move the NHS toward a separation of payment and provider responsibilities. Individual health authorities will be responsible for buying appropriate services for their populations within a given budget allocation. These services will be produced locally by NHS units or purchased from other health authorities or the private sector.

To stimulate the creation of such an "internal market", NHS hospitals will be allowed to opt for status as independent self-governing trusts. These trusts will determine the pay and working conditions of their staff (rather than being bound by national agreements as is currently the case). In addition, the trusts will be free to borrow on capital markets and will be able to retain their operating surpluses rather than remit them to the health authorities. Initially, the trusts will be single hospitals, but in the long term they may develop into more integrated health care providers of considerable size (Day and Klein, 1989; U.K. Secretaries of State for Health, 1989a).

The original proposal suggested that the self-governing hospitals would start operating in 1991 and would initially number about 200. These would all be medium to large acute care hospitals. More recent estimates indicate that fewer hospitals will make the initial transition to self-governing trusts. No one knows to what extent independent hospitals will become the norm, or to what degree self-governing trusts will be free to set their own strategic directions. This change does, however, augur an increase in the operating autonomy of at least some units of the NHS which had been to this point tightly bound by highly centralized authority and heavily bureaucratized policy directions.

In an article on the White Paper reforms, Day and Klein (1989) predicted that the principal beneficiaries of the new hospital status will be financial and managerial consultants and accountants, that is, those, as they see it, who profess expertise about efficiency, even if they do not necessarily add to it.

If carried out in more than a token fashion, the new reforms could further the long term goal of decentralization of considerable control to the local level. Such decentralization has been the object of earlier reforms, but has been resisted by the inertia of heavily centralized decision-making structures. The true measure of autonomy granted the new self-governing trusts will be seen only in practice, and this autonomy will be counter-balanced by the risks the trusts will take to assure their continued operation in a more competitive environment. The shift of reporting relationships for the trusts to the Regional Health Authorities from the District Health Authorities is one measure of the decreasing controls placed upon them.

The reforms also attempt to strike a balance between consumer demands for more services and the budgetary constraints of the NHS. Whether the reforms will lead to new efficiencies or will simply permit the government to transfer responsibility for program decisions to local levels is still another matter to be decided. At least some observers suggest that the move to create self-governing hospitals adroitly allows the NHS to pass the political pressures of wage demands and increased service needs to local units.

The British proposals suggest that the new boards of self-governing trusts will be composed of 10 members – five executive members of the authority and five non-executive members representing the community. The chair of the board will be appointed by the health secretary. Both the large number of insider directors and the relatively small size of the board reflect a pattern more similar to North American corporate boards than to traditional voluntary hospital boards.

The government has indicated that it wishes to grant the boards a substantial amount of freedom to run their own affairs. However, since in the short run the government will continue to be responsible for any losses incurred by the trusts, and since at least some observers believe that this situation will continue even after the initial stage, it is clear that the board will be faced with balancing its new freedom with a broader public accountability.

These recent NHS reforms provide an interesting counterpoint to current Canadian policy thrusts. While Canadian governments are examining how to link hospitals into area or regional planning authorities, the NHS is attempting to devolve those powers from the Regional and District Authorities to individual hospitals or groups of hospitals. These processes, although beginning in the British case from a heavily centralized system and in the Canadian from a system with centralized funding but largely autonomous providers, appear to be based on several similar health planning principles: first, that greater efficiencies are created by delegating control to local providers over production decisions, and second, that intermediary, regional bodies which mediate between centralized policy agencies and local providers are a necessary component of effective systems of care. Such regional bodies are best suited to assess local needs and coordinate the delivery of services of local providers.

CONCLUSION

The developments in governance structures and policies in the United States and Great Britain and the discussions now under way in various Canadian provinces demonstrate a number of similarities:

1. There is an increasing concern with inter-organizational forms and linkages balancing local and regional interests. In Canada, coordinating and resource allocation organizations such as DHCs in Ontario or the CRSSS in Quebec will likely assume greater powers. In the U.S., the integration stems from the development of multi-organizational structures such as the large for-profit hospital chains. The British reforms reflect innovations from a more centralized system, where self-governing hospitals are intended to increase responsiveness to local conditions, but remain accountable through the bureaucratic structure of the NHS. It is still too early to know whether the development of competition among providers will lead to strategic alliances or more formal linkages between hospitals in the U.K.

2. Continuing ascendance of health services administrators in the development of institutional policies is likely in all three jurisdictions.

3. A corresponding reduction in the power of physicians, both as individuals and as members of organized medical staffs, on the governance of health care organizations and the patterns of health care delivery in communities will also occur. Paradoxically, physicians may have greater opportunities to influence the decision-making of hospitals through program management and other administrative roles. These avenues to power may in the long run provide physicians with greater influence on organizational policy than did the traditional medical staff organization.

4. All three health care systems appear to be balancing the roles of individual provider organizations, regional or multi-institutional agencies, and central government. The differences in the roles of government in health care in Canada, the U.S., and the U.K. and the structure of their health care systems mean that such changes are developing in quite different ways, but there are interesting similarities in the emergence of coordinating bodies and the balancing of government regulation with market forces.

If the changes in Britain hold, there will be a diminution of the direct government role in the management of the NHS, and a shift to reliance on pressures generated by the creation of internal markets for services. Regional Health Authorities will continue to maintain their role in coordinating local services and health policy, but will be unable to exert the detailed administrative controls District Health Authorities have wielded. Self-governing trusts will develop more autonomy to identify and serve local needs and manage their affairs.

In the U.S., the regulatory impact of the federal government on hospitals has grown over the last decade. Hospital prospective payment policies for Medicare patients have altered the markets and structures of hospital services. Formulating outcome measures and assessments of hospital quality of care will create additional responses. The development of large hospital chains in the U.S. may be seen, in part, as a means of buffering the impacts of these financial and quality regulatory initiatives. Multi-hospital systems provide a resource base for initiating financial control and quality improvement initiatives, and the corporate offices of these systems have become intermediary and coordinating bodies for individual hospitals facing these external demands. Governance responsibilities for members of multi-institutional systems have shifted toward corporate offices in dealing with broader strategic issues, while local hospitals retain responsibilities for decisions on budgets and service changes required. Given the geographic spread of individual hospitals in multi-institutional systems, only a few systems (such as the Henry Ford Health System in Detroit) have sufficient concentration in any market to attempt to serve as a "regional coordinating body". But such coordination efforts may be served in other ways, such as the emerging efforts between individual hospitals and other agencies in a number of communities, including Cleveland, Ohio, Rochester, New York, and Kingsport, Tennessee.

In Canada, there is still only limited evidence that provincial governments will act on provincial commission recommendations to create regional bodies which take on major strategic and operational roles for health care. As noted above, however, the Quebec government tabled legislation in the spring of 1991 which would greatly increase the powers of regional councils over local hospitals and greatly diminish the operating authority of local institutions. Discussions in Ontario have focused on re-examining the roles of DHCs and, to a lesser extent, their relationships to government and hospitals. While the shape of future hospital governance remains to be decided, there is considerable interest in many provinces in creating more effective regional planning mechanisms which will advise on or, in some provinces, manage the allocation of resources across the hospitals in specific geographical areas.

In all three health systems, then, there has been a movement toward greater coordination and the development of governance arrangements which link individual hospitals into larger networks or (as in the British case) provide a mechanism to unbundle a formerly undifferentiated service delivery system. The era (in Canada and the U.S.) when hospital governance was a function of individual boards (acting with administration and medical staffs) appears to be evolving into more complex patterns which balance local institutional interests with broader health care needs and the regional service delivery network.

REFERENCES

Alexander J, Morlock L: Multi-institutional arrangements: relationships between governing boards and hospital chief executive officers. *Health Services Research* 19(6 Part 1):675-699, 1985.

Alexander JA, Morlock LL, Gifford B: The effects of corporate restructuring on hospital policy-making. *Health Services Research* 23(2):311-338, 1988.

Alexander JA, Morrisey MA, Shortell S: Effects of competition, regulation and corporatization on hospital-physician relationships. *Journal of Health and Social Behavior* 27:220-235, 1986.

Alexander JA, Schroer K: Governance in multi-hospital systems: an assessment of decision-making responsibility. *Hospital and Health Services Administration* 30:9-20, 1985.

American Hospital Association: *Hospital Statistics.* Chicago: American Hospital Association Publishing, 1988.

British Columbia Health Association: Models of Health Care Governance (mimeo). Victoria, B.C.: BCHA, 1988.

Croll K: Results of a Hospital Board Survey (mimeo). Fredericton, N.B.: New Brunswick Hospital Association, 1988.

Day P, Klein R: The politics of modernization: Britain's National Health Service in the 1980s. *Milbank Quarterly* 67(1):1-34, 1989.

Day P, Klein R: *Accountabilities: Five Public Services.* London and New York: Tavistock, 1987.

Day P, Klein R: Central accountability and local decision-making: towards a new NHS. *British Medical Journal* 290:1676-1678, 1985.

Delbecq AL, Gill SL: Developing strategic direction for governing boards. *Hospital and Health Services Administration* 33(1):25-35, 1988.

Eakin JM: Survival of the fittest? The democratization of hospital administration in Quebec. *International Journal of Health Services* 14(3):397-412, 1984.

Fennell ML, Alexander JA: Governing boards and profound organizational change in hospitals. *Medical Care Review* 46(2):157-187, 1989.

Griffith JR: Voluntary hospitals: are trustees the solution? *Hospital and Health Services Administration* 33(3):295-310, 1988.

Institute of Health Services Management, Healthcare Financial Management Association, KPMG Peat Marwick McLintock: *Making Contracts Work: The Practical Implications.* London, 1990.

Jabbari D: Laying down the law. *The Health Service Journal* 100:1180-1181, 1990.

Kaufman K et al: The effect of board composition and structure on hospital performance. *Hospital and Health Services Administration* 24 (Winter):37-62, 1979.

Klein R: *The Politics of the National Health Service,* second edition. London: Longman, 1989.

Knudson T: Models of board governance. *Hospital Trustee* March/April, 1990.

Kovner AR: Improving hospital board effectiveness: an update. *Frontiers of Health Services Management* 6(3):3-27, 1990.

Kovner AR: Improving the effectiveness of hospital governing boards. *Frontiers of Health Services Management* 2(1):4-33, 1986.

Manitoba Health Organizations: *A Guide to Self-evaluation of Your Governing Board.* Winnipeg: Manitoba Health Organizations, 1988.

Mintzberg H: *Power In and Around Organizations.* Englewood Cliffs, N.J.: Prentice-Hall, 1983.

Morlock L: Decision-making Patterns and Hospital Performance: Relationships between Case Mix, Admissions Rates and the Influence of Trustees, Administration and Medical Staff in 17 Acute Care General Hospitals. Paper presented to the annual meeting of the Association of University Programs in Health Administration, Toronto, May 1979.

Morlock LL, Alexander JA: Models of governance in multihospital systems: implications for hospital and system-level decision-making. *Medical Care* 24:1118-1135, 1986.

Morlock LL, Alexander JA, Hunter HM: Formal relationships among governing boards, CEOs and medical staffs in independent and systems hospitals. *Medical Care* 23(10):1193-1213, 1985.

Morlock LL, Nathanson CA, Alexander JA: Authority, power and influence. In: Shortell SM, Kaluzny AD (eds.): *Health Care Management: A Text in Organization Theory and Behavior* (second edition). New York: John Wiley and Sons, 1988, pp. 265-300.

Mott BJF: *Trusteeship and the Future of Community Hospitals.* Chicago: American Hospital Association, 1984.

Ontario Hospital Association: *Preliminary Submission on The Review of the Public Hospitals Act.* Don Mills, Ontario: OHA Publications, 1989.

Ontario Premier's Council on Health Strategy: *From Vision to Action: Report of the Health Care System Committee.* Toronto: Ontario Government Publications, 1989.

Pfeffer J: *Power in Organizations.* Marshfield, Massachusetts: Pitman, 1981.

Pfeffer J: Size, composition and function of hospital boards of directors: a study of organization and environment linkages. *Administrative Science Quarterly* 18:349-364, 1973.

Prichard JRS: *Liability and Compensation in Health Care. A Report to the Conference of Deputy Ministers of Health of the Federal/Provincial/Territorial Review on Liability and Compensation Issues in Health Care.* Toronto: University of Toronto Press, 1990.

Provan KG: Organizational and decision unit characteristics and board influence in independent versus multihospital system-affiliated hospitals. *Journal of Health and Social Behavior* 29:239-252, 1988.

Rehm JL, Alexander JA: Governing board-medical staff relations in the 80s. *Hospital Trustee* 39:24-27, 1986.

Robinson R: Self-governing hospitals. *British Medical Journal* 198:819-821, 1989.

Scott G: The Dubin Report: issues for hospital management. *Health Management Forum* 4 (Winter):3-12, 1983.

Seay JD, Sigmond RM: Community benefit standards for hospitals: perceptions and performance. *Frontiers of Health Services Management* 5:3-39, 1989.

Shapiro IS: Corporate governance. In: Williams HM, Shapiro IS (eds.): *Power and Accountability, The Changing Role of the Corporate Board of Directors.* New York: Carnegie-Mellon University Press, 1979, pp. 9-31.

Shortell S: New directions in hospital governance. *Hospital and Health Services Administration* 34(1):7-23, 1989.

Sinclair D: The Shape of Hospital Boards. Notes for a Speech to the Ontario Hospital Association, Toronto, Ontario, 1990.

Starkweather D: Hospital board power. *Health Services Management Research* 1(2):74-86, 1988.

Trypuc JM: *Hospital Trusteeship in Ontario.* Don Mills: Ontario Hospital Association, 1988.

U.K. Secretaries of State for Health: *Self-governing Hospitals.* Working Paper, no. 1. London: Her Majesty's Stationery Office, 1989a.

U.K. Secretaries of State for Health: *Working for Patients.* London: Her Majesty's Stationery Office, 1989b.

Umbdenstock RJ: *So You're on the Hospital Board,* second edition. Chicago: American Hospital Association, 1983.

Umbdenstock RJ, Hageman WM: The five critical areas for effective governance of not-for-profit hospitals. *Hospital and Health Services Administration* 35(4):481-492, 1990.

Wilson C: The board of the future. *Vision* (Ontario Hospital Association) (Summer):27-29, 1990.

Wilson CRM: *Governing with Distinction: Evaluation Models for Hospital Boards.* Ottawa: Canadian Hospital Association, 1988.

Wilson C: Roles for an effective board: a five finger exercise. *Hospital Trustee* 8 (January/February):16-17; 8 (March/April):6-7, 1984.

Witt JA: *Building a Better Hospital Board.* Ann Arbor, MI: Health Administration Press, 1987.

Working Party on Alternative Delivery and Funding of Health Services, Institute of Health Services Management: *Final Report.* London: Institute of Health Services Management, 1988.

INNOVATIVE FUND RAISING: THE ST. MICHAEL'S HOSPITAL HEALTH CENTRE

George H. Pink
Raisa B. Deber
Eric Aserlind
University of Toronto

Joe N. Lavoie
St. Michael's Hospital

INTRODUCTION

Until comparatively recently, most health service organisations in Canada did not seek funds from many sources besides government. However, because of limitations in funding, many Canadian hospitals have been seeking innovative methods of financing capital projects, new expensive technologies, and new programs and services. This study investigated innovative financing by Canadian health services organisations, defining innovative financing as any strategy, method, or technique used by a hospital to raise revenue for operating or capital purposes beyond the budgeted funds provided by government. The study consisted of a literature review and a case study of the St. Michael's Hospital Health Centre (SMHHC) in Toronto.

DESCRIPTION OF THE STUDY

The study included five components:
1. The Canadian health services management literature was critically examined to identify the state of existing knowledge about innovative financing in Canada.
2. The methods and techniques of innovative financing were analysed to identify similarities and differences and develop criteria for classification.
3. The case study described and analysed the management, decision-making, negotiation, marketing, financial, legal, and production processes that led to establishment of the SMHHC.
4. The case study then described and analysed the management, decision-making, marketing, financial, legal, and production outcomes of the SMHHC after one year of operation.
5. Finally, the findings from the literature review and the case study were synthesised to determine what internal and external conditions must exist for the identified types of innovative financing to be successful, and what criteria are important in determining whether a particular type of innovative financing will be successful for a particular hospital.

LITERATURE REVIEW

The innovative approaches discussed in the health care literature since 1980 were classified into six areas.

1. CLINICAL/DIAGNOSTIC INSURED SERVICES

This category includes radiology, laboratory, prosthetics, and other services for which hospitals are reimbursed on an output basis by a provincial health insurance plan. Much of the American literature has examined diversification into clinical and diagnostic insured services, such as outpatient surgery, freestanding emergency rooms, screening clinics, satellite clinics, urgent care facilities, and skilled nursing facilities. In Canada, however, there is little of this literature, except for some descriptions of hospital laboratories that have been able to use excess capacity to perform external work.

2. CLINICAL/DIAGNOSTIC NON-INSURED SERVICES

Much attention in the Canadian literature appears to have been focused on generating revenue by offering health services not reimbursed by provincial health insurance programs. Examples of these activities are elective cosmetic surgery, wellness centres, physical examinations for executives, lifestyle clinics (such as smoking cessation, fitness, stress, weight loss), nutrition counselling, inhalation therapy consulting, osteopathy clinics, sports medicine clinics, home oxygen, and occupational health services.

3. HOTEL SERVICES

Hotel services include support functions such as laundry, housekeeping, and food services. Examples cited in the literature were athletic facilities for staff, candlelight dinners for new parents, differential room charges, hostel facilities for (non-inpatient) out-of-town visitors, and meeting and conference room rental.

4. RETAIL

In addition to traditional hospital retail operations such as gift shops run by volunteers, the literature cited banking services, bakeries, beauty shops, car washes, flower shops, print and copy shops, pubs, retail pharmacies, and hospital uniform sales shops. Some hospitals, such as Ottawa Civic Hospital, have a retail mall that houses various retail services.

5. ADMINISTRATION

Some hospitals have tried their hands at contract management. Several hospitals have attempted to develop and market medical computer software, such as medical record-keeping systems. The Royal Victoria Hospital in Montreal entered into a joint venture to provide international health care consulting.

6. FINANCIAL

Some revenue generation activities, such as investments and sale and leasebacks, are paper transactions only. Some hospitals have generated income by leasing property. For example, in Winnipeg, a hospital leased out an operating room to doctors who needed space for day surgery.

GENERAL STRATEGIES

In addition to specific revenue generating activities, much of the literature deals with general strategies such as diversification.

THE ST. MICHAEL'S HOSPITAL HEALTH CENTRE

St. Michael's Hospital (SMH) is a tertiary care hospital located in downtown Toronto, Ontario. Founded in 1892, it maintains its role as the flagship institution of the Sisters of St. Joseph; its affiliation with the University of Toronto as one of 19 teaching hospitals in Ontario also means a continuing role as an important teaching and research institution.

The St. Michael's Hospital Health Centre (SMHHC) occupies a 9,264 square foot (853 m²) site approximately 300 feet southeast of the existing south wing of the main hospital. At the time the case study was written, SMHHC had the following occupants:

First floor – Elevator lobby, security desk, a non-hospital retail pharmacy, and space (currently vacant) for a deli-style takeout food shop.

Second floor – Rehabilitation services examining rooms, therapy rooms, and several offices.

Third floor – Family practice reception and waiting areas, medical records, doctors' offices, and examining rooms.

Fourth floor – Family practice and three programs related to family health – a walk-in breast-screening clinic, offices for the obstetrics-gynaecology department, and a travel clinic specialising in preventive care and vaccinations for travellers to overseas areas.

Fifth floor – The Women's Health Centre – a collection of hospital-run programs concerned with health maintenance, disease prevention, and treatment of health problems specific to women.

Sixth floor – Canada's first walk-in nutrition and risk-modification centre and the diagnostic imaging department, which provided professional services to the clinical departments in the building.

Seventh floor – Hospital administration, including finance, accounting, and human resources.

Eighth floor – Psychiatric daycare and outpatient facility, nuclear medicine (specifically, the bone mineral densitometer), and the department of occupational and environmental health.

Ninth floor – Nephrology and urology in a combination of office practices and clinics. As an adjunct to these departments, the offices for the renal transplant centre were located on the same floor.

REASONS FOR ESTABLISHING ST. MICHAEL'S HOSPITAL HEALTH CENTRE
Space

As an outgrowth of a comprehensive examination of the hospital's strategic planning, a study performed by a consulting group had concluded that, even with the planned completion of a new hospital wing, the hospital would still have a substantial space requirement deficit. The SMHHC building presented an opportunity to acquire space for existing and new services.

Revenue Generation

SMH identified three opportunities to generate revenue. First, by increasing the volume of certain insured services, the hospital could maximise Ministry of Health growth funding revenue. Second, revenue could be generated by providing non-insured health services paid by the patients/clients themselves or by a third party such as private insurance or employers. Third, revenue could be generated through ancillary services such as parking and leasing space to a pharmacy, a deli shop, and private practice physicians.

THE CATALYST

The catalyst was Joe Lavoie, then Vice President of Administration and Finance at Saint Michael's Hospital, who saw the opportunities inherent in the SMHHC.

LESSONS LEARNED
RISK

Assessment of risk is critical. In its broadest sense, risk takes two forms: *financial risk*, the variance of net revenue induced by leverage, and *business* or *economic risk*, the variance of net revenue induced by the general economic conditions of the industry. Assessment of business risk requires answering questions such as: Are we going into the right business? Is the market ready for us? What do we do if we don't succeed with this effort? How do we get out if we have to? Assessment of financial risk requires answering questions such as: How will we meet our loan payments if interest rates change? In general, assessing business risk means asking where we might go wrong, and assessing financial risk means asking how much it will cost us to go wrong.

If SMH had merely leased the space in a building owned by another party instead of purchasing a building, the hospital would be carrying very little financial risk. By purchasing the building, the hospital has assumed financial risk because, regardless of the revenue generated by SMHHC, SMH must pay debt service. Of course, in return for assuming this risk the hospital, rather than a third party, reaps any financial benefits such as capital appreciation and net revenue.

REVENUE GENERATING VS. NON-REVENUE GENERATING PROGRAMS

Originally, SMHHC was supposed to include only programs that would be revenue generating and self-supporting. However, among the final building occupants were programs that could not meet this requirement. These programs were selected because they were adjuncts of other programs selected, or because they were high priority programs. An example is the family practice program which, although currently not self-supporting, is believed by the hospital to be important in fulfilling its community services mission. At the same time, family practice may also be a "loss leader", a program that operates at a loss but brings in patients to other programs that are profitable.

RELATIONSHIP WITH MEDICAL STAFF

Revenue generation activities may change the relationship between a hospital and its physicians. For example, if a hospital decides to lease space in a new building to doctors who were previously given office space free of charge, in addition to the traditional professional relationship there now exists a landlord/tenant business relationship. In other types of revenue generation activities, physicians may need to be educated about the activity's operations and their role in the activity.

EVALUATION

Ongoing business evaluation of revenue generating activities is very important. Without this process, the tendency is to look only at the service aspects and conclude that the program is operationally successful although, in fact, it may be financially unsuccessful. Financial and marketing evaluation are particularly important.

MARKET ANALYSIS

Before introducing a new product, companies usually undertake market research to ascertain what the consumer wants, how to package it, and how to price it. Hospitals contemplating revenue generation activities should follow the same process. Targeting a specific market can avoid inappropriate product choices. Market analysis can help decide how best to attract patients/clients.

FINANCIAL RESOURCES

Most revenue generating efforts should probably be viewed as long term investments. Treated as such, hospitals must have the financial resources to sustain the operation and growth of these programs during the start up phase when expenses may be high and revenues low.

SMH arranged its financing prior to negotiating for the SMHHC building. This allowed the hospital to bargain from a solid financial position and allowed the Board of Directors to make informed decisions quickly. Although not needed, the hospital also had alternative financing in the event the chosen plan was not approved. In such an event, the alternative funding could have preserved the timing of the deal, which was crucial in the case of SMHHC.

PUBLIC RESISTANCE

The image the public holds about a particular service or program may determine its ultimate success. There may be consumer resistance to a revenue generation activity if the public thinks it should be an insured service. Assessment of public perception is particularly important when a revenue generation activity departs from the traditional role of the hospital.

THE HUMAN ELEMENT

The development or expansion of revenue generating services may require additional professionals and skilled technicians. Shortages of these human resources could inhibit the success of revenue generating ventures. As an example, it took months for the SMHHC to recruit an ultrasonographer.

The agents of change, usually managers, are as important as the change itself. In addition to having the skills and authority to implement a revenue generating activity, managers must have a sincere desire to make the changes succeed, particularly at the higher levels of management. Without commitment, there is little chance of effective change being made.

PRIVATE SECTOR

Hospitals that engage in revenue generation activities that compete with the private sector may incur the wrath of local business, particularly in small communities. Business often argues that hospitals are unfair competition because hospital prices do not include the cost of the corporate income taxes the private sector must bear. If local business is disenchanted, a hospital may realise less in corporate charitable donations, obtain fewer price discounts from business, and experience a loss in general business good will. Therefore, hospitals should assess the impact on these relationships carefully before proceeding with a revenue generation project.

PLANNING

Success of new revenue generating programs is more likely if they are implemented into the hospital's strategic plan. It is probably best to designate someone early on as a project coordinator with the authority to expedite action. Key players, such as department heads and program directors, should be involved in planning at an early stage. This can reduce the number of times that plans are rewritten or blueprints redrawn. With a shortage in some health occupations, the human resources department should be included at an early stage, rather than waiting until a new program is in place before searching for the people to fill the newly created slots.

Finally, planning must address the role of management. Specifically, management must ask itself some brutally honest questions, such as: Do we have the business skills needed to take on this revenue generation activity?

CONCLUSION

The conclusions of this literature review and case study are sixfold:

1. Innovative approaches discussed in the health care literature since 1980 can be classified into six areas: clinical/diagnostic insured services, clinical/diagnostic non-insured services, hotel services, retail, administration, and financial.

2. Many Canadian hospitals are engaging in innovative revenue generation activities. These activities will probably continue to be an important source of hospital discretionary funds and may increase as the fiscal crunch continues and hospitals achieve greater marketing expertise.

3. The success of revenue generation activities has been mixed. Most of the successful activities have been in programs and services closely related to the primary business of the hospital – clinical/diagnostic insured services, such as laboratory services, and clinical/diagnostic non-insured services, such as wellness centres and smoking cessation clinics. Less success has been reported with other activities, particularly retail.

4. There are many factors to consider when selecting revenue generation activities, such as the business and financial risk of the activity, the effect of the activity on the existing hospital and medical staff, the potential market for the activity, the profitability of the activity, and the competition.

5. Many aspects of innovative revenue generation involve sophisticated business and risk management skills not traditionally required in hospital management, including business management, negotiation, marketing, financial, legal, and production skills.

6. Implementation of revenue generation activities requires support from the hospital board, hospital staff, and medical staff. If any of those parties does not support the activities, the revenue generation goal may be obscured by organisational conflict and may ultimately not be realisable. For example, the decisions as to who would occupy space in SMHHC often sacrificed revenue generation goals to space needs of other programs, with likely consequences to ultimate financial returns. Although at the time the case was written, SMH considered SMHHC to be a success overall, the jury was still out on its financial success.

ACKNOWLEDGEMENT

We thank the National Research and Development Program, Health and Welfare Canada, for its support of this project (6606-3989-HT). The full case study and an annotated bibliography are contained in the project's Final Report. The results of the study are also reported in:
Pink GH, Deber RB, Lavoie JN, Aserlind E: Innovative revenue generation. *Healthcare Management Forum* 4(4), (Winter), 1991.

PURCHASING HOSPITAL CAPITAL EQUIPMENT: WHAT ROLE FOR TECHNOLOGY ASSESSMENT?*

Raisa B. Deber
Gail G. Thompson
Department of Health Administration
University of Toronto

Technology is often pointed to as a major cause of increased costs. But what is the money buying? How sure can we be that it is going to be used wisely to improve health? And what suggestions could we make for improvement?

This presentation draws from the Ontario portion of a larger study of technology acquisition in hospitals. We first surveyed hospitals in Ontario, and are currently completing a national study, including a resurvey of Ontario to examine possible changes. These results come from three sources: a) 120 completed Ontario hospital questionnaires; b) 415 surveys of key decision makers involved in capital acquisition decisions from 89 Ontario hospitals; and c) 74 request forms used by Ontario hospitals for capital expenditures or new or expanded programs.

CAPITAL EXPENDITURES

The 115 hospitals for which we had 1986-87 financial data spent between $4,198 and $44.8 million for capital expenditures, with a mean of $2.1 million. About 55% went for replacement of existing equipment. On average, 50% went for medical equipment, 25% for non-medical equipment, 22% for building and grounds, and the remaining 3% for other expenses (primarily renovations).

As can be seen in Figure 1, hospitals were moving towards setting up criteria for evaluating their requests for capital spending, but a quarter still had no criteria, and most of the ones that did tended to have informal ones.

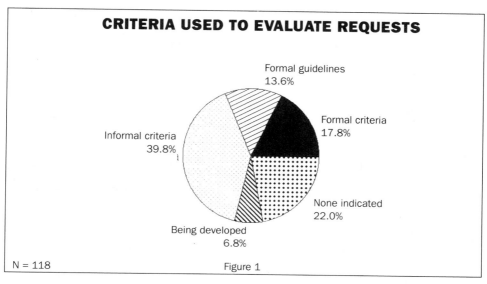

CRITERIA USED TO EVALUATE REQUESTS

Formal guidelines 13.6%

Formal criteria 17.8%

Informal criteria 39.8%

None indicated 22.0%

Being developed 6.8%

N = 118

Figure 1

INFORMATION SOURCES

What information did hospitals say they were using to make decisions about capital acquisitions? All hospitals indicated at least one source of information (Figure 2). This information, however, may not be impartial. The source most often named was presentations made by the staff who wanted the equipment; the next most frequent was information from the manufacturers. Just over half indicated some type of written technology assessment – it is not quite clear what – and 38% named the request form itself as a source of information.

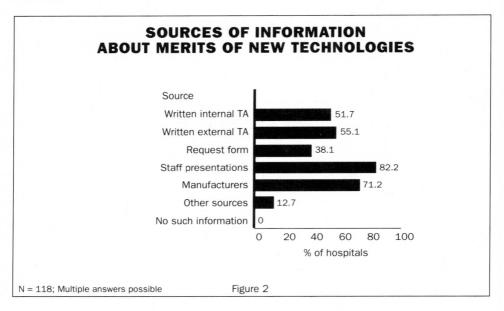

SOURCES OF INFORMATION ABOUT MERITS OF NEW TECHNOLOGIES

Source	% of hospitals
Written internal TA	51.7
Written external TA	55.1
Request form	38.1
Staff presentations	82.2
Manufacturers	71.2
Other sources	12.7
No such information	0

N = 118; Multiple answers possible   Figure 2

The interesting thing about the request form is that it is the only systematic way of obtaining consistent information, since presentations may not all provide the same information. So we developed a coding scheme to see what was included in these request forms – what information was being asked for.

We identified 90 possible pieces of information which might have been requested, and classified them as:

DESCRiption of the item (e.g., description, manufacturer, model number, quantity requested, purpose, new or replacement)

REASON for purchase (e.g., priority, fit with hospital goals)

COST (e.g., total cost, installation, additional staff, supplies)

SERVICing (e.g., warranty, availability of parts)

REVENue potential

EVALuation and assessment

OPTIONs to purchase (e.g., leasing, fabricating internally)

SCREENing (e.g., had it been scrutinized internally, or externally?)

EFFECTs (e.g., patient benefit, coordination with other departments, changes in case mix)

PREVious equipment (e.g., age of old equipment, depreciation/current value).

Seventy-four hospital request forms were analyzed. The proportion requesting each piece of information was calculated, and the information divided into quartiles (Table 1).

Table 1

PROPORTION OF HOSPITALS INCLUDING SPECIFIED ITEMS ON REQUEST FORMS, BY QUARTILE

Variable	Category	Mean score
First Quartile (≥75%)		
Description of item	DESCR	0.97
New/replacement/upgrade	DESCR	0.95
Total cost	COST	0.95
Unit cost	COST	0.88
Second Quartile (50% – 74.9%)		
Reason for purchase	REASON	0.70
Cost of adding staff	COST	0.69
Cost of training staff	COST	0.68
Priority	REASON	0.66
Supplies cost	COST	0.66
Installation cost	COST	0.65
Who will maintain?	SERVIC	0.65
Name of manufacturer	DESCR	0.62
Effect on operating costs	COST	0.62
Savings	COST	0.61
Need for renovation	EFFECT	0.59
Quantity requested	DESCR	0.51
Purpose of equipment	DESCR	0.50
Third Quartile (25% – 49.9%)		
Is price increase expected soon?	COST	0.45
Fate of old equipment	PREV	0.43
Model number	DESCR	0.42
Needed to maintain existing level of service, improve, or offer new service	DESCR	0.41
Existing power and other services adequate?	EVAL	0.32
Volume new unit can handle	EFFECT	0.32
Description of what is being replaced	PREV	0.32
Will service contract be required?	SERVIC	0.31
Other manufacturers	DESCR	0.30
Will equipment generate revenue?	REVEN	0.30
Prior approval from within hospital	SCREEN	0.30
Impact on efficiency, workload, process time	EFFECT	0.27
Age of old equipment	PREV	0.27
Date needed	REASON	0.26

Fourth Quartile (<25%)

Programs supported by purchase	DESCR	0.24
CSO and Hydro approvals	EVAL	0.24
Impact on other departments	EFFECT	0.24
Need for new space	EFFECT	0.24
Source of funds to pay for equipment	REVEN	0.22
Depreciation/current value of old equipment	PREV	0.20
Consequences of refusing request	REASON	0.19
What is being replaced?	PREV	0.19
How service is currently provided	DESCR	0.18
Has equipment been legislated, or recommended?	REASON	0.18
Service record of old equipment	PREV	0.18
Life expectancy of equipment	DESCR	0.16
Has request been coordinated with other departments?	EFFECT	0.16
Impact on working conditions	EFFECT	0.16
Does warranty exist?	SERVIC	0.15
Alternatives to purchase (e.g., leasing)	OPTION	0.15
Approval by external body (e.g., province, DHC)	SCREEN	0.15
Patient benefit	EFFECT	0.15
Current volume of work of present unit	EFFECT	0.15
Justification of choice of manufacturer	DESCR	0.12
Current program expense of requesting department	DESCR	0.12
Previously requested	REASON	0.12
Evidence of need	REASON	0.12
Is service provided elsewhere?	DESCR	0.11
Date to be purchased	REASON	0.11
Amount item will depreciate in value	COST	0.11
Current capacity of present unit	EFFECT	0.11
Results from technology assessment within hospital	EVAL	0.09
Need for add-ons in next few years	SERVIC	0.08
Results from technology assessment outside hospital	EVAL	0.08
Departments with which equipment will be shared	EFFECT	0.08
Could old equipment be repaired?	PREV	0.08
Demand projections	DESCR	0.07
Fit with hospital goals	REASON	0.07
Availability of parts	SERVIC	0.07
Have requesters seen item demonstrated?	EVAL	0.07
Assessment by present users of equipment	EVAL	0.05
Type of patient (target population)	EFFECT	0.05
Has equipment been tried in hospital?	EVAL	0.04
How will equipment be evaluated after purchase?	EVAL	0.04
Justification of purchase vs. lease or other options	OPTION	0.04
Who will use equipment?	EFFECT	0.04
Original cost of old item	PREV	0.04

How much of the old equipment is there now?	PREV	0.04
Justification for timing	REASON	0.03
Alternative plans if request denied	REASON	0.03
Cost of exact replacement (if upgrade)	COST	0.03
Feasibility of upgrading	SERVIC	0.03
Results from being out of service	PREV	0.03
Unused capacity of new equipment at other institutions	DESCR	0.01
Length of time equipment has been needed	REASON	0.01
Date by which purchase becomes essential	REASON	0.01
Availability of exact replacement (if upgrade)	COST	0.01
Payback analysis performed	COST	0.01
What are quality assurance mechanisms?	EVAL	0.01
Could hospital fabricate item?	OPTION	0.01
Impact on teaching programs	EFFECT	0.01
Changes in case mix	EFFECT	0
Impact on physician recruitment	EFFECT	0

Table 1 shows that what was being asked for was very simple: "What do you want, and how much does it cost?" Only four items were asked for by almost all hospitals: a description of the item (97%), whether it was new or replacement (some also asked about upgrades) (95%), the total cost (95%), and the unit cost (88%).

About 2/3 of the forms asked something about what priority the requester was giving the request, how much would have to be spent on training or adding staff, or how much on supplies. It's rather striking that a third of the institutions weren't even asking those questions.

Clearly, putting in a piece of equipment is going to affect other departments. Yet fewer hospitals were asking such broader impact questions as: "Do you need to renovate the place?" "Do you need more space?" "What is this equipment going to do to working conditions?" "What is it going to do to other departments?" "Have you coordinated with those other departments?" Still smaller numbers were asking about benefit to patients, evidence of need, and even whether the service was already being provided. Few asked for assessments to answer such questions as, "Is this thing going to do what it's supposed to?" or "What has been the experience of people who have tried it?", and only 4% asked how the technology would eventually be evaluated.

In general, decision makers would not have much information on the potential impact of the technology on other departments (even within the same institution) or on the merits of the expenditure. It appears that, to a large extent, the presumption was made that such "homework" had been performed by the requesting department.

DECISION MAKERS

Since committees usually made the final decision about what would be purchased, we looked closely at their structure. These committees drew their membership from a very limited group. They almost always had administrators and they almost always had medical staff, but they very rarely had nurses. Any representation of nursing usually came only from the senior nursing officer on the administrative team. There were almost never technical experts to give advice on whether the equipment was going to work, and community involvement came only through the board.

The decision makers we surveyed had been identified by their CEO as being involved in decision making within their institution, so the number per institution varied. We asked them, among other things, to rate the importance to decision making about capital budgeting in their institution of 25 different items on a scale from 1 (not at all important) to 5 (extremely important). It is not surprising that the highest rated items were quality of care, need, and compatibility with role and mission, with cost also rated pretty highly (Table 2). Such items as availability of similar services elsewhere in region, formal technology assessment, and priorities of provincial government or regional planning bodies also ranked above the mid-point, but were given lower mean importance ratings.

Table 2
PERCEIVED IMPORTANCE OF VARIOUS ITEMS TO DECISION MAKING ABOUT CAPITAL EXPENDITURES IN THEIR INSTITUTION

Item	Score
Quality of health care	4.70
Need	4.55
Compatibility with institution's role and mission	4.45
Total cost of item	4.22
Net cost of item	4.21
Revenue potential	3.96
Patient demand	3.89
Availability of similar services elsewhere in region	3.87
Completeness of services	3.77
Formal technology assessment	3.57
Priorities of provincial government	3.56
Reimbursement regulations	3.49
Completeness of application	3.40
Priorities of regional planning bodies	3.35
Fear of malpractice/liability	3.32
Previous allocations of funds	3.10
Community pressure	3.09
Cohesiveness of requesting group	3.05
Desire to please medical staff	2.89
History of institution	2.64
Priorities of university (if teaching hospital)	2.60
Power of requesting department	2.54
Sense of equity (effort to give everyone something)	2.52
Prestige of proposed item	2.23
Prestige of requesting unit	2.21

Measured on scale from 1 (not at all important) to 5 (very important)

Fifty-three percent of respondents indicated that "quality of health care" was the most important factor; 18% suggested "need", and 13% suggested "compatibility with institution's role and mission". Fourteen other possibilities each received less than 3% of responses.

WHAT MAKES A GOOD DECISION?

We also asked the decision makers to what extent they thought the current process of technology acquisition in their institution usually led to the right decision for a variety of stakeholders: the patients, doctors, staff, department, institution, community, and province as a whole. On the whole, the respondents thought that the current process for technology acquisition at their institution resulted in the right decision for all parties. They felt more strongly that the decisions were the right ones for patients (mean 4.2 on a scale of 1 to 5). They felt next most strongly that these were the right ones for the institution, the doctors, and the community (these responses tended to cluster). It is interesting to note that respondents felt least certain that the current process usually resulted in the right decision for the province (mean 3.4).

Most people felt that their institution met the needs of the community they served slightly better than others of the same type and size (mean 3.8 - i.e., between "about the same" and "slightly better").

Using the Ministry of Health's classification of hospitals, the data were sorted into responses from large hospitals and small hospitals and then compared. There were no very significant differences in how respondents from the two groups rated the importance of the 25 variables. However, prestige of the proposed item, revenue potential, prestige of the requesting unit, and formal technology assessment tended to be rated more highly by the larger hospitals, and history of the institution, community pressure, and desire to please medical staff rated more highly by the smaller ones.

A factor analysis of these 24 variables (omitting priorities of the university, since it was not applicable to many of the responding institutions) revealed three underlying factors. Those variables with factor loadings of 0.5 or higher on each are shown below.

Factor 1 links (factor weights shown in parentheses):
- priorities of regional planning bodies (0.60)
- availability of similar services elsewhere in region (0.51)
- formal technology assessment (0.51)
- priorities of provincial government (0.55)
- reimbursement regulations (0.50)
- completeness of application (0.61)
- community pressure (0.52)
- cohesiveness of requesting group (0.55)
- previous allocations of funds (0.52)

and can be thought of as the EXTERNAL FORCES/PLANNING factor.

Factor 2 links:
- power of requesting department (0.76)
- prestige of requesting unit (0.69)
- prestige of proposed item (0.67)
- desire to please medical staff (0.62)
- need (inversely related) (-0.57)

and therefore can be thought of as the INTERNAL HOSPITAL POLITICS AND

PRIORITIES factor, which, interestingly, is inversely related to the respondent's perception of need for the item. (More optimistically, this can be interpreted as meaning that as need is seen as being more important, these other factors are seen as less so.)

Factor 3 links:
- total cost of item (0.71)
- net cost of item (0.73)

and can be thought of as the COST factor.

These three factors were then included in a linear regression, with the dependent variable being the extent to which the respondent perceived that the current process of technology acquisition resulted in the right decision for: the patients, the doctors, the institution staff, the individual department, the institution, the community, and the province. Other independent variables were dummy variables for: hospital size, whether the respondent was a physician, whether the respondent was a nurse, whether the respondent was in a senior management position, plus a constructed variable indicating the degree to which the respondent was involved in "network" activities (meetings, conferences, etc.) outside his/her own job or institution.

Table 3

REGRESSION COEFFICIENTS: DETERMINANTS OF "RIGHT" DECISIONS FOR:

Variable	Patients	Doctors	Staff	Department	Institution	Community	Province	Needs Met
R^2	0.14*	0.06#	0.13*	0.07#	0.13*	0.16*	0.20*	0.06@
Beta weights:								
Intercept	0 *	0 *	0 *	0 *	0 *	0 *	0 *	0 *
External factor	0.23*	0.18#	0.21#	0.14#	0.16#	0.27*	0.37*	n.s.
Internal factor	-0.27*	n.s.	-0.16#	n.s.	-0.23*	-0.24*	-0.13@	n.s.
Cost factor	n.s.	n.s.	n.s.	-0.14@	n.s.	n.s.	n.s.	0.15@
Hospital size	n.s.	n.s.	n.s.	n.s.	n.s.	n.s.	n.s.	n.s.
Senior manager (Y/N)	n.s.	n.s.	0.22#	0.15@	n.s.	n.s.	n.s.	n.s.
Nurse (Y/N)	n.s.	n.s.	n.s.	n.s.	n.s.	n.s.	n.s.	n.s.
Physician (Y/N)	n.s.	n.s.	n.s.	n.s.	n.s.	n.s.	n.s.	n.s.
Networking	n.s.	n.s.	n.s.	n.s.	n.s.	n.s.	n.s.	0.16#

Note: First 7 columns are responses to question sequence: "To what extent do you think the current process of technology acquisition in your institution usually results in the right decision for: The patients? The doctors? The institution staff? The individual department? The institution? The community? The province?" Response scale was from 1 (not at all) to 5 (very much). Last column is response to "On the whole, how well do you feel your institution is meeting the needs of the community as compared with others of the same type and size in this area of the country?" Response scale was from 1 (much worse) to 5 (much better).

Table entries denote standardized beta coefficients in OLS regressions in SAS-PC; statistical significance of unstandardized coefficient denoted as follows:
- * = .0001 or less
- # = between .01 and .0001
- @ = between .05 and .01
- n.s. = not statistically significant

The results of these regressions supported advocates of multi-institutional coordination (Table 3). All equations were statistically significant, although they rarely explained more than 15% of the variance. The most statistically significant variables were Factors 1 and 2. Respondents felt that decisions were better when higher weights were placed on external/planning factors, and that they were worse (i.e., the regression coefficient had a negative sign) when higher weights were placed on internal factors. Those respondents who were more likely to feel that such considerations as power and prestige or desire to please medical staff were important in decision making about capital budgeting in their institution were also less likely to think that the decisions made were the "right" ones for anyone, with the possible exception of the medical staff. The importance of cost was unrelated to perceived quality of decisions, although it was weakly related to how well the respondent felt their institution was meeting community needs. It is noteworthy that respondents who perceived that more weight was placed on external factors in their institutions also perceived that the results were better *internal* decisions for almost all parties involved.

DISCUSSION AND CONCLUSIONS

So what can we conclude? This plus our other data suggested that institutions seemed to be paying the closest attention to initial costs, but tending to miss two factors which, in the aggregate, could turn out to be very costly. First, although the individually expensive purchases received intensive scrutiny, the less expensive ones tended to be under-scrutinized (data not shown). These less expensive items had lower individual capital costs but, when taken together, made up the bulk of the budget. Secondly, comparatively little attention was paid to the ongoing implications and costs of a technology once it had been purchased. Impact analysis, which is now being looked at in decisions about medical staffing, may also have a role in capital budgeting.

We also suspect there is too little use of both impact and assessment information. Rational decision making would imply that if you're going to make a rational decision about a purchase, you should at least know whether it works and what its impact is likely to be. Our results suggest that there should probably be systematic ways of ensuring that that information is made available and that there is probably a need for broader representation on the committees that make acquisition decisions.

Our third conclusion is a rather hopeful one – that decision makers find that paying more attention to implications beyond the walls of their institution results in better decisions for everybody, presenting the possibility of a win-win situation. Broader multi-hospital planning could benefit not only the province and the community, but also the individual institution and the patients who seek care from that institution. And particularly in a world where rugged individualism and competition and all of these things are getting so much attention, I find it rather comforting to see that possibly compromise, consultation, and working together may lead to better results for everybody.

NOTE
* edited transcript of talk by Raisa Deber

ACKNOWLEDGEMENTS

We thank NHRDP for funding our studies of technology acquisition (6606-2964-46 and 6606-3841-57), in what we really hope will not be their last such acts of generosity. We also thank our co-investigators, Peggy Leatt and George Pink. Our advisory committee and the participating hospitals have made invaluable contributions. We are grateful to our part-time research assistants and our support staff – Ahmed Bayoumi, Louise Castellan, Jennifer Chow, Alfred D'Sa, Amol Deshpande, Pamela Ko, Ann Pendleton, Celeste Superina, Mary Wiktorowicz, and Cynthia Wong – who have worked on pieces of the studies over time, usually during medical elective or summer student programs.

REFERENCES

Deber RB: Translating technology assessment into policy: conceptual issues and tough choices. *International Journal of Technology Assessment in Health Care* (in press).

Deber RB, Thompson GG, Leatt P: Technology acquisition in Canada: control in a regulated market. *International Journal of Technology Assessment in Health Care* 4(2):185-206, 1988.

Institute of Medicine, Committee for Evaluating Medical Technologies in Clinical Use, Division of Health Sciences Policy, Division of Health Promotion and Disease Prevention: *Assessing Medical Technologies.* Washington, D.C.: National Academy Press, 1985.

DISCUSSION
Chair: John Horne
Health Science Centre, Winnipeg

Peter Ruderman (Toronto)

I want to address one part to Raisa, one part to George Pink. For Raisa, it's simply this. Do you think there's any special role for study, and if so what have you found out, about the major capital items, where it isn't so much the institutions you'd study, but the province's right of veto that comes into account? And for George, a cautionary tale. One of my former health administration students got a job as personal assistant to the president of a large metropolitan hospital, a very entrepreneurial president. When I saw him a year later, it turned out that this guy was so busy wheeling and dealing that he turned over the actual administration of the hospital to a 24-year-old kid with no previous experience. How general is that risk?

Raisa Deber (University of Toronto)

The question you asked, Peter, is an interesting one. It depends on the province how much is handled centrally and how much is delegated down to the individual institution. I think it's extremely difficult for micro-management, which requires knowing what the needs are in a locality, to be handled at a more central level. I think that's an extraordinarily difficult thing for a province to do. It's probably more manageable in smaller provinces, where you have that type of oversight. In a province like Ontario, Quebec, or British Columbia, I think it's an extraordinarily difficult thing to do, and there is a tendency to delegate it down. I think one of the weaknesses is that there isn't that middle structure where the regional coordination of these sorts of things can easily happen. Hospitals are much more into individual competition, and it's interesting to note how many of the commissions and reports have called for some sort of regional body, precisely to give an organizational mechanism for this type of thing. I think that's one of the gaps in our current system.

George Pink (University of Toronto)

I guess the only comment I would have is I think, obviously, there has to be some concern about how administrators spend their time. I don't think Vic Stoughton should be out on University Avenue selling used cars or doing things that are totally unrelated to his job. On the other hand, I think a lot of the things that have been done in the last few years have been good. I think hospitals, for example, have a lot of unused capacity within their four walls. They have dietary, laundry, and so on. Why not use some of the excess capacity – unused capacity – to generate money? That, to me, is just good business management. I don't think anyone would argue that managers should be wheeling and dealing all the time, and spending time away from their main jobs, but I think there is a role for judicious management of resources and maximizing revenue.

Carl Roy (Sudbury General Hospital)

Raisa, specific to your suggestion that the decision making for capital equipment acquisition be broadened, did your instrument attempt to measure at all any subcommittees that may support the decision making process, specifically around nursing input or technical assessment of some of the requests?

Raisa Deber

Part of our study, which I haven't reported today, asks what the committees are that are involved in decision making, what the composition is, and what they do. And my statement that there was probably an underuse of technical expertise and nursing came from that piece of the analysis.

Don MacNaught (Health and Welfare Canada)

George, in your case study, did you encounter the public policy issue of the privileged position that hospitals have with respect to tax policy, i.e., exemptions from federal and perhaps in some instances provincial sales tax, compared to, obviously, competitive business enterprises in somewhat the same nature of business? And if you did, what was the resolution of the issue?

George Pink

We did. It was actually quite interesting, because at the time we were undertaking this study, I believe it was the Public Trustee of Ontario was taking Scarborough Centenary Hospital to court for the medical mall that it wants to build. In fact, the hospital has now actually won that court case. And so a lot of those issues were occurring at the same time in the legal forum, and a lot of those issues were resolved as the Public Trustee lost that court case. With respect to specific legal questions, the legal process was a very long and negotiated one, and the hospital's always very careful to obey the provisions of the income tax act and so on. Without going into long discussion about all the individual specifics, yes it was addressed, yes it was resolved, but it was primarily resolved by the Public Trustee court decision that allowed hospitals, I think, to engage in these types of things.

Cope Schwenger (University of Toronto)

Another question for George. George, what are we talking about in terms of money actually brought in by these innovations? Is it big bucks or little bucks, in total amount and relative to the total budget of the hospital?

George Pink

Relative to the total budget of the hospital, it is still relatively small. I believe the latest figure I've seen – at least, what Peter Coyte told me a few months ago – was 81% in Ontario. The average Ontario hospital receives 81% of its revenue from the Ministry of Health, 5-6% from other government sources. But it varies enormously. The University of Western Ontario in London gets millions and millions and millions of dollars in non-governmental private revenue, as it were. I think the thing that makes it of so much interest to managers, and again I'd welcome correction by managers in the audience, but the thing, I think, that makes it so important, and why managers are spending so much time addressing it, is that it is marginal revenue. It's revenue that you can do stuff with, versus the public – Ministry of Health – global budget, which is really, as Peter Carruthers described in my class a few months ago, the minimum wage for providing health services. And the discretionary revenue really allows the hospital to do the things that it wants to do.

Raisa Deber

Another interesting source of additional revenue, incidentally, tying in with our morning session, is providing insured services to uninsured people, namely Americans. And another potential revenue source, where there is excess capacity, is to market to American institutions as a cheaper form of provision. And I know that that's another place that's being eyed by some places.

Richard Edwards (University of Toronto)

My question comes, I guess, out of the theme of the whole thing, which is, "How do we get there from here?" And it is a question that comes out of the "What is the there?" And so my question really is, "Is there an explicit concept of the hospital in the system that is driving some of these innovations?" For instance, your remark about setting up hospital malls. There are some people who could argue, in fact, that hospitals perhaps should be restricted to more acute care. Now, I guess the question is, is there an explicit concept driving some of this stuff? If there is – or if not – what is it? And do you see, for instance, governance structures being determined by what the explicit concept of a hospital should be? Do you see governance structures being related to that?

G. Ross Baker (University of Toronto)

I think the issue of what the governance structure is is obviously going to be a very complex one. What I was trying to identify is the various underlying trends that I see emerging, not only in the Canadian system but in other systems as well, and the kind of pressures that we will have to respond to in the governance structures that we develop. Hospitals have a niche in the system. The question is really, "Do we want to see the hospital broaden to take in other parts – other activities? Or do we want to see those other activities essentially broadened, with the hospital brought in as more of a liaison?" And I think we're going to see all of those models evolving in this system. So I don't think there's one answer as to what the role of the hospital will be.

Maurice McGregor (Le Conseil d'évaluation des technologies de la santé)

Two questions that have come up repeatedly in the extra fund raising debate. Surely any health ministry would look extraordinarily unfavourably towards our deploying the limited resources of a hospital to raising revenue from Americans who haven't got as good a system. And I'm surprised that it comes up to issue, because as a taxpayer I would want my ministry to put a finger on that one. The second point is, is it not very likely that – and this I don't favour – that the large and enterprising hospital that manages to raise substantial revenues will have that taken into account when their budget is being considered by a health ministry? Ministries have to keep everybody going. And if you're showing the ability to go it on your own, you're going to get a little bit less help. And isn't the debate very much damaged by these two issues?

George Pink

Well, in response to the first question, as a taxpayer I see absolutely nothing wrong with a hospital's using excess capacity to generate revenue.

Maurice McGregor

What if it's not excess?

George Pink

Well, if it's not excess, then as a taxpayer I'm opposed to it. Canadians would always come first. And at least in the circumstance that Raisa is referring to, the people that I have talked to about it – the hospital has a policy that Canadians will always get first come, first served service. But given that there are physical, capital investments idle part of the time, why shouldn't the hospital use that to generate revenue from Americans? If the Americans are willing to pay for it, I think there is absolutely nothing wrong with that.

Raisa Deber

There is a political angle to it, also, which is, if there is excess capacity, another way to handle it is to shut down some of that capacity. But then you get into the regional reality. And it's very difficult to say, "No, we won't have these services in Hamilton, because there's not going to be enough volume to justify them in Hamilton." So you can provide facilities in regions where there's not a patient base to justify them, and you then fill the excess space by marketing them somewhere else. There is a possibility, to some extent, of a win-win situation, with the only ones hurt being the taxpayers, because the Americans are not going to pull in all of the money needed to pay for those facilities.

George Pink

In response to your second question, you're quite right. That's been a fear of hospital managers I've talked to, that if you are successful in raising money they're going to subtract it from your global budget. And I guess the only answer I have to that is that the Ministry of Health in Ontario, at least under the BOND [Business Oriented New Development] program, has always encouraged hospitals to generate more revenue. In fact, if the Ministry is taking a long term view, it is in the long term interest of the Ministry for hospitals to be financially successful. If they are going to turn around and penalize financially successful hospitals, then what incentive do hospitals have to generate revenue? There isn't any. So I would hope that Ministry bureaucrats are sufficiently long sighted that they would see it as in the interests of everyone to give incentives to hospitals to generate revenue, and not penalize them.

**QUALITY
TIME**

ASSESSING THE QUALITY OF MEDICAL CARE

Jane E. Sisk
Office of Technology Assessment, U.S. Congress

INTRODUCTION

Several factors have coalesced to produce a widespread call for better information on the quality of medical care. Some of the impetus comes from trends in our overall society – to promote consumerism and to question authority. People increasingly wish to become better informed and to participate in decisions that affect them. These developments have had their counterpart in medical care: Polls have found that 95% or more of respondents want their physicians to answer their questions and to provide more information about their medical conditions.

The recent upsurge of U.S. interest in the quality of medical care has been associated with attempts to contain medical expenditures. Especially after the Medicare program began to use diagnosis-related groups as the basis for paying for inpatient services, concern grew that third-party payers, hospitals, and physicians facing cost pressure would skimp on services to the detriment of people's health. Although threats to quality may arise from the overuse as well as the underuse of medical services, people seem to worry much more about underuse. This concern led people in the medical community, consumer advocates, policymakers, employers, and unions to call for better information on quality. The rationale has been that, with better information on quality, individual consumers and organizations that act on their behalf – employers, insurers, unions, and government programs – could use their leverage from the purchase and use of services to promote good quality care and avoid poor quality providers. It has also been postulated that with better information on quality, clinicians and administrators could improve the bases on which they refer patients and credential physicians.

Moreover, some within the medical and policymaking communities expect better information on quality to result in cost savings. Although they have not completely elucidated the rationale, they believe that poor quality care is more expensive care and that better information on quality can enable managers to identify problems, improve care, and save money.

Whatever the potential of better information on quality, its achievement depends on having valid measures of assessment. We examined whether there are valid indicators of the quality of medical care that consumers could use to choose physicians and acute-care hospitals. We found, not surprisingly, that every measure has some problems, but in the process we identified the shortcomings of currently-available measures and steps needed to improve them.

BEYOND WEBSTER: DEFINITION OF TERMS

Like other intangible concepts, the quality of medical care is difficult to define. Indeed, quality acquires concrete properties only when one measures it. Attempts to define quality in the medical field are plagued not only by the abstract nature of quality but also by particular characteristics of medical care.

The quality of medical care has many dimensions, a fact that reflects the diversity of acceptable outcomes for patients and the complexity of the medical care process. Since medical care is intended to benefit individuals, it is appropriate to evaluate the quality of care from the perspective of how it benefits them. Depending on their medical conditions and preferences, patients may vary widely in the health outcomes they desire. Although the consumer, the provider, and the overall society may emphasize different aspects of quality, each from its own perspective, all view both the technical and interpersonal aspects as important (Donabedian, 1980).

The framework that Donabedian proposed in the 1960s to measure quality continues to provide the best conceptual basis (Donabedian, 1966). According to his triad, the *structure* of care refers to the resources and organizational arrangements in place to deliver care, such as medical personnel and facilities; the *process* of care to the activities of physicians and other health professionals engaged in providing medical care; and the *outcomes* to the intended effects of medical care, including dimensions of patient health and satisfaction (Donabedian, 1980).

As Donabedian stated, assessing quality via structural indicators, such as physician specialization, presupposes that the presence of certain structural conditions increases the likelihood that providers will perform well, and their absence the likelihood that providers will perform poorly. This assumption in turn raises the question of whether specific structural characteristics are, in fact, associated with better performance. In evaluating the process of medical care, one should limit evaluations of providers' performance to measures that are known to improve or harm patients' health and satisfaction (Donabedian, 1966). The problem is that the link between the process of care and patient outcomes has been established for relatively few procedures. In addition, medical knowledge and what is considered appropriate care are constantly evolving. The major problem with using patient outcomes to evaluate quality is that attributing changes in outcomes to medical care requires distinguishing the effects of medical care from the effects of the many other factors that influence patient health and satisfaction (Donabedian, 1966; McAuliffe, 1978; Brook and Lohr, 1985).

Incorporating these and other considerations, we developed the following definition of quality: The quality of medical care is the degree to which the process of care increases the probability of desired outcomes and reduces the probability of undesired outcomes, given the state of medical knowledge. This definition reflects the probabilistic nature of patients' outcomes even when medical knowledge and technology are applied well, the evolution of medical knowledge, and possible differences in the outcomes desired. The definition also points out that valid assessments of quality require linking the process of care with effects on patients' health and satisfaction.

These concepts relate to the assessment of quality. They may also be applied to promote "continuous improvement" in quality and to undertake quality assurance. Some have argued that an atmosphere of continuous improvement should pervade medical practice (Berwick and Batalden, 1987; Rubin, 1975). Rather than depending on external assessments and perhaps penalties for wrongdoing, advocates of this approach conceive of routine quality assessments being used by providers and organizations to identify problems, which would then be addressed. Quality assurance programs, whether in hospitals or government programs, also use the results of quality assessments. Although these programs have often fallen short of their objectives, they are intended to set up mechanisms to forestall problems and to identify and address those that do occur.

Another concept often confused with quality assessment is technology assessment. In health policy, technology assessment connotes any form of policy analysis concerned with medical technology. Medical technology in turn encompasses the drugs, devices, and medical and surgical procedures used in medical care plus the organizational and support systems within which such care is provided. Technology assessments, especially of efficacy and safety, should underlie quality assessments related to the process of care. A great deal of medical practice has not been evaluated, and even routine procedures may lack efficacy or entail undue risk in the circumstances in which they are used. In deciding how to evaluate the process of a provider's care, one should therefore select technologies and conditions for which evidence on efficacy and safety exists.

EVALUATING THE VALIDITY OF QUALITY INDICATORS

We selected 10 possible indicators of quality to exemplify different dimensions of quality, approaches to measuring quality, and measures being used. Based on a synthesis of the literature and principles of research methodology, we evaluated the validity of each indicator (Sisk et al, 1990; US Congress, OTA, 1988). In general, assessments regarding quality are hampered by the lack of an accepted criterion or "gold standard" against which to validate possible indicators of quality. In the absence of such a criterion, more weight is given to associations among possible indicators, that is, to convergent validity. In fact, the use of Donabedian's three approaches to measuring quality illustrates the application of this principle.

ASSESSMENT OF PATIENT OUTCOMES: HEALTH AND SATISFACTION

Using patient outcomes to measure quality commands great interest within the policy and research communities. By far the most prominent public information related to quality has been the Health Care Financing Administration's release annually since 1986 of mortality rates experienced by Medicare beneficiaries in specific hospitals throughout the United States.

Based on an evaluation of hospital mortality rates and other adverse events experienced by patients, we concluded that quality assessment techniques have not progressed to the point that one can rely on data on outcomes, such as hospital mortality, alone. Although researchers have identified characteristics of patients at high risk of dying in intensive care units, techniques to adjust for patient risk across the hospital for all conditions are still being developed and tested. Recent research results emphasize the importance of a two-step process involving first the collection of data about a bad outcome, such as hospital mortality, and second, the examination of medical records or other sources of information to determine whether a quality problem exists.

Studies using medical record review or other techniques to try to validate hospital mortality analyses have repeatedly found quality deficiencies in under 10% of the cases or hospitals, and sometimes identified fewer quality problems in high-mortality hospitals than in others (Hannan and Yazici, 1988; New York State, 1987; US Congress GAO, 1988). A recent study by Park and colleagues confirmed those results. Differences in the quality of the process of care could not explain differences between hospitals with higher-than-expected mortality rates and other hospitals (Park et al, 1990). An exception to this pattern was Dubois' findings that for two of three conditions evaluated by physicians using implicit criteria based on their professional judgment, high-mortality hospitals were significantly more likely than low-mortality ones to have preventable deaths (Dubois et al, 1987).

ASSESSMENT OF THE MEDICAL CARE PROCESS

Evaluation of how physicians take care of specific patients has been the traditional method used by physicians to assess their peers. The College of Physicians and Surgeons of Ontario and the College of Family Physicians of Canada, for example, have been applying this method to review charts in physicians' offices (Borgiel, 1987; Davis et al, 1990).

Evaluations of a physician's performance for a specific condition can produce valid assessments of quality if, as is the case with hypertension screening and management, the assessment criteria have been linked to changes in patients' outcomes. These may be immediate outcomes, such as physiologic effects, or more long-term aspects of patients' health and satisfaction.

To assess physicians' management of a condition, the most reasonable approach is to review the process of care using a combination of explicit criteria and implicit judgments of experts. Patient outcomes might also be used to select cases for review. This combination approach has not been well evaluated, however (US Congress, OTA, 1988), nor has the validity of criteria and standards developed by expert panels been established.

Furthermore, an evaluation of a physician's performance for one condition is not necessarily generalizable to other conditions or to the physician's overall practice (Sanazaro and Worth, 1985). Reflecting this fact, evaluations by the College of Family Physicians review a range of conditions typical of office-based practice.

ASSESSMENT OF STRUCTURAL CHARACTERISTICS

Many of the measures of quality discussed by policymakers and the lay press relate to providers' structural characteristics. We reviewed six structural measures: the volume of services in a hospital or performed by a physician, malpractice awards, disciplinary actions by state medical boards, sanctions taken by the U.S. Department of Health and Human Services on the recommendation of peer review organizations (PROs), physician specialization, and accreditation guidelines for specialized hospital services.

Although many of these measures have strong face validity, that is, they make sense as measures of providers' quality, few have been validated by confirming an association with process or outcome measures. Such research has been performed for physician specialization. Based on medical record reviews, researchers have concluded that physicians practicing in the area of their training are more likely to deliver care of higher technical quality than physicians practicing outside their training (Palmer and Reilly, 1979). On the other hand, certification by a medical specialty board has not been associated with the quality of a physician's care (Palmer and Reilly, 1979). This finding may reflect problems such as shortcomings in the methods that specialty boards use to assess physician clinical competence (Payne, Lyone, and Neuhaus, 1984).

The association between volume and outcome has also been the subject of considerable research, but the conclusions are less definitive. For certain procedures, such as coronary artery bypass surgery and total hip replacement, researchers have found lower hospital volumes to be associated with higher inhospital mortality rates or other adverse patient outcomes (Luft et al, 1987). In contrast, researchers have reported mixed results for the volume of services performed by physicians or for all the services studied (Luft et al, 1987; Hannan et al, 1989). Nor has the association between lower volumes and worse outcomes been validated by linking lower volume to deficiencies in medical care. Because the relationship is between volume and patient outcome, adjusting data for patients' risk poses the same problems here as for hospital mortality rates.

Malpractice compensation is a poor indicator of technical quality and exemplifies the pitfalls of structural measures. Of the 1% of patients who experience a negligent injury that leads to a longer hospital stay or to disability at discharge, only a small subset file malpractice claims (Harvard Medical Practice Study, 1990). Furthermore, for a substantial portion of claims litigated under the tort system, preliminary data indicate that there may have been no adverse event related to negligence (Harvard Medical Practice Study, 1990). A malpractice suit more clearly indicates a patient's dissatisfaction with a provider's care, especially the interpersonal aspects. Once a suit is filed, many factors besides a provider's negligence, especially judicial and insurance procedures, determine the disposition of the case.

IMPLICATIONS FOR POLICY

Although none of the indicators examined provides definitive information on the quality of a hospital or physician across the range of medical care, this conclusion is hardly surprising given the complexity of medical care and the many dimensions of quality. Several of the indicators can provide useful information. Organizations and individuals can use some of the indicators as screens, to flag areas that merit further examination. Information about unacceptable care justifies more attention than information that ranks good quality providers because of the greater risks posed by poor quality and because of the current state of quality assessment techniques.

People would also be well advised to combine information from more than one indicator (e.g., hospital mortality rates and volumes of hospital procedures) and from more than one year, to increase the likelihood that the relationship identified is accurate.

As third-party payers and accrediting bodies attempt to incorporate quality measurements into their decisions, it becomes increasingly important to improve the validity of those measurements. Particularly needed are better methods to take into account patient characteristics that affect outcomes independently of quality, better methods to assess care in ambulatory settings, and better evaluations of the efficacy and safety of medical technologies as bases for assessing their appropriate use.

Besides the validity of quality measures, their financial implications also merit comment. Even if certain measures produce valid results, they may not be the most efficient way to assess quality. Suppose 5% of hospitals with mortality rates higher than expected have quality problems. Is this yield sufficient, or are there other methods, perhaps other adverse events, that offer greater specificity/sensitivity for the cost? Neither the validity nor the efficiency of the screens that PROs used to target reviews of hospitals has been studied. Similarly, the Health Care Financing Administration, which administers the U.S. Medicare program, is planning to require myriad clinical data on each patient, but has assessed neither the validity nor the efficiency of using these data.

The United States has recently created a new agency, the Agency for Health Care Policy and Research, to assess the effectiveness of medical technologies and the quality of providers. At least part of the political support for the agency came from the expectation that developing guidelines for physicians' practice and assessing providers' quality will control medical expenditures. Some clinicians have noted that poor quality care tends to be expensive care: to cope with the aftermath of poor quality may require longer hospital stays, readmissions, more extensive diagnostic workups, or additional procedures and medications. Much, maybe most, poor quality care, however, has no remarkable consequences and does not result in higher expenditures. Moreover, many studies that have evaluated physicians' practices according to specific criteria have faulted them for not providing many services. Acting on quality assessments thus has the potential to increase use and expense.

In the United States, we have embarked on a course of making more information on the quality of physicians and hospitals available to the public. One can argue that meaningful external evaluation of providers' quality is long overdue. Inevitably, some providers will unjustly be labelled as poor quality, some patients will needlessly change providers, and some payers and regulatory groups will waste money on inaccurate or inefficient assessment methods. These negative effects are more likely when assessments are still being refined and people are learning to interpret new information. But ultimately, the validity of the assessments is key. Assessments of quality require the active participation of physicians and other health professionals. At a minimum, their participation depends on their acceptance of the validity of the assessments and the fairness of the process.

NOTE

This paper was based on a report by the Office of Technology Assessment, *The Quality of Medical Care,* and an article in *Inquiry* (Sisk JE, Dougherty DM, Ehrenhaft PM, Ruby G, Mitchner BA: Assessing information for consumers on the quality of medical care. *Inquiry* 27:263-272, 1990). The views expressed here are the author's and do not necessarily represent those of the Office of Technology Assessment or its Technology Assessment Board.

REFERENCES

Berwick D, Batalden P: *Toward an Alternative Theory of Quality*. Harvard Community Health Plan (Cambridge, Massachusetts) and Hospital Corporation of America (Nashville, Tennessee), 1987.

Borgiel AEM: Assessing the Quality of Care in Family Physician' Practices by the College of Family Physicians of Canada. Presented to the Institute of Medicine's Health Care Technology Forum, Washington, DC, May 15, 1987.

Brook RH, Lohr KN: Efficacy, effectiveness, variations, and quality. *Medical Care* 23:710-722, 1985.

Davis DA, Norman GR, Painvin A, Lindsay E, et al: Attempting to ensure physician competence. *Journal of the American Medical Association* 263:2041-2042, 1990.

Donabedian A: Evaluating the quality of medical care. *Milbank Memorial Fund Quarterly* 44(3, Part 2): 166-203, 1966.

Donabedian A: *Explorations in Quality Assessment and Monitoring, Vol. I: The Definition of Quality and Approaches to its Assessment*. Ann Arbor, MI: Health Administration Press, 1980.

Dubois RW, Rogers WH, Moxley JH, et al: Hospital inpatient mortality: is it a predictor of quality? *New England Journal of Medicine* 317:1674-1680, 1987.

Hanft RS, Sisk JE, White CC: Measuring health care effectiveness: use of large data bases for technology and quality assessments. *International Journal of Technology Assessment in Health Care* 6:181-303, 1990.

Hannan EL, O'Donnel JF, Kilburn H Jr, Bernard HR, Yazici A: Investigation of the relationship between volume and mortality for surgical procedures performed in New York State hospitals. *Journal of the American Medical Association* 262:503-510, 1989.

Hannan EL, Yazici AA: *Critique of the 1987 HCFA Mortality Study Based on New York Data*. Albany, NY: Office of Health Systems Management, New York State Department of Health, 1988.

Harvard Medical Practice Study: *Patients, Doctors, and Lawyers: Medical Injury, Malpractice Litigation, and Patient Compensation in New York*. Report to the State of New York. Boston: Harvard University, 1990.

Luft HS, Garnick DW, Mark D, et al: *Evaluating Research on the Use of Volume of Services Performed in Hospitals as an Indicator of Quality*. Contractor Document. Washington, DC: Office of Technology Assessment, U.S. Congress, 1987.

McAuliffe W: Studies of process-outcome correlations in medical care evaluations. *Medical Care* 16: 907-930, 1978.

New York State Department of Health, Office of Health Systems Management, Bureau of Healthcare Research: *Investigation of Quality of Care in Hospitals*. Albany, NY, 1987.

Palmer RH, Reilly MC: Individual and institutional variables which may serve as indicators of quality of medical care. *Medical Care* 17:693-717, 1979.

Park RE, Brook RH, Kosecoff J, Kessey J, et al: Explaining variations in hospital death rates: randomness, severity of illness, quality of care. *Journal of the American Medical Association* 264:484-490, 1990.

Payne BC, Lyone TF, Neuhaus E: Relationships of physician characteristics to performance quality and improvement. *Health Services Research* 19:307-322, 1984.

Rubin L: *Comprehensive Quality Assurance System: The Kaiser-Permanente Approach*. Oakland, CA: The Permanente Medical Group, Inc., of Northern California, 1975, reprinted 1987.

Sanazaro PJ, Worth RM: Measuring clinical performance of individual internists in office and clinical practice. *Medical Care* 23:1097-1114, 1985.

Sisk JE, Dougherty DM, Ehrenhaft PM, Ruby G, Mitchner BA: Assessing information for consumers on the quality of medical care. *Inquiry* 27:263-272, 1990.

U.S. Congress, General Accounting Office: *Medicare: Improved Patient Outcome Analyses Could Enhance Quality Assessment*. Washington, DC.: U.S. Government Printing Office, 1988.

U.S. Congress, Office of Technology Assessment: *The Quality of Medical Care: Information for Consumers*. Washington, DC: U.S. Government Printing Office, 1988.

ASSESSING THE QUALITY OF MEDICAL CARE*
Discussant: Geoff Anderson
University of British Columbia

Dr. Sisk opens her excellent presentation by suggesting that two factors – consumerism and cost control – have led to increasing interest in the United States in quality assurance. I think that's probably true in Canada, though I'm not sure of the importance of the role of consumerism. I still have trouble getting a real handle on that one, but it seems clear to me the cost control debate in Canada can be characterized by two statements. One side says, "Under-funding has led to a decrease in the quality of care." The other side says, "There are inefficiencies in the existing system, and quality can be maintained while costs are controlled or reduced." And we've been having that debate on and off for the last 10 or 15 years. And it seems to me that we're never going to make any progress on that debate until we start to measure quality. The concepts "funds" and "quality" are in both statements. We can measure funds pretty accurately, but what we can't measure is quality. And unless we start measuring quality, we are not going to be able to resolve that very important argument.

Dr. Sisk then goes on to provide with us with, I think, a very good definition of the quality of care, I won't bother repeating it. The major point I want to make in relation to that definition is that you can now think of quality assurance as a process designed to help to ensure the quality of care. So if you think quality of care is a goal that should be pursued, then you have to be in support of quality assurance. That's sort of stating the obvious, but that's a good thing to do. And it seems clear to me, and it seems clear to probably everybody in this room, that quality assurance is an integral part of any health care system, or should be. Improvement in quality assurance is something that's worth striving for. So I think the definition really highlights it. Once you see that definition, you realize that it is sort of the essence of medical care summed up there.

Dr. Sisk then goes on to discuss various measures of quality. And I'm just going to touch briefly on each one of those, because she did a much better job of going through them than I possibly could. But I just want to make some interesting points, or what I think are interesting points.

The first one is that hospital mortality, as we now measure it, may not be a very good tool for assessing the quality of care. This is an important thing. It is so easy to measure that people – Health Care Financing Administration is a great example – have taken it and sort of run with it. And I think it is very important to realize that it may not be a great measure. And I also think it is important to remember that, while valid process measures should be related to outcomes, it is not necessarily true that bad outcomes are related to bad processes. We have got to be able to make that distinction, that simply having a bad outcome does not mean that you did something wrong. There are problems in trying to rank hospitals in terms of what in essence may be very random events – certainly over short periods of time, rare events, like hospital mortality, do show a lot of randomness.

She does point out the importance of developing process measures on the basis of evidence of effectiveness and efficacy. And I think that's very important, that when you are developing criteria, whether they be implicit or explicit, they should somehow be tied to evidence or a knowledge base or something logical – there should be some way to support each one of the criteria that you use. And evidence is the best, but if all we did was to look at things that we had evidence of efficacy for, we wouldn't be looking at very much. I think you are all very aware of that. So at some point we have to say, "Well, we just have to base that on underlying logic." But whatever that is, it has to be made explicit. So when you are making up process criteria, you have to be explicit about how they are linked to evidence – if not evidence of effectiveness, at least the logic that you have behind them.

Finally, she points out that structural characteristics, especially things such as specialty certification, are relatively poor measures of quality. I think this is an important lesson for people in Canada, or certainly for our concept of quality assurance, which has relied to a large part, I think, in recent years on certification or licensure as a guarantee of quality. It seems clear that the evidence is pretty well in, or is very strong, that licensure or certification alone is not a guarantee of high quality care. It may be a prerequisite, but it certainly is not a guarantee. So that we are certainly going have to move forward from just looking at certification.

Now at this point Dr. Sisk enters the discussion of policy implications for the United States. I'd just like to take a few minutes and try to set this in a Canadian context, of where we are now and where we want to be. Let me begin by defining where the "there" is that we want to be at. What is our goal? I think most people would agree that all the major stakeholders in healthcare – providers, patients, governments, the public – are very supportive of the idea of quality of care, or quality assurance. As suggested earlier, it's like apple pie – it is the essence of medicine. It is what the system is supposed to do. So everybody is very supportive of it. So our goal is clear. The "there" we want to get to is a system that provides high quality care.

So with that in mind, let's try and think about where the "here" is. Where are we now in Canada? And I'm certainly not going to attempt to do that in two or three minutes in a comprehensive sense, but I just want to touch a few important things. Let me begin by saying that I think there are two main types of quality assurance. I think there is a very complex informal system of quality assurance. I think you will all agree that the vast majority of providers of care are committed to providing high quality care, that it is part of what they do, that there is an essential element of all provider-professions that is involved in trying to provide high quality care, that people make extensive efforts within their own practice to ensure the quality of care. So this is a generally unrecognized, informal system which I think serves us very well. There is, on the other side, a formal system which has structures and lines of reporting, etc. etc. And in Canada I would say that we are at a fairly rudimentary level in that sort of system. We have colleges that have licences, we have professional bodies that give licences, we have legislation that has the term "quality assurance" in it, but we really haven't developed the formal side, although I think we have a very strong informal side. So that's a sort of picture of where we are.

How about how we are doing? Well, that's very difficult to answer. On sort of the general level, people have expressed concerns about the quality of care in Canada. On the other hand, there are no riots in the streets, and there's not a huge line-up of people getting sued, so on a very general level, it seems like the quality is not terrible.

What do we have in the way of studies? Well, I think there are a lot of pretty good studies in Canada. We have the work of Alex Borgiel and Jack Williams, who have done a marvellous study of the level of quality of care in Canada. There's some nice work out of McMaster by Dave Davis and his group. There's the work by Les Roos. And I think it all shows that the quality of care in Canada is not at the level we'd like it to be, that there is clearly room for improvement in the quality of care. When you take out explicit criteria and you find that people don't meet those criteria, that's an indication that care is not at the highest level, the level that you might like it at. So I think it would be fair to say that there is room for improvement in the quality of care. I think that most people would agree with that; that is not a shocking statement.

Now, what can we do to move from that system of where we are now to where we would like to be? Well, I think there are two paths by which we can do that. I think the important one, and the one I think keeps getting neglected, is to provide increased support for that informal network that I mentioned earlier, that we've got to be able to provide an environment in which practitioners feel that they get support in following quality of care issues, that that part of their normal professional activity is one that's acknowledged, is credible, is rewarded. So we have to make it easy for all sorts of providers to provide high quality care – things like having a reimbursement system that certainly has incentives for high quality care, or at least doesn't have incentives for low quality care. I think the other major thing in the informal system is to get back to medical school. Getting more material in the curriculum in medical schools is like getting a camel through the eye of a needle or something, but I think we've got to get residents, medical students, nursing students, and all provider students used to the notion that quality of care is just part of their profession. And it should be done at the earliest possible time.

Now how about for the formal stuff? Well, as an academic, of course I should argue that there should be increased training and expertise in the formal side of quality assurance. My latest bugbear is this notion of the consensus conference. We have in Canada this sort of Spanky and Our Gang attitude towards guidelines. We'll get a group of good people together, and we will put on a consensus conference, right? Unlike Spanky and his gang, who always ended up with Broadway calibre shows, we end up with a lot of very poor guidelines. The cholesterol debacle is a great example. We have five blue ribbon panels recommending things that are all over the map in terms of what should be done. So I think we need to think about the basic methodology that's involved in quality assurance.

The second thing, I think, besides the training and expertise, is that we need to develop more formal structures in Canada for quality assurance that bring all those parties together. It seems to me that we have the licensure colleges in every province, we have the Royal College and other professional societies, we have professional associations, we have the public. We have to find some forum where they can all get together and deal with this initiative that they all agree should be dealt with and that I think is to the benefit of all of them to deal with.

NOTE

* edited transcript of talk

DISCUSSION
Chair: Mark Wheeler
Health and Welfare Canada

J. Ivan Williams (Sunnybrook Health Sciences Centre)

Jane, I'd like to make an observation and then ask two questions. I'm wondering whether we aren't paying undue attention to mortality as an outcome. To be a little bit cheeky, a preventable death is a contradictory concept. Death is never prevented, unless one is Shirley MacLaine or another such individual who lives in the land of reruns. We can influence the timing of death and the conditions under which it occurs. And indeed now, it seems that some of the consumer demands are for more control of the conditions under which one dies. Now, how does that factor in when one is using mortality as a crude indicator of outcome? And, indeed, one can even argue that some of the most inappropriate forms of care are given within the last year of life, over a succession of hospital stays and medical interventions. So I'm wondering whether we shouldn't be rethinking mortality as an outcome if we're looking at quality assurance. That's kind of a rhetorical question. Now the two questions are as follows: When thinking about quality of care in your group, are you thinking about the lowest denominator that one would expect in hospital care, or optimal care? Optimal care could be described as fulfilling as many of the professional and public expectations as possible, whereas safe care could be defined as that which is deemed necessary to achieve appropriate outcomes. And then, related to that in part is how much should we be expecting to spend per hospital day on quality assurance activities? And I raise the question because we have been looking at what it would take to collect all of the data necessary for the APACHE ratings of critical care units within one hospital, and it boils down to pretty close to, as a conservative estimate, $100 per critical care bed per year. Now, should we not be thinking of some guidelines when we start this quest for information, as to how much information we can afford, let alone use?

Jane Sisk (Office of Technology Assessment, U.S. Congress)

Well, you've obviously made some really good points. I have a lot of misgivings about using mortality data as a measure of quality, and I tried to express some of them. As we were doing our study, people raised the fact that in those mortality statistics were certainly some people who had been allowed to die, given their poor state and the expense and misery of merely keeping them alive a little bit longer. But the sense was that that was likely to be a small percentage of deaths in any institution, so that there was unlikely to be a systematic bias that would affect the ranking of a particular institution. But I think the fact of the matter is that nobody really knows. I don't know of any study that's really gone through and tried to look at any of those issues and tried to separate out different kinds of deaths. So that's a short answer to the provocative questions you raised about that particular measure.

As far as whether we were thinking of quality as the lowest common denominator or the lowest acceptable level, or the optimal level, we recognized that those were issues that people implementing any kind of a quality assessment or assurance process had to deal with, but we didn't have to deal with them. So we mentioned them, and then we went on. What we were about was looking at whether there were valid indicators, and ones that were maybe not quite on the shelf, but available, or the information to create them was readily available.

And the third question about how much you spend, well of course there's no answer to how much you spend. That's a value judgment, with all the tradeoffs. But I had a lot of misgivings as we were finishing up our study a couple of years ago and certain states were mandating hospitals, every hospital in their state – I'm thinking specifically of Pennsylvania – to use a particular commercial product to report data that may be relevant to measuring quality. What that entailed was a large investment on the part of each hospital in the state to buy a software package that some researchers in the field have misgivings about. It was MedisGroups in the case of Pennsylvania. At least up until that point, there had not been a description or an evaluation of it in the peer review literature. The system is proprietary. It's put out by a profit-making entity, and they for obvious reasons did not want to make the nuts and bolts of what was in their black box available publicly. Not only were there those concerns about the validity and the efficiency of using some of these hospital data, but there was also the question of what the most efficient way to do this was, and the problem of the fact that not just the state of Pennsylvania, but the national system in the United States, the Joint Commission on the Accreditation of Health Care Organizations, is simultaneously coming up with additional requirements for these institutions. The federal government has got a laundry list of things that they're considering. So what this very easily added up to was very big bucks that hospitals, in particular, are going to be expected to undertake, all from the requirements of a lot of diverse entities.

Carol Kushner (Health Concepts Consultants)

Dr. Sisk, I just wanted to ask about the role of the consumer and the public's use of the information that is becoming available on the quality of hospital care, and in particular whether it has been possible for your office or others who are publishing this data, including reporters, to make some of the measurement caveats that you've highlighted today available to the public? What's been the response from consumers, and how has that data been used? Are they voting with their feet?

Jane Sisk

As far as I know, nobody has looked at that, at what the effects of the availability of this information have been. We did collect some press reports about the – I guess it was 1987 – release, and the range of the quality of the reporting was tremendous. There were some articles that were terrifically perceptive and they had all of the caveats, proper wording that you would most like in your dreams to see in a press article, and there were others that were just terrible, as far as giving what seemed like a very inaccurate impression of what the statistics meant. And that's – journalism, at least in the United States – democracy or something. The feeling of consumer advocates such as Sid Wolfe or Ralph Nader's Health Group, who are very very strongly in favour of this kind of public information, is that even in the short term, if there are mistakes made, if there are inaccuracies put out, that's not nearly so important as what he or they hope will happen over the long run, which is that there will be this external pressure for providers to improve, and people will somehow get more familiar with how to use the information, not perhaps put as much stock in it as they might have when they first saw the information in the initial release. But all of that is just speculative. Who knows?

Robert Evans (University of British Columbia)

Mark, as a point of information, a study by Bruce Vladeck from the United Hospital Fund of New York, published in *Health Affairs* about 18 months ago, split his hospitals into three groups – high, medium, and low on the HCFA Report, and then looked to see whether, over time, there had been any differential change in occupancy in the low-quality, medium-quality, and high-quality hospitals. In the report in *Health Affairs,* he found zip effect.

Jane Sisk

There was a recent Luft article – was it in *JAMA?* – that used some measures, I think they were mostly structural – sort of an *ex post facto* sort of thing going back into the 1980s – and I think they concluded that they thought there was some suggestion that people had gone towards what they might have considered higher quality, but as far as I could see in that article, they didn't ask – they didn't test out their theories on the consumers. It may have been that those people went to those hospitals for totally different reasons.

METHODOLOGY FOR ECONOMIC EVALUATION: GIVE US THE TOOLS

IMPLICATIONS OF BASING HEALTH CARE RESOURCE ALLOCATIONS ON COST-UTILITY ANALYSIS IN THE PRESENCE OF EXTERNALITIES

Roberta J. Labelle
Jeremiah E. Hurley
Centre for Health Economics and Policy Analysis
McMaster University

INTRODUCTION

Economists have long recognized that utility derives, at least in theory, from a variety of sources and that the benefits and costs of a program or service can accrue to more than only the users (for example, Mishan, 1971a; Sugden and Williams, 1978; Boadway and Bruce, 1984). A comprehensive program evaluation therefore requires that, in addition to user-specific costs and benefits, external costs and benefits be included. As Mishan (1971a) points out, "A conscientious cost-benefit study, it is hardly necessary to remark, cannot ignore any spillover effect, positive or negative, that is of social concern." The practical problems, however, of identifying and measuring externalities for program evaluation have challenged economists for decades. In response to the challenge, a number of methods have been devised for measuring people's willingness-to-pay for external benefits, including travel costing models, hedonic price equations and, more recently, contingent valuation methods. The context for these methodological developments has been almost exclusively cost-benefit analysis (CBA), rather than cost-utility analysis (CUA) or cost-effectiveness analysis (CEA).

The importance of externalities (particularly external benefits) in the health sector has been acknowledged by a number of economists (Mishan, 1971b; Culyer, 1976; Evans and Wolfson, 1980). Culyer (1976), for example, points out that the "humanitarian spillovers" from health care are sufficiently large to provide a case for subsidizing health care consumption and have been used as a justification for the publicly-financed National Health Service in the U.K.

In health care applications, however, the difficulties (and, some would argue, the inappropriateness) of quantifying health-related benefits within a willingness-to-pay paradigm have led to a shift from CBA to CEA and CUA. Currently, applications of CEA and CUA to health care interventions and programs dominate the relatively infrequent uses of CBA. Although CEA requires less demanding information than does a comprehensive CBA, there are also stricter limitations on the use of the results. These limitations arise because the objectives, and hence the scope of inquiry, of CEA are more narrow than those of CBA. In particular, CEA is a useful analytic approach for evaluating technical efficiency, but it cannot be used for determining allocative efficiency. Accordingly, it can provide only part of the information for health policy decision-making (Cullis and West, 1979). As early as 1971, Klarman cautioned that, "One must recognize that CEA cannot provide rankings or priorities across diverse avenues of public expenditure." (Klarman, 1982).

Although these limitations of CEA have generally been acknowledged and accepted, there has been some debate about whether they apply to CUA. Because CUA, by definition, attempts to incorporate individuals' valuations of health outcomes, it shifts the focus of the evaluation from issues of purely technical efficiency to those of allocative efficiency. As noted, CUA emerged in part as a response to the difficulty of quantifying benefits in monetary terms, as is required by a CBA, and the conceptual underpinnings of CBA have been held to apply to CUA (Feeny and Torrance, 1989; Drummond, Stoddart, and Torrance, 1987).[1] But what was recognized in the CBA context – the notion that externalities are potentially important and hence should be included – has not been pursued in the development and application of CUA. Cost-utility ratios, as currently constructed, do not include external benefits or costs. Although the same is true for cost-effectiveness ratios, we focus on CUA because there are few examples of CEA's being used to determine efficiency across a broad range of services and programs within the health care sector. Its application has been restricted primarily to assessments of technical efficiency. CUA, in contrast, is increasingly being advocated as a means of providing information for setting priorities and allocating resources within (and to) the health care sector.

ROLES FOR CUA

Cost-utility analysis, which is a comparison of the costs of two or more alternatives and the health-related quality of life associated with them, has had two primary applications: to guide clinical decision making and to provide information relevant to health (care) policy decisions[2] (Drummond, 1989). The first refers to decision making regarding optimal treatment, in a technical sense, for a given disease (e.g., what is the most efficient treatment for chronic renal failure?) or for a particular patient population (e.g., what is the most efficient approach to improving the quality of life of nursing home residents?). The analysis is used to aid clinical decisions that focus exclusively on the costs and outcomes incurred by a defined set of patients, and hence does not take into account the effects (either positive or negative) of an intervention on other individuals. Examples include CUA conducted as part of a clinical trial (e.g., Bombardier et al, 1986), or studies of the effects of the introduction of a new program (e.g., Boyle et al, 1983). When applied in this context, CUA provides essential information on patients' quality of life – an outcome dimension that historically has been largely ignored because of the emphasis on purely clinical outcomes.

The second application, the use of CUA to guide health (care) policy decisions, is increasingly evident. Applied in this context, CUA is used to inform the process of resource allocation, both within the health care sector and between the health care sector and other sectors. Because the focus is on system-level decisions, the potential beneficiaries and conditions (either to be treated or prevented) are diverse; for example, requests for funding of prenatal care programs may compete with requests for programs to reduce the incidence of stroke or with calls for increased funding for long term care institutions. In an even broader sense, if the objective of public sector resource allocations is the maximization of societal wellbeing, it is possible that demands for higher levels of income assistance or improved housing might be assessed against demands for more health care.

Several of the advocates of CUA argue that the results can be used to assist decision makers in allocating health care resources (Sackett and Torrance, 1978; Williams, 1985; Gudex and Kind, n.d.; Drummond, 1989; Cairns and Johnston, 1990). Cost-utility analyses commissioned by public health authorities actually have contributed, in varying degrees, to health care resource allocation decisions (Gudex, 1986; Dept. of Health and Social Security (UK), 1986; Allen, Lee, and Lowson, 1989). Perhaps the most visible evidence of the expanded role given to CUA is the emergence and proliferation of "league tables". A league table provides a cardinal ranking of the cost per quality-adjusted life year (QALY) of various health care interventions, with the intervention yielding the lowest cost/QALY seen to be the "best", that is, the most (technically) efficient means of producing QALYs.

Table 1, an example of a league table, provides a ranking of the cost/QALY results from various studies, in ascending order. These summary tables are increasingly included when interpreting the results of specific studies. (See, for example, Torrance and Zipursky, 1984; Williams, 1985; Drummond, Teeling Smith, and Wells, 1988; Torrance and Feeny, 1989; Goel, Deber, and Detsky, 1989). Although several criticisms and caveats have been raised with regard to the compilation and interpretation of league tables (Drummond, Teeling Smith, and Wells, 1988; Drummond, 1987; Loomes and McKenzie, 1989), the tables continue to be proffered as a means of directly comparing the value of various programs.

Practitioners of economic evaluations have argued convincingly that if the evaluations are to be used for setting resource allocation priorities, the analysis should be conducted from the "societal perspective", which requires that all costs and benefits be included, regardless of to whom they accrue (Drummond, Stoddart, and Torrance, 1987; Mulley, 1989). In the case of CUA, although great effort has been taken to identify, measure, and value all social costs (see, for example, Boyle et al, 1983), less emphasis has been placed on identifying, measuring, and valuing all sources of society's utility.

As currently measured, the utility included in a CUA pertains to the utility of health states associated with the programs or services being evaluated. These health state utility values are obtained from a variety of sources, often raising the question of whose values should count (Mooney, 1986; Mulley, 1989). Patients are typically the source of utility values (McNeil, Weichselbaum, and Pauker, 1981; Bombardier et al, 1986; Churchill et al, 1987), although caregivers (Mohide et al, 1988), researchers (Goel, Deber, and Detsky, 1989), health care providers (Williams, 1985), the general public (Ciampi, Silberfeld, and Till, 1982), or a combination of the above (Rosser and Kind, 1978) have also been used. When the values are elicited from non-patients, in most if not all cases respondents are asked to reply as if they were a patient with the condition of interest.[3] They are often asked explicitly to "put yourself in the patient's position" and respond accordingly, regardless of whether the choice is posed in the first person (e.g., "I prefer health state A to health state B"), the third person ("Mrs. Smith's health state (A) is preferable to Mrs. Jones' health state (B)"), or without explicit reference to a specific individual ("Health state A is preferred to health state B"). As a result, when utility assessments have been conducted on the general public, often for the purpose of increasing sample size, the responses have been used as proxies for patient responses (Torrance and Feeny, 1989). Utility to non-patients, in the form of external benefits and costs, is omitted.

EXTERNALITIES

We focus on two types of external benefits that may be particularly important in the health sector: benefits derived from interdependent utility with respect to health and health care and benefits associated with option demand. Other types of externalities undoubtedly exist, but the two analyzed herein have been the types most frequently associated with health care provision.

Table 1
EXAMPLE OF A LEAGUE TABLE

Program	Cost-utility ratio, $/QALY gained •
Screening for phenylketonuria	< 0
Postpartum anti-D therapy	< 0
Antepartum anti-D therapy	1,480
Coronary artery bypass surgery for left main coronary artery disease	5,100
Neonatal intensive care for infants weighing 1000 to 1499 g.	5,460
Screening for thyroxine deficiency	7,650
Treatment of severe hypertension (diastolic pressure ≥ 105 mm Hg) in men aged 40 yr.	11,400
Administration of new contrast media to 30% of population at highest risk, with 10-fold reduction in relative risk	23,000
Treatment of mild hypertension (diastolic pressure 95 to 104 mm Hg) in men aged 40 yr.	23,175
Estrogen therapy among postmenopausal women who have not had hysterectomy	32,760
Neonatal intensive care for infants weighing 500 to 999 g.	38,580
Coronary artery bypass surgery for single-vessel disease in patients with moderate angina	44,400
Tuberculin testing in school	53,000
Continuous ambulatory peritoneal dialysis	57,100
Complete conversion to new contrast media, with 10-fold reduction in relative risk	64,000
Hemodialysis in hospital	65,500
Administration of new contrast media to low-risk patients, with 10-fold reduction in relative risk	220,000

• Values adjusted to 1986 US dollars.
Reprinted, by permission of publisher, from Goel V et al: Nonionic contrast media: economic analysis and health policy development. *Canadian Medical Association Journal* 140:393, 1989.

INTERDEPENDENT UTILITY AS A SOURCE OF BENEFITS

An interdependence of utility functions creates external effects because one person's consumption of health care affects another person's utility. This type of external benefit of health care interventions has been recognized at least since the late 1950s and was initially associated with immunization against communicable diseases (e.g., Weisbrod, 1961). In the last 30 years, however, the conceptualization of the nature of the interdependence has expanded (Culyer and Simpson, 1980; Evans and Wolfson, 1980). Evans and Wolfson (1980) identify three main types of interdependence: selfish, paternalistic, and altruistic. Selfish interdependence exists when individual A cares about individual B's consumption of health services because B's consumption directly affects A's health status. An example is treatment for a communicable disease: when B is treated for hepatitis, thereby decreasing the probability that A will get the disease, for purely selfish reasons A's utility increases. Paternalistic interdependence exists when B's consumption of health care, B's level of health status, or both, directly enter A's utility function. That is, A cares about B's consumption of health care not because of its effects on A's health but because of its effects on B's health. Finally, altruistic interdependence exists when B's level of utility (as opposed to health status) enters A's utility function. How B obtains this utility does not matter to A; the only thing that matters to A is B's level of utility, which is determined only in part by B's health status. Although the exact nature of the interdependence has important implications for the role of government in the health care sector (see Evans and Wolfson, 1980), it is less important for our purposes. If only selfish interdependencies exist, the class of programs for which external benefits exist is limited. But if one admits of either paternalistic or altruistic interdependencies, then external effects exist for a broad array of health care interventions, and economic evaluations conducted from the societal viewpoint should include these benefits (or costs).[4]

There is considerable empirical support for the proposition that interdependent utilities exist for many goods, and for health care in particular. In the U.S., for example, the charitable sector accounts for over 2% of GNP, over 85% of all households make donations to charities, and in 1981 health organizations and hospitals raised over $7 billion in contributions (Andreoni, 1988). The amount of voluntary labour in the health sector is substantial, and a large portion of blood products is provided through voluntary donations. Paternalistic and altruistic interdependencies are perhaps best evidenced by the fact that every industrialized nation has attempted to remove barriers to care by undertaking some form of public financing of health services. Undoubtedly all these actions could be explained by a sufficiently ingenious model of purely self-interested utility maximizing individuals, but such elegant models should not obscure the motivation for giving: people care about others. The importance of this observation has been noted by a number of economists (Collard, 1978; Margolis, 1982; Etzioni, 1989; Sugden, 1985; Phelps, 1975). Indeed, it is ironic that the benefits accruing from one of the primary motives for public intervention in the health sector have been excluded from evaluations of services provided through such systems.

OPTION VALUE AS A SOURCE OF BENEFITS

In his seminal paper, Arrow (1963) identified two types of uncertainty associated with health care: (1) uncertainty regarding illness and the need for care; and (2) uncertainty regarding the effectiveness of care. Whenever uncertainty is present, there is potential to improve welfare by reducing or eliminating the uncertainty. The second source of non-user benefit, termed option value when first discussed by Weisbrod (1964), is present because of the uncertainty regarding future need for health care. When future need, and hence demand, is uncertain, there exist current non-users who, given the uncertainty regarding their future demand, are willing to pay an amount in the current period (an option value) to ensure that the service will be available at a later time. Option demand thus exists even though some (or possibly even most) individuals may never actually need or use the service. Conventional evaluation methods that count only the benefits to users, even if the entire future stream of user benefits is incorporated, will exclude this option value. Option value theoretically may exist for almost any good, but the benefits associated with it are likely to be significant compared to user benefits only for goods for which use is infrequent and for which there is considerable uncertainty regarding future demand. National parks and hospitals (or specific health services) are two examples that have been cited (Weisbrod, 1964; Culyer, 1971).

Since Weisbrod's original paper on option value, there has been considerable development and clarification of the concept, particularly its relationship to conventional benefit measures used in cost-benefit analysis (Cicchetti and Freeman, 1971; Schmalensee, 1972; Graham, 1981; Bishop, 1982, 1986; Smith, 1983). Of particular interest is the relationship between option price, defined as the total amount a current non-user is willing to pay today to ensure the future supply of a good at a specified price (Weisbrod's original option value), and expected consumer surplus, defined as the expected value of the consumer surplus obtained in alternative future states of the world. The difference between option price and expected consumer surplus is termed option value. Option value is analogous to the difference between an actuarially fair premium (expected value of a loss) and the maximum premium an individual is willing to pay to purchase insurance and thereby eliminate uncertainty.

There has been much debate in the cost-benefit literature regarding the most appropriate measure of benefits in the presence of uncertainty, but a consensus is emerging that option price is the best measure because it incorporates both expected consumer surplus and the benefits associated with risk reduction. Graham (1981) concluded that, given the constraints of actually measuring benefits, option price is the best measure of welfare under uncertainty. Bishop (1986) also supports the use of option price.

Attempts to measure option prices in other applied fields indicate that the contribution of such benefits can be large relative to user benefits. Greenley et al (1981) concluded that non-user benefits of preserved water quality were approximately 40% of user benefits; Walsh et al (1984) estimated that the non-user preservation value of wilderness in the state of Colorado was 60% of recreational-use value; and Brookshire et al (1983) obtained positive non-user option prices for the preservation of grizzly bear and bighorn sheep in the Wyoming wilderness.

Most of the development of this concept, both theoretical and empirical, has occurred in natural resource economics. But clearly, as Weisbrod noted, such non-user benefits may also be quite large for health services. There is considerable uncertainty regarding the future need (and demand) for many health services and, given the consequences of not receiving needed care, the option value associated with service availability may be considerable relative to user benefits. For example, at any given time only a small fraction of the population are in need of, and use, emergency room services, but most people are at some risk for future use.

MODELLING THE EFFECTS OF OMITTING NON-USER UTILITY

The omission of non-user benefits does not necessarily invalidate program rankings based on economic evaluations, as currently reported in league tables. If, for example, non-user benefits are always proportional in size to user benefits, then the inclusion of externalities would not alter the ordinal rankings. Even when this is not the case, it is possible to correct for the omission if it can be determined, *a priori,* that the underestimate varies consistently with certain characteristics of the program (e.g., the size of the target population). If it is not possible, however, to predict the effect of the omission on the cost-utility ratio, it becomes necessary to measure the externalities directly to incorporate their impact on both users and non-users.

To explore the effect of the omission of non-user benefits on measures of economic efficiency, we develop a simple model for calculating the incremental total societal utility and the incremental cost-per-util-gained associated with a hypothetical program. We employ cost-per-util rather than the more common outcome measure, cost-per-quality-adjusted life year (QALY), for several reasons. First, utility measures must be based on a valid and accurate representation of individual preferences, and there is concern that the QALY fails in this regard (Mehrez and Gafni, 1989; Loomes and McKenzie, 1989). An alternative utility-based measure, Healthy Years Equivalent (HYE), overcomes some of the methodologic difficulties with QALYs (Mehrez and Gafni, 1989). Although as a preference measure the HYE has an intuitive appeal and interpretation when applied to patients, it makes less sense when applied to non-patients. Therefore, in the context of both user and non-user utility, we represent utility in units of "utils". We do not propose the cost-per-util as an alternative outcome measure for cost-utility analysis, but use it merely to illustrate the main points of the model.

Using the model, we then compare the incremental cost-per-util-gained when external benefits are excluded versus when they are included. Of particular interest in this comparison is the relationship between the prevalence of a disease and the magnitude of the discrepancy between the cost-per-util-gained with and without the inclusion of non-user benefits. The impact of prevalence is important because one characteristic of league tables is that they compare interventions aimed at diseases with dissimilar prevalence rates. This can be seen, for example, in Table 1. Treatment of severe hypertension, which has a prevalence of approximately 4.0% in adult males, is compared directly with treatment for mild hypertension, which has a prevalence of approximately 12.2% in the same population (Gunning-Schepers, 1989). Thus the construction of ratios to report results means that issues such as cost-of-illness, burden of illness, and total impact of treatment, which are all functions of prevalence, are ignored.[5]

THE MODEL

To construct the model, we assume that a program has been proposed for the treatment of a specific condition and that it is to be evaluated from the societal viewpoint. The baseline for the comparison is the "no program" (i.e., no treatment) alternative, and we assume that all individuals with the condition receive treatment. The standard assumptions found either implicitly or explicitly in CUA studies are made: that individuals have measurable cardinal utility functions and that societal utility is additive in each individual's utility. In addition, we assume that the utility function is additively separable in each of its components.

The following notation is used to represent the variables that enter the analysis:

N = total population (assumed to be constant during the period under analysis);

P = prevalence rate[6] of the condition/disease being treated;

NP = number of people in society who have the condition;

U_P = mean increment in **patient** utility resulting from treatment,

$$\frac{\sum_{i=1}^{NP} U_{P,i}}{NP},$$

where $U_{P,i}$ is the incremental utility for the ith patient;

U_{PID} = mean increment in **patient** utility resulting from treatment of **other patients**,

$$\frac{\sum_{i=1}^{NP} \sum_{\substack{k=1 \\ k \neq i}}^{NP-1} U_{PID,i,k}}{NP(NP-1)},$$

where $U_{PID,i,k}$ is the incremental interdependent utility for the ith patient from the treatment of the kth patient;

U_{NPID} = mean increment in **non-patient** utility resulting from the treatment of **patients**,

$$\frac{\sum_{j=1}^{N-NP} \sum_{i=1}^{NP} U_{NPID,j,i}}{(N-NP)NP},$$

where $U_{NPID,j,i}$ is the incremental interdependent utility for the jth non-patient from the treatment of the ith patient;

$U_{OV}(P-P^2)$ = mean increment in option value for a **non-patient**,

$$\frac{\sum_{j=1}^{N-NP} U_{OV,j}(P-P^2)}{N-NP},$$

where $U_{OV,j}$ is the incremental option value for the jth non-patient;

b = incremental cost of treatment per patient (constant);

TC = total incremental cost = $b(NP)$.

The utility variables are specified as means because the analysis is not affected by the distribution of utility values across individuals. The use of means also simplifies the algebra. We make a distinction between the interdependent utilities of patients (U_{PID}) and non-patients (U_{NPID}) because it is possible that the mean values of the interdependencies may differ. On average, an individual with the condition who receives treatment may get a different level of utility from the treatment of others with the same condition than would an individual who does not have the condition.

Prevalence enters directly into the model. Option value is explicitly made a function of prevalence (P) because, for a given degree of risk aversion, option value varies systematically with the degree of uncertainty regarding future demand. (U_{OV} is simply a scaling factor.) As such, prevalence can be interpreted as a proxy measure of the probability of needing the program.[7] The functional form for option value, $U_{OV}(P-P^2)$, was chosen to reflect the fact that when there is no uncertainty (P = 0 or P = 1.0), option value is zero; when P = 0.5, an individual's uncertainty is greatest and, other things equal, option value is at its maximum. Option value accrues only to non-patients, since patients with the disease do not face uncertainty about acquiring the illness. Constant marginal cost is assumed for simplicity.

TOTAL BENEFITS

Because it is assumed that total societal utility is additive in each individual's utility, and that each individual's utility is additive in its components, the total societal utility associated with the program is the sum of utilities across individuals and utility components. If non-users are excluded and only the utility accruing directly to patients is measured, the increment to total utility associated with the program is:

$$U_{NE} = NP(U_P) \tag{1}$$

where the subscript NE denotes that only user utility is measured (i.e, there are no externalities).

If non-user utility is also measured (i.e., when externalities are included), the increment to total utility is:[8]

$$U_E = NP(U_P) + NP(N-NP)U_{NPID} + NP(NP-1)U_{PID} + (N-NP)U_{OV}(P-P^2) \tag{2}$$

Equations (1) and (2) demonstrate that the difference between the two benefit measures, $U_E - U_{NE}$, varies systematically with prevalence. For $U_{NPID} > 0$, $U_{PID} > 0$, and $U_{OV} > 0$, this difference is greater than zero and increases over the interval $0 < P \le 0.33$; for $P > 0.33$ the difference is still positive ($U_E - U_{NE} > 0$), but depending on the relative values of U_P, U_{PID}, U_{NPID}, and U_{OV}, it may increase or decrease as P increases.

COST-PER-UTIL

The incremental cost-per-util-gained when non-user utility is excluded is:

$$C/U_{NE} = \frac{C}{U_{NE}} = \frac{b(NP)}{NP(U_P)}$$

$$= \frac{b}{U_P} \tag{3}$$

With no externalities, the cost-per-util-gained does not vary with the prevalence of a disease, because prevalence cancels out of the C/U ratio. Consequently, two programs for which the cost-per-util-gained is the same would be ranked as equal, regardless of whether or not the prevalence rates of the underlying diseases differed markedly.

When non-user utility is included, the incremental cost-per-util-gained becomes:

$$C/U_E = \frac{b(NP)}{NP(U_P) + NP(N-NP)U_{NPID} + NP(NP-1)U_{PID} + U_{OV}(P-P^2)(N-NP)}$$

$$= \frac{b}{U_P + N(1-P)U_{NPID} + (NP-1)U_{PID} + (1-2P+P^2)U_{OV}} \tag{4}$$

and the cost-per-util-gained varies systematically with the prevalence of the disease.

The primary concern that motivated this paper is that using CUA to allocate resources when non-user utility is excluded may unknowingly lead to recommending a non-optimal allocation. This possibility is addressed by using the model to examine possible biases. Specifically, we attempt to identify situations in which the omission of externalities has the greatest likelihood of changing program rankings. The analysis focuses in particular on the relationship between prevalence and the amount by which cost-per-util-gained for a program is overestimated by the exclusion of externalities.

The relationship can be examined by subtracting equations (4) from (3) and taking the derivative with respect to P. This yields the following conditions:

i) if P >

ii) if P =
$$1 + \frac{N(U_{NPID} - U_{PID})}{2(U_{OV})}, \quad \text{then} \quad \left(\frac{C}{U_{NE}} - \frac{C}{U_E}\right)$$

iii) if P <

increases with P;

is constant with respect to P;

decreases with P.

The expressions indicate that the critical determinant of the relationship is the relative values of U_{PID}, U_{NPID}, and U_{OV}. Theoretically, each of U_{PID}, U_{NPID}, and U_{OV} could be positive, negative, or zero for any given disease. Because the purpose of this paper is to examine the impact of excluding externalities, when they in fact exist, we restrict our attention to the situation in which U_{PID}, U_{NPID} and U_{OV} are all positive (on net). In this case, the relative values of U_{PID} and U_{NPID} alone determine which of the above conditions hold. Three relationships are possible:

a) $U_{PID} > U_{NPID}$; this assumes that an individual with the condition derives more interdependent utility from the treatment of others with the same condition than does an individual who does not have the condition. In this case, $(U_{NPID} - U_{PID})$ is less than zero, and the gap between C/U_E and C/U_{NE} becomes a function of the size of the term $\frac{N(U_{NPID} - U_{PID})}{2U_{OV}}$, hereafter referred to as Z^*. If $Z^* < -1$, then $(C/U_{NE} - C/U_E)$ increases with P over the whole range of P $[0 \leq P \leq 1]$. This situation is depicted in Figure 1a, where the gap between the two cost-utility ratios widens as prevalence increases. If, however, $-1 < Z^* < 0$, then $(C/U_{NE} - C/U_E)$ is decreasing in P over the interval $[0, P^*]$ and increasing over the interval $[P^*, 1]$. This case is shown in Figure 1b.

b) $U_{PID} = U_{NPID}$; this is a situation in which the amount of interdependent utility received is the same for patients and non-patients. In this case, Z^* is zero and $(C/U_{NE} - C/U_E)$ decreases with P over the whole range of P. This is illustrated in Figure 1c, where the gap narrows as prevalence increases.

c) $U_{PID} < U_{NPID}$; in this final scenario, non-patients receive greater interdependent utility from the treatment of a disease than do the patients with the disease. Here, Z^* is positive and hence $(C/U_{NE} - C/U_E)$ again decreases with P, as in Figure 1c.

The above conditions demonstrate that it is not possible to determine, *a priori*, either the magnitude or the direction of the bias introduced by omitting externalities from a cost-utility analysis. To do this requires knowing the relative values of U_{PID} and U_{NPID}. But does this imply that, even under certain assumptions, it is not possible to estimate the impact of the omission? This question is important because it may be that there are assumptions that could be made which would preserve the relative rankings of programs, even if externalities were included. Consider, for instance, the simplest case, in which the values of U_{PID}, U_{NPID}, and U_{OV} are identical across two programs. Even with this restrictive (and unrealistic) assumption, it is impossible to predict in advance the direction of the bias introduced by the omission of non-user utilities without knowledge of the specific values of the U_{NPID} and U_{PID}. That is, any of the relationships in Figure 1 could hold. If, for example, a disease with high prevalence was compared with one of lower prevalence, and the

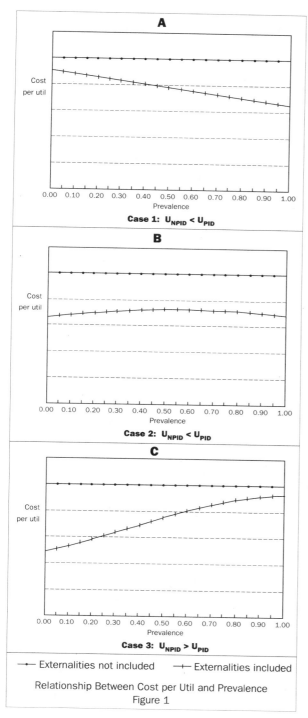

A

Cost
per util

0.00 0.10 0.20 0.30 0.40 0.50 0.60 0.70 0.80 0.90 1.00
Prevalence

Case 1: U$_{NPID}$ < U$_{PID}$

B

Cost
per util

0.00 0.10 0.20 0.30 0.40 0.50 0.60 0.70 0.80 0.90 1.00
Prevalence

Case 2: U$_{NPID}$ < U$_{PID}$

C

Cost
per util

0.00 0.10 0.20 0.30 0.40 0.50 0.60 0.70 0.80 0.90 1.00
Prevalence

Case 3: U$_{NPID}$ > U$_{PID}$

—•— Externalities not included   —+— Externalities included

Relationship Between Cost per Util and Prevalence
Figure 1

situation as in Figure 1a prevailed, then the inclusion of externalities would result in a smaller C/U ratio for the higher prevalence disease. If, however, the situation was as in Figure 1c, the inclusion of externalities would favour the low prevalence program, and the rankings would be reversed. Therefore, there is no way of knowing whether, and how, the relative rankings in a league table would be affected.

DISCUSSION

The significance of omitting externalities depends crucially upon what one believes to be the appropriate theoretical basis for allocating society's resources and what one believes the theoretical foundations of CUA to be. If the common economic view of allocating resources in a manner that maximizes technical and allocative efficiency (as defined within the welfare theoretic tradition) is accepted, then externalities should be included in the evaluation of health care programs. The methods employed to conduct the evaluation should conform to the principles of welfare theory, with respect both to what is measured and to how the values are obtained. Currently there are differing views in the CUA literature regarding whether welfare theory does, or even should, form the basis of CUA (Williams, 1981; Feeny and Torrance, 1989). Yet most CUA studies are conducted and interpreted as if the technique were capable of evaluating allocative efficiency. If the theoretic foundations of welfare economics are germane, then the deficiencies of CUA in this regard are an issue. Omitting externalities is a shortcoming of the technique, and the validity of CUA is compromised because it cannot, at least as currently structured, measure the theoretical constructs that are held to underlie it.

A second question then arises as to whether externalities are large enough (relative to user-specific costs and benefits) to affect allocation decisions. Evidence from studies outside the health sector strongly suggests that this might be the case, but there is little empirical information on the magnitude of health-care related externalities *per se*. The nature of the commodity health, however, coupled with the experiences from other sectors, indicates the need to explore these issues further.

Can the existing CUA methodology be adapted to measure externalities? It might be possible, but it will certainly not be a straightforward task; we outline some of the difficulties that are likely to be encountered. First, the respondent sample would have to be expanded from patients (users of care) to the community at large (non-users). Patients would be represented in this sample only in proportion to the prevalence of their disease in the population. The second modification would involve the information that would have to be conveyed to respondents. Typically, in a CUA, respondents are given information about the health outcomes, or states (e.g., functional ability, mental ability, pain, dependence) associated with the alternatives being evaluated. They are then asked to choose amongst options based on their preferences for the health outcomes. A much broader range of information is required, however, for capturing externalities. In addition to the information on health status improvements for those treated (including long term sequelae and prognosis), to evaluate the program respondents would have to be provided with data on prevalence, incidence, and communicability of the disease and on the distribution of its impact across population sub-groups. Particularly important for assessing option demand might be information on risk factors and future patterns of illness. This list is not comprehensive, but it illustrates the types of information that respondents would require to estimate external benefits and costs. It appears that the greatest challenge for researchers who attempt to move from measuring individual utilities to societal utilities will be in obtaining and conveying the requisite information. Much of the information listed above is not known, or not known with precision. Nor will it be easy to present the information to respondents in a meaningful way. A second challenge will be to determine whether the existing utility measurement tools of standard gamble, time-trade-off, or category scaling could be modified to incorporate the information, if available.

Given the methodological obstacles to modifying CUA techniques for resource allocation purposes, it may be useful to reconsider cost-benefit analysis. There are several recent examples of CBAs in the health care field, and considerable work is being directed at revising traditional CBA methodology for health care-related applications. Contingent valuation methodology, which has been used to value externalities in other sectors, is an approach that has the potential to incorporate the information needed for a full evaluation and which can be modified in light of the criticisms levied against standard CBA methods applied to the analysis of health care. Willingness-to-pay techniques can be replaced by more relevant approaches such as willingness to reallocate public funds and willingness to be taxed (Donaldson, 1990). The advantage of moving (back) to a CBA approach is that the theoretic underpinnings, and hence the attendant value judgments, are well understood. Moreover, the approach would provide more comprehensive information on the sum total of benefits to society, not just to a sub-sample of patients. Much work needs to be done refining CBA measurement techniques for the health care context, but such efforts may prove worthwhile if they help form a solid basis for resource allocation decisions. As Mishan (1971b) has emphasized,

> In view of the existing quantomania, one may be forgiven for asserting that there is more to be said for rough estimates of the precise than precise estimates of economically irrelevant concepts.

ACKNOWLEDGEMENTS

The authors thank George Torrance, Amiram Gafni, Tony Culyer, and members of the Health Utilities Group at McMaster for valuable comments on earlier versions of the paper. Research for this paper was supported in part by a Career Scientist Award from the Ontario Ministry of Health (RL).

NOTES

1. It should be acknowledged that the notion of using the Paretian Principle to identify socially optimum allocation does not necessarily imply the simultaneous objective of maximizing social utility, as measured by ΣU_i. As Mishan (1971a) emphasizes, "...the rationale of the conventional cost-benefit analysis is not to be interpreted as having an affinity with a social goal of maximizing or increasing aggregate utility. No interpersonal comparisons of utility are to be invoked."

2. A third application, that of guiding decisions at the individual patient level, is advocated by some (Williams, n.d.), while strongly discouraged by others (LaPuma and Lawlor, 1990). Because the focus of the present paper is on decisions made at the health system level, we subsume the patient-level application in "clinical decision making".

3. Detailed descriptions of procedures for measuring health state utilities can be found in Furlong et al (1990), Gudex and Kind (n.d.), and Torrance (1986).

4. In a recent paper, Jones-Lee has argued that within a utilitarian framework externalities should be measured only if they are of the selfish or paternalistic type, i.e., they are directly tied to a good and are not purely altruistic in the sense defined above (Jones-Lee, 1991).

5. The inherent limitations of basing allocation decisions on any ratio measures have been well documented in the CBA literature (Birch and Donaldson, 1987).

6. More specifically, for purposes of this analysis, we employ the notion of "period prevalence", which is defined as the number of people known to have the disease over a specified time period divided by the number of people at risk over that period.

7. This is true in the sense that the prevalence rate for a specified population or sub-population is, in fact, the pre-test likelihood (of having the disease) for an individual (from that same population) undergoing a diagnostic test. But if, at any given time, an individual knows with certainty whether or not he/she has the disease, future demand is likely to be a function of the rate of *new* cases arising in the population. Accordingly, option demand will be determined by the incidence of a disease, or the rate of new cases arising in the population, rather than the prevalence rate. To simplify the model, however, and to avoid cumbersome notation, we have not distinguished between prevalence and incidence, since this refinement does not affect the results in a qualitative way.

8. A more general specification of the total utility function is:
$$U = N \times F(U_P, U_{PID}, U_{NPID}, U_{OV}, P).$$

This general specification allows for the interaction of utility components and option value, which has intuitive appeal. (Consider, for example, the potential relationship between U_{PID} and U_{NPID}.) To facilitate the mathematics, however, we made the simplifying assumptions listed in the text.

REFERENCES

Allen D, Lee RH, Lowson K: The use of QALYs in health service planning. *International Journal of Health Planning and Management* 4:261-273, 1989.

Andreoni J: Privately-provided public goods in a large economy: the limits of altruism. *Journal of Public Economics* 35:57-73, 1988.

Arrow K: Uncertainty and the welfare economics of medical care. *American Economic Review* 44:941-973, 1963.

Birch S, Donaldson C: Applications of cost-benefit analysis to health care: departures from welfare economic theory. *Journal of Health Economics* 6:211-226, 1987.

Bishop R: Option value: an exposition and extension. *Land Economics* 58:1-15, 1982.

Bishop R: Resource valuation under uncertainty: theoretical principles for empirical research. In: Kerry Smith VK (ed.): *Advances in Applied Microeconomics: Risk, Uncertainty, and the Valuation of Benefits and Costs.* Greenwich, Conn.: JAI Press, 1986.

Boadway RW, Bruce N: *Welfare Economics.* Oxford: Basil Blackwell, 1984.

Bombardier C, Ware J, Russell IJ, Larson G, Chalmers A, Reid JL: Auranofin therapy and quality of life in patients with rheumatoid arthritis. *American Journal of Medicine* 81:565-578, 1986.

Boyle MH, Torrance GW, Sinclair JC, Horwood SP: Economic evaluation of neonatal intensive care of very-low-birth-weight infants. *New England Journal of Medicine* 308:1330-1337, 1983.

Brookshire D et al: Estimating option prices and existence values for wildlife resources. *Land Economics* 59:1-15, 1983.

Cairns JA, Johnston KM: Developing QALYs from condition-specific outcome measures. Paper presented at the Health Economics Study Group Meeting, Dublin, 1990.

Churchill DN, Torrance GW, Taylor DW, Barnes CC, Ludwin D, Shimizu A, Smith EKM: Measurement of quality of life in end-stage renal disease: the time trade-off approach. *Clinical and Investigative Medicine* 10:14-20, 1987.

Ciampi A, Silberfeld M, Till JE: Measurement of individual preferences: the importance of "situation-specific" variables. *Medical Decision Making* 2:483-495, 1982.

Cicchetti C, Freeman M: Option demand and consumer surplus: further comment. *Quarterly Journal of Economics* 85:528-539, 1971.

Collard D: *Altruism and Economy: A Study in Non-selfish Economics.* New York: Oxford University Press, 1978.

Cullis JG, West PA: *The Economics of Health, An Introduction.* Oxford: Martin Robertson, 1979.

Culyer AJ: The nature of the commodity "health care" and its efficient allocation. *Oxford Economic Papers* 23:189-211, 1971.

Culyer AJ: *Need and the National Health Service: Economics and Social Choice.* Oxford: Martin Robertson, 1976.

Culyer A, Simpson H: Externality models and health: a rückblick over the last twenty years. *Economic Record* 56:222-230, 1980.

Department of Health and Social Security: *Breast Cancer Screening* (The Forrest Report). London: HMSO, 1986.

Donaldson C: Willingness to pay for publicly-provided goods: a possible measure of benefit? *Journal of Health Economics* 9:103-118, 1990.

Drummond MF: Resource allocation decisions in health care: a role for quality of life assessments? *Journal of Chronic Diseases* 40:605-616, 1987.

Drummond MF: Output measurement for resource allocation decisions in health care. *Oxford Review of Economic Policy* 5:59-74, 1989.

Drummond MF, Stoddart GL, Torrance GW: *Methods for the Economic Evaluation of Health Care Programmes.* Oxford: Oxford University Press, 1987.

Drummond M, Teeling Smith G, Wells N: *Economic Evaluation in the Development of Medicines.* London: Office of Health Economics, 1988.

Etzioni A: *The Moral Dimension: Toward a New Economics.* New York: The Free Press, 1989.

Evans RG, Wolfson AD: *Faith, Hope, and Charity: Health Care in the Utility Function.* Discussion Paper 80-46, University of British Columbia, 1980.

Feeny DH, Torrance GW: Incorporating utility-based quality-of-life assessment measures in clinical trials: two examples. *Medical Care* 27:S190-S204, 1989.

Furlong W, Feeny G, Torrance G, Barr R, Horseman J: *Guide to Design and Development of Health-State Utility Instruments.* Working Paper #90-9. Hamilton, Ontario: Centre for Health Economics and Policy Analysis, McMaster University, 1990.

Goel V, Deber RB, Detsky AS: Nonionic contrast media: economic analysis and health policy development. *Canadian Medical Association Journal* 140:389-395, 1989.

Graham D: Cost-benefit analysis under uncertainty. *American Economic Review* 71:715-725, 1981.

Greenley D et al: Option value: empirical evidence from a case study of recreation and water quality. *Quarterly Journal of Economics* 657-673, (November), 1981.

Gudex C: *QALYs and Their Use by the Health Service.* Discussion Paper 20, Centre for Health Economics, University of York, 1986.

Gudex C, Kind P: *The QALY Tool Kit.* Discussion Paper 38, Centre for Health Economics, Health Economics Consortium, University of York, n.d.

Gunning-Schepers L: The health benefits of prevention: a simulation approach. *Health Policy* 12:1-2, 1989.

Jones-Lee MW: Altruism and the value of other people's safety. *Journal of Risk and Uncertainty* 4:213-219, 1991.

Klarman HE: The road to cost-effectiveness analysis. *Milbank Memorial Fund Quarterly* 60:585-603, 1982.

La Puma J, Lawlor E: Quality-Adjusted Life-Years: ethical implications for physicians and policymakers. *Journal of The American Medical Association* 263:2917-2921, 1990.

Loomes G, McKenzie L: The use of QALYs in health care decision making. *Social Science and Medicine* 28:299-308, 1989.

Margolis H: *Selfishness, Altruism, and Rationality.* New York: Cambridge University Press, 1982.

McNeil BJ, Weichselbaum R, Pauker SG: Speech and survival: tradeoffs between quality and quantity of life in laryngeal cancer. *New England Journal of Medicine* 305:982-987, 1981.

Mehrez A, Gafni A: Quality-Adjusted Life Years, utility theory, and Healthy Years Equivalent. *Medical Decision Making* 9:142-149, 1989.

Mishan EJ: *Cost-benefit Analysis.* London: George Allen and Unwin, 1971a.

Mishan EJ: Evaluation of life and limb: a theoretical approach. *Journal of Political Economy* 79:687-705, 1971b.

Mohide EA, Torrance GW, Streiner DL, Pringle DM, Gilbert R: Measuring the wellbeing of family care-givers using the time trade-off technique. *Journal of Clinical Epidemiology* 41:475-482, 1988.

Mooney GH: *Economics, Medicine and Health Care.* Brighton: Wheatsheaf Books Ltd., 1986.

Mulley AG: Assessing patients' utilities: can the ends justify the means? *Medical Care* 27:S269-S281, 1989.

Phelps E (ed.): *Altruism, Morality, and Economic Theory.* London: Penguin, 1975.

Rosser R, Kind P: A scale of valuations of states of illness: is there a social consensus? *International Journal of Epidemiology* 7:347-358, 1978.

Sackett DL, Torrance GW: The utility of different health states as perceived by the general public. *Journal of Chronic Diseases* 31:697-704, 1978.

Schmalensee R: Option demand and consumer's surplus: valuing price changes under uncertainty. *American Economic Review* 62:813-824, 1972.

Smith VK: Option value: a conceptual overview. *Southern Economic Journal* 49:654-688, 1983.

Sugden R: Consistent conjectures and voluntary contributions to public goods: why the conventional theory does not work. *Journal of Public Economics* 27:117-124, 1985.

Sugden R, Williams A: *The Principles of Practical Cost-Benefit Analysis.* Oxford: Oxford University Press, 1978.

Torrance GW: Measurement of health state utilities for economic appraisal: a review. *Journal of Health Economics* 5:1-30, 1986.

Torrance GW, Feeny D: Utilities and Quality-Adjusted Life Years. *International Journal of Technology Assessment in Health Care* 5:559-575, 1989.

Torrance GW, Zipursky A: Cost-effectiveness of antepartum prevention of Rh immunization. *Clinics in Perinatology* 11:267-281, 1984.

Walsh R et al: Valuing option, existence, and bequest demands for wilderness. *Land Economics* 60:14-29, 1984.

Weisbrod B: *Economics of Public Health.* Philadelphia: University of Pennsylvania Press, 1961.

Weisbrod B: Collective consumption services of individual consumption goods. *Quarterly Journal of Economics* 78:471-477, 1964.

Williams A: *Medical Ethics: Health Service Efficiency and Clinical Freedom.* Folio 2, Nuffield/York Portfolios. Oxfordshire: Nuffield Provincial Hospitals Trust, n.d.

Williams A: Welfare economics and health status measurement. In: Van der Gaag J, Perlman M (eds.): *Health, Economics, and Health Economics.* Amsterdam: North-Holland, 1981.

Williams A: Economics of coronary artery bypass grafting. *British Medical Journal* 291:326-329, 1985.

Roberta J. Labelle
(September 21, 1957 - July 9, 1991)

During her too-short career,
Roberta J. Labelle touched
many with her intelligence,
humor, and vitality. She will
be sadly missed by all her
friends and colleagues.

CONDUCTING COMPREHENSIVE COST ASSESSMENTS: A CASE STUDY OF AN ASSERTIVE MENTAL HEALTH COMMUNITY TREATMENT PROGRAM*

Nancy Wolff
Thomas Helminiak
Burton Weisbrod
Ronald Diamond
University of Wisconsin – Madison

Today I'm presenting results from a comprehensive costing study of the Mobile Community Treatment program. The cost results I'll be featuring are for direct mental health care and law enforcement services. In addition, I'll be highlighting several methodological problems that plague all costing studies. What you can expect to learn from my presentation can be summarized in three 'south of the border' lessons; I hope these lessons will be permitted to clear Canadian customs.

Lesson one: One can never be too skeptical of use and cost numbers or of the data sets from which those numbers were obtained.

Lesson two: One can never over-estimate the amount of time, effort, and money necessary to complete a costing study.

Lesson three: Non-obsessive researchers should not attempt to sail the murky waters of use and cost data, especially if they don't have an economist on board the ship.

With that brief introduction, let me turn to the details of our study.

My colleagues Ron Diamond, Tom Helminiak, and Burt Weisbrod and I have been applying a comprehensive costing model to the Mobile Community Treatment Program. Our study entails the retrospective tracking of resources used by 94 study subjects over a 12-month period. Our motivating research questions are:

1. What are the absolute costs associated with the treatment of the severely mentally ill through the Mobile Community Treatment Program?, and

2. What is the relative distribution of these absolute costs across the following cost categories:
   • mental health treatment,
   • indirect treatment,
   • law enforcement,
   • maintenance, and
   • family burden?

We also felt that it was time to revisit the comprehensive costing framework developed by Weisbrod, Test, and Stein in the late 1970s and later refined by Barbara Dickey and her colleagues.

It is our assessment that more considered thought needs to be given to several methodological issues. Our first such question is: "What resource areas should be included in the costing framework?" There is general agreement in the literature that these major categories of: mental health treatment, indirect treatment, law enforcement, maintenance, and family and community burden should be included in the comprehensive societal costing framework. There is, however, considerably less agreement about the sub-categories to be included under these major categories. This is especially true under law enforcement and family burden, two areas on which we have focused a considerable amount of our research effort.

The next question is, "What is the definition of a service unit, or contact?" At first blush, this may appear to be a rather trivial question, but practically speaking, it has proven very difficult to answer in many cases. We found four different service unit definitions in one data set alone, and the data specialists weren't even aware that they had four service unit definitions in their data set. For example, are we talking about an hour of billable services or an hour of client time? More specifically, how is an hour of co-therapy defined in the unit measurement? The issues get even thornier when we look on the law enforcement side. What is a contact with police? Is this a telephone contact with the dispatcher, an arrest, an incident that leads to a written report, or any incident? Does it matter the role of the individual in the incident, that is, if the person is a suspect, a victim, or a reporting person? Moreover, is a unit of service the same for a chronically mentally ill person as a non-chronically mentally ill person? These are just a few of the questions that we've struggled with.

The last question is, "Are the use and cost data what they purport to be?" Our experience with other private and public data sets has conditioned us to assume the data are dirty until proven clean through a series of rigorous investigative tests. Our investigative inquiry into the accuracy and reliability of management information systems on this study has confirmed our concern about the indiscriminate use of computer information systems. In a moment I will convince you of this through a series of illustrations. It is very difficult to ascertain that the data in fact represent the variable they purport to represent, that they are complete and unbiased, and that they are, in all senses, reasonably accurate. In cases where the data do not meet these characteristics, this needs to be recognized and acknowledged. Let me be clear. The problem is not the presence of data problems – that goes with the territory – but rather the amount of staff time necessary to diagnose and then treat the data problems.

Before getting to the numbers, let me tell you a little bit about MCT. MCT (or Mobile Community Treatment Program) is a community support program based on the Training in Community Living Model and is a unit of the Mental Health Center of Dane County. The two key programming features are assertive community outreach and strong case management. There are 12 full-time staff providing services from 8:00 A.M. to 10:30 P.M. seven days a week, with the midnight shift covered by Crisis Intervention. MCT is designed specifically to provide services to the most difficult to treat, most severely mentally ill residents in Dane County. Candidates for MCT mainly have psychotic disorders – schizophrenia, manic-depression, schizoaffective, or other similar disorders. They all have a long standing mental illness, are generally non-compliant with medication, and are at high risk of rehospitalization. We consider MCT our caboose program.

Ninety-four of the 181 clients active in MCT in 1988 agreed to participate in our study. For those 94 study subjects, we collected a wide assortment of data.

Table 1 shows the direct mental health treatment costs for the Mental Health Center in 1988. Over all, the Mental Health Center provided roughly 10,000 hours of billable services to the 94 study subjects, estimated at a total cost of $411,000. The average cost, which appears in parentheses, is about $4,400. Roughly 85% of the total estimated cost represented services provided directly by MCT.

Oft-times a researcher conducting a costing study has a choice of using primary or secondary data sources to collect use and cost data. We were faced with this choice to collect the Mental Health Center data. The choice we had was to get the data directly from the Mental Health Center itself or to go to a secondary source – the Unified Services Board. The Unified Services Board is the county agency that contracts with the Mental Health

Table 1

DIRECT MENTAL HEALTH TREATMENT COSTS

	% of sample	# of hour units	Estimated $ costs
MCT	100%	7,563	$348,405
		(80)	($3,706)
Support network	19	2,065	35,455
		(20)	(377)
Crisis intervention	47	157	10,652
		(2)	(112)
Alcohol/drug	15	168	7,488
		(2)	(80)
Other programs	11	143	9,361
		(2)	(100)
Mental Health Centre	*100%*	*10,096*	*$411,361*
		(106)	*($4,376)*

Center to provide services to the chronically mentally ill. The Unified Services Board data had one compelling advantage. The Board is a clearing house source. Every agency that is contracted by the county to provide services to the mentally ill reports its use and cost data directly to the Unified Services Board. That is, we could have gotten information from 30 agencies by going to the Unified Services Board as opposed to going to each one of those 30 agencies independently. We resisted the obvious temptation of using the Unified Services Board data, and instead decided to do a comparative analysis of the primary and secondary data sources to look at comparability in the unit measurements as well as the cost.

Table 2 shows the result of this comparison for those two data sets for MCT. As you can see, the Unified Services Board was missing data on one client for whom data were available from the Mental Health Center records. Also note that the number of units reported in the Unified Services Board data is about 20% less than reported in the Mental Health Center data. We were able to uncover two reasons for this discrepancy. First, the Mental Health Center records report hours of billable service, whereas the Unified Services Board reports hours of client time. This is a case in point where one does have to struggle with the unit definition issue. The second reason has to do with incomplete reporting. For at least two clients, we found that the Unified Services Board data indicated only a modest fraction of the reported utilization appearing in the Mental Health Center data. We still are not sure how this happened. As you can see from the last line of the table, the Unified Services Board reported cost figures that are significantly larger than those for the Mental Health Center, even though the opposite relationship held for the unit measurement. To the best of our knowledge, the reason for this discrepancy has to do with the misapplication of contract rates within the Unified Services Board data, which led to the overinflation of the rates in those data. The point of this illustration is that we would have over-estimated the cost of MCT services had we succumbed to the temptation of using a secondary data source. Without this comparative analysis we would not have known the direction or the cause of the bias in either the use or the cost estimates. Let me assure you that these anomalies are not unique to these two data sources. We have yet to find one management information system that provided accurate and reliable information to the degree purported by the agency archiving that data.

Table 2
ALL MCT SERVICES

	MHCDC data	USB data
Clients with recorded utilization	94	93
Units (hours) of service	7,563	6,135
(average)	(80)	(65)
Costs of service	$348,405	$511,278
(average)	($3,706)	($5,439)

Next I would like to turn our attention to the law enforcement side. This particular area is of growing concern, because the law enforcement sector is becoming – or at least it is argued that it is becoming – the *de facto* custodial care provider for the chronically mentally ill who are placed in the community. Our study extends both the breadth and the depth of law enforcement information included in the costing framework and includes costs for:

1. Police and sheriff departments
   Police department contacts
   Sheriff department contacts
   County jail (including medical costs)
2. Judicial system
   Court costs
   Litigation
3. Penal system
   Prison
   Probation/parole
4. Fire department

The unit costs for each of these agencies were independently derived by us, and they reflect the average resources used to provide specific services to the chronically mentally ill population. Table 3 shows our estimates for the major categories. As you can see for 1988, the law enforcement sector provided approximately $122,000 worth of services to the 94 study subjects. These figures are roughly 1/3 the size of the total estimated Mental Health Center costs in Table 1. The largest cost component is for the police and sheriff, representing about 70% of the total law enforcement cost.

Table 3
ESTIMATED LAW ENFORCEMENT COSTS

	$ Total	$ Average
Police and sheriff departments	$ 85,316	$ 908
Judicial system	29,567	314
Penal system	6,786	72
Fire department	828	9
Total	*$122,497*	*$1,303*

The police and sheriff costs are disaggregated in Table 4. For 1988, roughly 61% of our study subjects had at least one contact with the police department. A contact means that a written report was actually submitted by an officer. The total cost of the 235 contacts was $66,000, or approximately $704 per person. If our unit costs had not been adjusted to reflect the differential resource utilization of the chronically mentally ill, these numbers would be about 17% lower. I think it's interesting also to note in passing that of those 235 contacts, 3% involved our study subjects as victims.

Table 4

LAW ENFORCEMENT COSTS

	% of sample	# of units	Estimated $ costs
Police dept. contacts (average)	60.6 %	235	$ 66,158 ($704)
Sheriff dept. contacts (average)	11.7	19	1,486 (16)
County jail			
Jail days (average)	17.0	184	16,869 (179)
Medical care provided (average)			803 (9)

The last item I would like to talk about from this table is jail days. Sixteen of our study subjects had spent at least one night in the county jail in 1988. A total of 184 jail days were provided to study subjects, at a total cost of $17,000 dollars. Again I would like to illustrate how important it is to scrutinize the data obtained from any agency. Over the course of several months we received five different jail record printouts from the Sheriff's Department. Each earlier printout was rejected because subjects were missing, citations were incomplete, or aliases were not cross-referenced. Once we got our "best" printout, we decided to validate the booking and release dates which are used to determine the number of jail days, as each individual jail day is a costly event. Table 5 shows you the result of this comparison. The naive estimates are based on our "best" printout. Note the naive estimates showed that 17 clients were booked a total of 36 times, and they spent a total of 491 days in jail. After our investigation we found, however, that only 16 clients were booked a total of 31 times, and they spent only 184 days in jail. Let me assure you that this discrepancy is not the result of that one extra person or those five extra bookings. In fact, there are a number of reasons, but the two most important ones include human error in inputting jail record data and the variability of the definition of a release date. Had we not conducted this investigative test, we would have inadvertently reported total jail day cost of $44,000, a 160% increase over our final total cost estimate. Again, this investigation led to the discovery of non-trivial differences in use and costs of resources to the studied population.

Table 5

DANE COUNTY JAIL DAYS DATA

	Naive estimates	Final estimates
Number of clients booked	17	16
Total jail bookings	36	31
Total jail days	491	184
Total jail days costs*	$43,866 ($467)	$16,869 ($179)

* includes bailiff costs

Table 6 shows a comparison of average law enforcement costs reported in the literature. These are all comprehensive costing studies. They all use basically the same costing framework, and they focus on a similar mentally ill population. The reported average law enforcement cost ranges from a low of $316 to a high of $1,300. What accounts for the wide variation? Good question, but not answerable. Because of the lack of methodological standardization in documentation, it is unclear whether and to what extent these variations are attributable to differences in the definition of cost categories or sub-categories, definition of service units, definition in calculation of unit prices, data collection techniques, programmatic anomalies or attributes, or population characteristics.

Table 6
COMPARISON OF LAW ENFORCEMENT COSTS

	$ Average [*]	n
Wolff, Helminiak, Diamond, Weisbrod, 1990	$ 1,303	94
Shern, Saranga-Coen, Nelson, Wilson, Vasby, 1990	316	198
Dickey, McGuire, Cannon, Gudeman, 1986	680	43
Weisbrod, Test, Stein, 1980	987	130

[*] adjusted to 1988 prices

I do have a few conclusions. I've been reporting on our attempts to identify, quantify, and value the various forms of social costs associated with the seriously mentally ill and their treatment in the Mobile Community Treatment Program. To provide useful, meaningful, and comparable use and cost numbers, researchers have to make sure that:

1. All important cost categories are included in their framework,
2. Units and prices are consistently and accurately defined, and
3. Data sources used provide reliable and complete measures of the desired variables.

Our experience with computer information systems leads us to believe that they should be used only after a great deal of inspection. The burden should be placed on the researcher to demonstrate through cross-validation that his/her numbers are accurate and reliable measures of the desired use and cost variables. We do not find that the discrepancies in these data sources are trivial, nor do we think they can be counted on to average out over large numbers of people or a large number of programs. Our research has led us to believe that without vigorous review of the validity of data systems, study conclusions are at least as likely to be determined by the net inaccuracy of the data as by the true state of the world. Let me again be clear. These computer based information systems can and should be used in costing studies. However, their biases and measurements should be investigated and formally acknowledged so that policy makers and other researchers can adjust their confidence in the numbers.

NOTE
* edited transcript of talk by Nancy Wolff

REFERENCES
Dickey B, McGuire T, Cannon N, Gudeman J: Mental health cost models: refinements and applications. *Medical Care* 24:857-867, 1986.

Shern D, Saranga-Coen A, Nelson L, Wilson N, Vasby O: Innovative Service Delivery Models and the Cost of Chronic Mental Illness. Unpublished Final Report to Robert Wood Johnson Foundation, 1990.

Weisbrod B, Test MA, Stein L: Alternative to mental hospital treatment: II. Economic benefit-cost analysis. *Archives of General Psychiatry* 37:400-405, 1980.

DISCUSSION
Chair: Andrea Baumann
McMaster University

Charles Wright (Vancouver General Hospital)

I'd like to address a comment to Roberta Labelle and Jeremiah Hurley. I'll try and do this politely but still get the juices flowing. I used to think that surgery was an inexact science. Correct me if I'm wrong, but it seems to me that you are completely confusing the necessity for the objective aspects of a cost-utility analysis – and heaven knows that even that is very difficult, because a lot of subjectivity comes into that 'objective' analysis when you go on to QALYs and so on – but you are confusing that area with the second, entirely different process, which is to take the cost-utility analysis and make decisions as to whether to apply it or not, which is entirely a subjective process, and there is never any way to objectify that. That will always depend on who you are, what your GNP is, what your country is, who thinks what, what are the basic values. Just to take an example with which I am very personally familiar, any debate about whether you do mammography for breast cancer screening would be utterly ridiculous in any developing country in the world. And yet we do it, because we're in an extremely wealthy country. So when you speak of the interdependent utility and the option value, aren't you really getting into the area of the subjective decision as to whether or how to use that cost utility analysis in making a decision about whether to do a program or not?

Jeremiah Hurley (McMaster University)

In some sense, yes, it is bringing in some subjective elements, but we're trying to include the value of non-users in conducting an analysis, because a basic perspective of economics would be that when you're doing an analysis for resource allocation decisions, to choose, "What should we do with the money, let's say, in the public sector? Should the government spend – allocate its money among health care programs?", the basis for that allocation should be, in some sense, society's values as expressed through the benefits and costs that accrue to all members of society. And that will reflect values. What we're suggesting is that as it has been done in the past, it has restricted the measurement of benefits of a program to simply the users and that, if we want to expand the use of not just QALYs but any method of economic evaluation, we have to expand also the benefits that we measure to include both users and non-users if we truly want to reflect the preferences of society.

Roberta Labelle (McMaster University)

Contrary to the title of our paper, we're not advocating that cost-utility analysis should be used for any particular purpose. We are saying that when you use it – and it has been used for this purpose – you are excluding these sorts of things. Now people might decide that that's irrelevant, that those types of benefits should not be included in the evaluation. I think what we're saying is that those people should at least be cognizant of the fact that those benefits are excluded. And I don't think we're prescribing in any way how then to use the cost utility analysis. We're just holding up a mirror.

Frank Markel (St. Joseph's Health Centre, Toronto)

One quick technical question. You didn't leave the equations on very long, but since you mentioned prevalence in the second-order effect, doesn't it make sense to think about putting the prevalence factor in with the first order, that is, that the individual unit QALY is important, but the prevalence of the disease in society in the first instance may also be important. Your mention of the word "prevalence" made me start thinking about that.

Jeremiah Hurley

In fact, that is one of the things which got us thinking along these lines, because on some of the league tables – for instance, the one that Roberta put up – very high on the list was a disease that has a prevalence of about .000003 or something. And we got thinking about that. And in fact, prevalence doesn't enter as first or second order, it simply is one of the factors that affect how important these non-user benefits are. What happens is that once you include these non-user benefits, other things constant, the cost per util will vary with the prevalence rate of a disease and in fact – well, we can't say – sometimes it will depend upon the various relationships and interdependencies. It may increase with the prevalence of a disease, it may decrease. That's one of the problems – we can't say *a priori* what the direction – or how it will vary with prevalence. We know only that if externalities are positive, by excluding externalities you will be overestimating costs per util. But prevalence is a crucial aspect of the model, yes.

V.J. Kulkarni (University of Toronto)

This is a question for Nancy Wolff about the patients who have agreed to participate in the program. How similar are they to the hospital population? How generalizable is this data?

Nancy Wolff (University of Wisconsin – Madison)

I took out those slides that did a sample to population comparison. We did a passive review of those who did not agree to participate in our study, and we found no significant difference across any of the variables that we looked at. We also arranged through the Mental Health Center to have a passive review of law enforcement use by those clients who did not agree to participate in the study. And we also found out that their utilization of the law enforcement services didn't seem to differ either. So we're reasonably confident that our population is generalizable, for that group.

ECONOMIC EVALUATIONS OF HEALTH PROGRAMS: COSTS AND CONSEQUENCES

DETERMINANTS OF MEDICAL MALPRACTICE: THE CANADIAN EXPERIENCE

Peter C. Coyte
Department of Health Administration

Donald N. Dewees
Department of Economics

Michael J. Trebilcock
Faculty of Law
University of Toronto

INTRODUCTION

Since the 1980s there has been a perception among Canadian health care providers that health care professionals and the institutions that assist in the delivery of health care are facing a malpractice crisis. This perception has a substantial basis in reality, since the number of claims, the number of paid claims, and the amount of the average paid claim have all risen dramatically since 1971.

Between 1971 and 1989, the number of malpractice writs issued against physicians increased seven-fold, from 130 to 878. The size of an average paid claim grew from $8,000 in 1971 to $150,600 in 1989, almost doubling between 1980 and 1983, and doubling again in 1984. The average malpractice fee increased more than ten-fold between 1976 and 1989, doubling between 1983 and 1985, then doubling again by 1987.

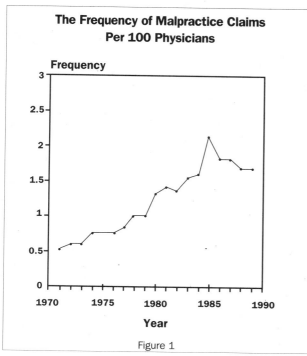

Figure 1

These data, however, greatly overstate the true magnitude of the increases by failing to account for increases in the volume of medical services performed and by ignoring inflation, which reached rates over 10% per year during this period. The number of writs filed per 100 practising physicians increased on average at 6.4% per year between 1971 and 1989 and has actually declined steadily since 1985 (Figure 1). After adjusting for inflation, the size of an average paid claim, expressed in 1989 dollars, increased at an annual rate of 9.7% between 1971 and 1989 (Figure 2). After adjusting for inflation, the average malpractice fee paid increased by 14.7% per year between 1976 and 1989 (Figure 3). Furthermore, a significant portion of this fee increase resulted from a changeover from pay-as-you-go to funded insurance, which required a one-time increase in reserves which had by 1988 been accumulated. The actual trends, while significantly upward, are far less alarming than suggested by the raw data.

Although the frequency with which malpractice claims are initiated is significantly lower in Canada than in the United States, the growth rate in both frequency and severity is similar in the two countries. Furthermore, average payments to successful litigants are also not significantly different. Consequently, success in accounting for the determinants of the trends in the frequency and severity of malpractice claims in Canada may provide insight into the trends in malpractice claims in the U.S.

This paper tests various hypotheses shaping the increase in malpractice claims in Canada. This exercise requires data on the trends in malpractice and their determinants. Although empirical research of this kind has progressed further in the U.S., the complexity of the exercise continues to present analysts with severe problems (Danzon, 1985;

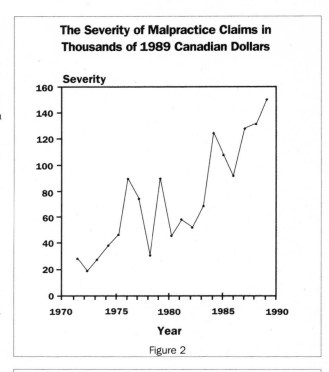

The Severity of Malpractice Claims in Thousands of 1989 Canadian Dollars

Figure 2

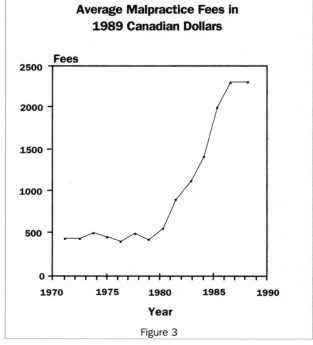

Average Malpractice Fees in 1989 Canadian Dollars

Figure 3

Law and Contemporary Problems, 1986). Our data gathering has fortunately been facilitated by two factors. First, most malpractice claims against physicians in Canada are dealt with by a single organization, the Canadian Medical Protective Association; in the U.S., many insurers are involved. Second, since Canada has universal health insurance, provincial government health insurance plans contain very detailed data on changes in patterns of medical practice and procedures. Access to both sets of data has allowed us to perform analyses that could not have been performed in the U.S. and have not been performed in Canada. We believe that we have had sufficient success in gathering the necessary data to allow us to illuminate a number of central issues.

We present an outline of the hypotheses frequently advanced in the literature to explain the increase in malpractice litigation, a brief description of the data and methodology employed, and, finally, our major empirical results.

POSSIBLE EXPLANATIONS FOR TRENDS IN MEDICAL MALPRACTICE

The literature suggests a large number of hypotheses explaining the increase in frequency and severity of malpractice awards against physicians, which may be organized into three categories: the professional environment, the social environment, and the legal environment.

THE PROFESSIONAL ENVIRONMENT

Increases in the volume of medical procedures performed, and particularly of inherently risky and technologically sophisticated procedures in which inadequate medical care gives rise to obvious and observable adverse outcomes, might explain the liability trends. More specifically, much of the increase in the severity of awards might be attributed to an increase in the number of very large claims arising from life-saving procedures that were not available in the past, despite the relative infrequency of such claims. The quality of health care professionals, measured by both training and experience, and the exercise of professional discipline by professional bodies may also affect the frequency of incidents giving rise to malpractice claims. Increasing specialization might increase the frequency with which patients are treated by a physician on a single occasion, a situation more conducive to litigation than treatment by a family physician with whom the patient has a continuing relationship. On the other hand, increasing specialization might increase the quality of care provided.

THE SOCIAL ENVIRONMENT

Society may have become more litigious, and this trend may have been accentuated in the medical context by increasingly impersonal and perhaps transitory relationships between patients and physicians and by rising public expectations regarding the successful outcome of medical treatment. Patients may be more inclined to pursue financial compensation for injuries than previously, regardless of their belief about the culpability of the physician's conduct. Furthermore, to the extent to which different individuals and demographic groups have different propensities to litigate, changes in the age-sex structure of the population may partially account for the trends in physician liability.

THE LEGAL ENVIRONMENT

It might be argued that judicial determination of grounds for liability and quantification of damages have changed substantially in the medical context so as to increase the expected value of a malpractice claim, thus encouraging more litigation. Specifically, changes in the tax implications of interest on settlements, claims by family members, and prejudgment interest may have increased the size of awards for particular types of injuries. Changes in the doctrine of informed consent or in statutes of limitation may have increased the number of injuries that give rise to actionable claims.

SOURCES OF DATA
PHYSICIAN LIABILITY DATA

Data on physician liability were provided by the Canadian Medical Protective Association (CMPA), a non-profit organization which represents over 90% of all active civilian physicians in Canada and which has been in existence for over 50 years (Canadian Medical Protective Association, 1989). The CMPA sets fees for universal, comprehensive, and unlimited coverage for each physician specialty; hires and provides payment to lawyers to defend physicians named in malpractice cases; and ultimately compensates the victims of medical misadventure if a claim proves successful.

The CMPA allowed us to analyze three data sets: *closed claims,* reported to the CMPA since January 1, 1976 which closed with or without payment by December 31, 1987, and which comprise claims filed against 6,680 defendant physicians; *open claims,* reported to the CMPA since January 1, 1976, but which remain open as of December 31, 1987, and which comprise claims filed against 5,332 defendant physicians; and *large paid claims,* a subset of the closed claims comprising 107 claims resulting in payments to plaintiffs exceeding $100,000 in 1976 Canadian dollars. The CMPA data sets report the type of injury alleged; the specialty of the physician named; and other information about the patient, the physician, the event, and the disposition of the claim.

PROVINCIAL HEALTH INSURANCE DATA

Since at least 1971, each of the 10 provinces and two territories has had a public health insurance plan which covers all necessary medical and hospital services. Federal government funding of 50% of all health expenditures has led to similar plans across Canada, providing reasonable access by all residents to the full range of insured services. Funding for the provision of health care services is derived from both general taxation and insurance premiums; patients do not pay directly for health care. The overwhelming majority of Canada's practising physicians are self-employed, but reimbursed by provincial health insurance plans on a fee-for-service basis. These fees are determined by negotiation between each province's government and its medical association.

The provincial health insurance plans generate data on the amount billed for various medical services. After obtaining the permission of each provincial and territorial government, the Health Information Division of Health and Welfare Canada provided us with these data, which we have used, after adjusting for changing fee levels, as measures of the activity level of physicians.

ANALYSIS OF MEDICAL MALPRACTICE

Using both the open and the closed claim data sets, we constructed the *semi-aggregate* data set. This data set was formed by allocating each defendant physician to one of six groups according to his or her area of practice: anaesthesia, obstetrics and gynaecology, family practice, orthopaedic surgery, all other areas of practice, and missing cases (where a defendant's specialty designation was not reported). Construction of this data set provided the basis for an examination of the frequency of claims, the proportion of claims that resulted in payment, and the severity of these paid claims for each of the specialties.

FREQUENCY OF MALPRACTICE CLAIMS

The distribution among specialties of defendants named in malpractice claims is shown in Table 1, along with the percentage of all active civilian physicians who fall into the same practice categories. Anaesthetists, orthopaedic surgeons, and obstetricians and gynaecologists account for 25% of all defendant physicians and of all physicians involved in malpractice

Table 1

FREQUENCY DISTRIBUTION OF DEFENDANT PHYSICIAN SPECIALTIES, AND VARIOUS DIMENSIONS OF MALPRACTICE LIABILITY

Semi-aggregate Data (Open and Closed Claim Data)

	Anaesthesia	Obstetrics & Gynaecology	Family Practice	Orthopaedic Surgery	Other Areas of Practice	Missing Cases
Number of defendant physicians	617	1,101	2,788	1,201	5,736	569
Percentage distribution of defendant physicians	5.1	9.2	23.2	10.0	47.8	4.7
Defendant physicians in paid claims	141	215	541	221	942	179
Percentage distribution of defendant physicians in paid claims	6.3	9.6	24.1	9.9	42.1	8.0
Percentage distribution of practising physicians	3.4	3.0	42.6	1.7	49.3	-
Defendant physicians per 100 physicians 1976-1984	4.4[+]	9.1[+]	1.6[+]	18.0[+]	2.8	-
Percentage of defendant physicians in paid claims 1976-1984	41.5[+++]	36.4[+++]	36.5[+++]	33.2[+++]	33.5	-
Average paid claim in 000's of 1987 dollars 1976-1984	174.4[++]	71.2[+++]	118.3[+++]	81.6[+++]	107.4	-
Percentage of total paid damages 1976-1984	11.0	6.9	28.7	8.1	45.3	-

[+] Significantly different (p<0.001 by Student's t-test) from "Other areas of practice"
[++] Significantly different (p<0.01) from "Other areas of practice"
[+++] Not significantly different (p>0.05) from "Other areas of practice"

claims that resulted in payment to plaintiffs, but represent only 8% of physicians in Canada, revealing that these three categories of physicians are relatively frequent targets of malpractice claims and family practice physicians relatively infrequent targets.

Although malpractice frequency rates are available from 1968, incidents occurring before 1976 tend to be under-reported, since many of them would have been reported to the CMPA before January 1, 1976 and would therefore not appear in this data set. In addition, since a delay occurs between the incident and the reporting and closing of a claim, many incidents that occurred before 1987 would not appear in the data set. Consequently, our statistical analysis is confined to the incident years 1976-1984 to minimize any bias associated with this under-reporting.

The sixth row in Table 1 reports the malpractice frequency rate for each physician specialty for the years 1976-1984. The frequency rate for orthopaedic surgeons is twice that for obstetricians and gynaecologists, four times that for anaesthetists, and over 10 times that for family physicians. To test whether there are statistically significant differences in the malpractice frequency rate across each of the five physician categories, we employed the technique of multiple regression analysis (Kmenta, 1986). As reported in Table 1, the frequencies of litigation for each of the five physician specialties are found to be significantly different ($p<0.001$ by Student's t-test). Orthopaedic surgeons exhibit the largest claims frequency and family practice physicians exhibit the lowest.

PROPORTION OF MALPRACTICE CLAIMS THAT RESULT IN PAYMENT

The seventh row in Table 1 reports the proportion of physicians named as defendants who were also defendants in paid claims between 1976 and 1984. Although malpractice claims against anaesthetists result in payment more often than the others, and claims involving orthopaedic surgeons less often, regression analysis revealed that these small differences are not significant ($p>0.05$).

SEVERITY OF MALPRACTICE CLAIMS

The eighth row in Table 1 reports, in 1987 Canadian dollars, the severity (average dollar value) of malpractice claims between 1976 and 1984. Although the severity of malpractice claims involving anaesthetists is almost 50% greater than that for family physicians, which in turn is over 60% greater than that for obstetricians and gynaecologists, there is considerable variation in the severity of these claims from one year to another. To test whether there are significant differences in the severity of malpractice claims across each of the five physician categories, we used regression analysis. As reported in Table 1, only the severity of malpractice claims for anaesthetists was significantly different ($p<0.01$) from the benchmark of "all other areas of practice".

TOTAL MALPRACTICE CLAIM COSTS

Total malpractice claim costs are defined as the product of the frequency of malpractice claims, the proportion of paid claims, and the severity of malpractice claims. Since significant differences ($p<0.001$) among all physician categories were found only in frequency rates, specialties with significantly higher malpractice claim frequencies should figure more prominently than others in the share of total payments. Since the proportion of total payments attributable to anaesthetists, orthopaedic surgeons, and obstetricians and gynaecologists exceeds the proportion of these specialists in the stock of physicians (Table 1), these specialties are over-represented in the total payments by the CMPA by factors of 3.2, 4.8, and 2.3, respectively, and family practice is under-represented by 1/3. We conclude that total malpractice payments per physician differ significantly by area of practice.

DETERMINANTS OF PHYSICIAN LIABILITY

Table 1 reveals inter-specialty differences in malpractice liability, but neither explains these differences nor accounts for the time trends. We performed additional analyses, including multiple regression analysis, to distinguish between the competing explanations for the trends in physician liability. Regression analysis estimates the relationship between a dependent variable (such as the frequency of malpractice claims) and a number of independent variables (such as surgical utilization or legal doctrines). This procedure generates estimates of the impact of each independent variable when all other independent variables are unchanged. Estimates of two equations capturing the trends in malpractice liability are shown in Tables 2 and 3. We discuss the results of this analysis under the three broad headings: the professional environment, the social environment, and the legal environment.

THE PROFESSIONAL ENVIRONMENT
Utilization of Health Care Services

We tested two definitions of health care utilization: total medical billings per physician for health care services by specialty, and total billings per physician by specialty for major surgical procedures – musculo-skeletal, respiratory, cardiovascular, integumentary, digestive, and urinary surgery, as well as major operations on eyes and ears. Major surgical procedures were selected over total billings on the basis of intuitive appeal, data validity, and statistical significance.

Table 2

DETERMINANTS OF THE FREQUENCY OF MALPRACTICE CLAIMS BY INCIDENT YEAR, 1978-1984
Semi-aggregate Data (Open and Closed Claim Data)

(Variable)	(Point estimate	$\pm$ 2 x estimated standard error)
Major surgical utilization	0.2510 $\pm$	0.0234[+]
Predicted severity[*]	0.0158 $\pm$	0.0113[++]
Predicted proportion[**]	24.6450 $\pm$	19.6375[+++]
Informed consent dummy	3.1360 $\pm$	1.3459[+]
Constant	-10.4940 $\pm$	7.4690[++]
Unadjusted R^2	0.948	
Adjusted R^2	0.941	

Dependent variable: The number of defendant physicians in malpractice claims per one hundred physicians
[+] $p<0.001$ by Student's t-test
[++] $p<0.01$
[+++] $p<0.02$
[*] Derived from estimates of the severity of malpractice claims shown in Table 3
[**] Derived from estimates of the proportion of paid malpractice claims, not shown

Table 3

DETERMINANTS OF THE SEVERITY OF MALPRACTICE CLAIMS BY INCIDENT YEAR, 1978-1984

Closed Claim Data

(Variable)	(Point estimate	$\pm$ 2 x estimated standard error)
Severity (-1)	0.0013 $\pm$	0.325
Severity (-2)	0.2699 $\pm$	0.333
Percentage Canadian medical graduates	-9.8905 $\pm$	7.637 [++]
Percentage children under 5	5651.000 $\pm$	2379.368 [+]
Percentage women 18-44	6771.700 $\pm$	3023.080 [+]
Percentage elderly over 65	-6439.300 $\pm$	2811.921 [+]
Long bond yield (+3)	245.280 $\pm$	124.508 [+]
Real wages (+3)	42.335 $\pm$	21.435 [+]
Constant	-146950.000 $\pm$	67100.457 [+]
Unadjusted R^2	0.718	
Adjusted R^2	0.631	

Dependent variable: Average paid claim in '000s of 1987 Canadian dollars
[+] $p < 0.001$ by Student's t-test
[++] $p < 0.02$
Otherwise $p > 0.05$

Although the utilization of major surgery is significant neither in the determination of the proportion of paid claims ($p > 0.05$), which is not shown, nor in the severity of those paid claims ($p > 0.05$), it is the single most important variable explaining the variation, over time and across specialties, in the frequency of malpractice litigation (Table 2). Since, as Table 1 reveals, most of this variability occurs across specialties, this result primarily explains the inter-specialty variation rather than the general trend over time. The dominant role of major surgery is underlined by our analysis of the large paid claims data set in which 35% of the malpractice claims and 37% of the damages awarded arise from incidents occurring during the performance of major surgery (Table 4). These results suggest that a patient's exposure to iatrogenic injury is closely related to the performance of major surgery and that the inter-specialty differences in the frequency of malpractice litigation are largely accounted for by differences in the volume of major surgery performed.

Quality of Health Care Services

The age of a physician could be related to incidents of malpractice either because of the inexperience of young physicians or because of the failing skills of older ones. Since the frequency distribution of the age of physicians named as defendants in the large paid claims data set is relatively uniform over the interval 30 to 60 years of age, the data do not support the hypothesis that malpractice is a particular problem for those in their early or late years of practice.

The proportion of domestically-trained physicians is not significant ($p > 0.05$) in accounting for either the variation in the frequency to litigate or in the proportion of claims that result in payment, but it is significant ($p < 0.02$) in accounting for the variation in the severity of these claims (Table 3). The negative effect of domestically-trained physicians on the

Table 4
TREATMENTS GIVING RISE TO MALPRACTICE CLAIMS
Large Claims Data

Treatment Category	Number Mentions	Damages Associated (millions of 1987$)
Consultation	0	0.00
Complete examinations	1	0.51
Other office visits	8	3.03
Other hospital visits (including complete examinations)	16	6.40
Home and emergency visits (including home examinations)	10	2.60
Major surgery	54	24.40
Minor surgery	7	1.80
Surgical assistance	0	0.00
Obstetrical services	17	9.14
Anaesthesia	12	4.03
Radiology	5	1.63
Laboratory services	0	0.00
Other diagnostic/ therapeutic services/ special services	25	12.00
Miscellaneous services	0	0.00
Total	*155*	*$ 65.54*

severity of malpractice claims might be construed as indicating that these graduates provide higher quality health care than their foreign-trained counterparts. However, we could not confirm this result with the large paid claims data set.

Although specialists may offer the public higher quality health care than generalists, they may also be held to a higher standard of care and attract the more difficult cases. We found that the proportion of physicians who are specialists is not a significant determinant ($p > 0.05$) of the three dimensions of malpractice liability (frequency, severity, and proportion of claims resulting in payment); trends in malpractice liability therefore appear not to be caused by increasing medical specialization.

It has been suggested that advancing medical technology has increased the likelihood of malpractice claims by raising the possibility of saving previously hopeless cases, using techniques in which momentary inattention or mistakes could give rise to large losses. For example, premature infants who might earlier have died, giving rise to a negligible claim, might now be saved, but could require extremely costly lifetime care; kidney failure need not be fatal, but errors in diagnosis or treatment using renal dialysis could result in fatality. Our data do not allow a clear test of this hypothesis, but they are not inconsistent with it. Although not many of the large claims arose from cases involving high technology, many did arise in situations that are highly intrusive, such as major surgery or anaesthesia, in which a small error could result in serious injury.

THE SOCIAL ENVIRONMENT
General Propensity to Litigate

U.S. studies (Danzon, 1985) suggest that only a small fraction, perhaps 20%, of negligently caused injuries result in the filing of a malpractice claim. The much lower rate of malpractice litigation in Canada may reflect a still smaller proportion of malpractice incidents being litigated. Clearly, factors such as social attitudes that substantially change the propensity to litigate claims can have a dramatic effect on the frequency of claims filing even if the injury rate is unchanged. We found that over the past decade there have been marked increases in the frequency of claims against Canadian lawyers and against Ontario dentists, and somewhat less dramatic increases in third party bodily injury claims arising out of automobile accidents in Ontario and the Atlantic provinces. On the other hand, claims frequency has not increased for architects, engineers, and chartered accountants. These data suggest an increase in the general propensity to sue professionals providing services to individuals and therefore support the idea that individuals are increasingly reluctant to accept risk, as revealed in the post-war growth of the welfare state and a sharply increased regulatory role for governments (Aharoni, 1981; Douglas and Wildavsky, 1982). This reluctance to accept risk results in risk-shifting from patients to physicians, who are assumed to possess the necessary technical expertise to reduce or eliminate risk. Furthermore, increasing social distance between patients and physicians, arising from both increased mobility and specialization, may encourage this attitude and heighten claims consciousness. However, our data reveal no significant ($p>0.05$) positive relationship between interprovincial migration and immigration per capita and the frequency of malpractice litigation.

Demographic and Economic Factors

Increases in the severity of malpractice claims are expected to be positively related to those population groups that are significantly at risk of serious iatrogenic injuries. To examine this hypothesis, we divided the population into four mutually exclusive sets: children under 5, women 18-44, the elderly over 65, and all others. Although the demographic categories are unrelated both to the frequency of malpractice claims and to the proportion of paid claims, they are significant ($p<0.001$) in determining the size of the average paid claim. Specifically, an increase in the proportion of the population either under 5 or of women 18-44 raises the average paid claim, and an increase in the proportion of the population over 65 lowers the average paid claim (Table 3). These results are consistent with the hypothesis that the severity of claims is positively associated with a patient's foregone earnings. A further test of this hypothesis used average real wages three years after the incident date as an estimate of foregone earnings at the time the case closed. These wages were found (Table 3) to be significant ($p<0.001$) in the severity equation, supporting the hypothesis that foregone earnings play a major role in the determination of the average paid claim.

THE LEGAL ENVIRONMENT
Liability Rules

Both the severity equation (Table 3) and the proportion of paid claims equation (not shown) were specified with lagged dependent variables to capture the evolution of various legal doctrines. The lagged dependent variables were jointly significant ($p<0.001$) in both equations, supporting the view that considerable legal inertia exists in the determination of the proportion of paid claims and in the severity of malpractice claims.

The effect of liability rules (such as changes in both the customary practice and locality rules) on the frequency of malpractice claims is captured by the predicted proportion of paid claims. Since this variable is significant ($p < 0.01$) and positively related to the frequency of malpractice claims, we have support for the hypothesis that liability rules are important in the initiation of malpractice claims.

The effect of more stringent requirements for informed consent on the three dimensions of malpractice liability is captured by a dummy variable which is equal to unity after January 1, 1981 (the approximate date when informed consent requirements became more stringent) and equal to zero at other times. (Other events that took place at the same time, such as the move to apply real discount rates to future losses, are also captured by this variable.) Although the informed consent variable is not significant ($p > 0.05$) in either the severity or the proportions equation, it is significant ($p < 0.001$) in the frequency equation (Table 2). Consequently, there is evidence that these legal changes have significantly increased the frequency of malpractice claims.

Compensation Rules

The effect of compensation rules (such as those associated with the tax implications of interest on settlements, and claims by family members) on the frequency of malpractice claims is captured in part by the predicted size of the average paid claim. Since this variable is significant ($p < 0.01$) and positively related to the frequency of malpractice claims, we have support for the hypothesis that compensation rules play a significant role in the initiation of malpractice litigation.

Our results confirm that changing legal rules are important in accounting for the trends in malpractice liability. However, although most of the relevant legal changes in Canada occurred after 1979, half of the growth in frequency and severity occurred before this time (Figure 1). Clearly, other factors have been equally important in generating the trends identified here.

Miscellaneous Factors

The nominal rate of interest is expected to be positively associated with the severity of malpractice claims, because prejudgment interest is added to the calculated damages awarded to plaintiffs. To test this hypothesis, we included the yield on long term government bonds (10 years and above) lagged three years from the incident date to approximate the bond yield prevailing at the time the case closed. The results show a significant ($p < 0.001$) positive relationship between the bond yield and the severity of malpractice claims (Table 3), thereby supporting the hypothesis that prejudgment interest is an important determinant of the severity of malpractice claims.

The supply of lawyers per capita is insignificant ($p > 0.05$) in accounting for variations in the frequency to litigate, the proportion of paid claims, and the severity of those claims.

DISCUSSION

The large differences between specialties in the frequency of malpractice litigation can be largely explained by the differential performance of major surgery, reflecting intrusive treatment where error can result in large losses. Increases in the total number of malpractice claims are significantly explained by increases in medical activity, measured by the number of physicians or the performance of major surgery. We believe that increasing frequency is also attributable to an increased propensity of injured patients to sue, arising from a diminished patient-physician relationship and decreasing individual willingness to accept risks. It probably also arises from changes in medical technology and practice that yield more opportunities to save lives, but also yield an increase in the frequency with which physicians provide the types of care in which a momentary mistake or inadvertence can give rise to a large loss. Both the frequency and the severity of claims have increased in response to changes in legal doctrines that reduce barriers to suit or increase damages awarded. Increased incomes of victims also increase the incentive to pursue a claim. The supply of lawyers does not appear to be a factor in increased litigation. Finally, since malpractice trends in Canada and in the U.S. are similar, we believe that many of our results would apply in the United States as well.

NOTE

A more detailed version of this paper appears as:
Coyte PC, Dewees DN, Trebilcock MJ. Canadian medical malpractice liability: an empirical analysis of recent trends. *Journal of Health Economics* 10:2, 1991.

ACKNOWLEDGEMENTS

The research reported in this paper was conducted under the auspices of the Canadian Federal/ Provincial/Territorial Health Provider Liability Task Force and was supported by a grant from Health and Welfare Canada as well as a grant from the Social Sciences and Humanities Research Council of Canada. Special thanks are due to Pat Danzon, Greg Stoddart, and numerous other individuals who offered helpful comments on earlier drafts of the paper.

REFERENCES

Aharoni Y: *The No-risk Society.* Chatham, N.J.: Chatham House, 1981.

Canadian Medical Protective Association: *Eighty-eighth Annual Report.* Ottawa: Canadian Medical Protection Association, 1989.

Coyte PC, Dewees DN, Trebilcock MJ: Medical malpractice – the Canadian experience. *New England Journal of Medicine* 324:89-93, 1991.

Danzon PM: The frequency and severity of medical malpractice claims: new evidence. *Law and Contemporary Problems* 49:57-84, 1986.

Danzon PM: *Medical Malpractice: Theory, Evidence and Public Policy.* Cambridge: Harvard University Press, 1985.

Douglas M, Wildavsky A: *Risk and Culture.* Berkeley: University of California Press, 1982.

Kmenta J: *Elements of Econometrics* (second edition). New York, N.Y.: Macmillan Publishing Company, 1986.

Law and Contemporary Problems, Symposium Issue 49:2, 1986.

National Association of Insurance Commissions: *Medical Malpractice Closed Claims, 1975-78.* Washington, D.C.: NAIC, 1980.

U.S. General Accounting Office: *Medical Malpractice: Characteristics of Claims Closed in 1984.* Washington, D.C.: USGAO, GAO/HRD-87-55, April 1987.

U.S. General Accounting Office: *Medical Malpractice: Six State Case Studies Show Claims and Insurance Costs Still Rise Despite Reforms.* Washington, D.C.: USGAO, GAO/HRD-87-21, December 1986.

Weiler P: Legal Policy for Medical Injuries. American Law Institute Working Paper, 1988.

PRELIMINARY FINDINGS OF THE ECONOMIC EVALUATION OF AN ONTARIO GERIATRIC DAY HOSPITAL

D. Joan Eagle
School of Nursing

Ronald Wall
Centre for Health Economics and Policy Analysis

Fawne Stratford-Devai
Department of Clinical Epidemiology and Biostatistics

Gordon Guyatt
Department of Clinical Epidemiology and Biostatistics
Department of Medicine

Christopher Patterson
Division of Geriatric Medicine

Irene Turpie
Department of Medicine
St. Joseph's Hospital

Barbara Sackett
School of Nursing
McMaster University

INTRODUCTION

Elderly patients suffering from multiple medical problems often require comprehensive clinical investigations and treatments. Although these patients may not need hospitalization, ambulatory access to hospital-based diagnostic, therapeutic, and rehabilitative technology has not been available in Ontario (Eagle, 1985). Providing additional services to the growing number of elderly in the face of resource constraints necessitates initiatives aimed at improving healthcare system performance. Reductions in the numbers of inappropriately hospitalized elderly could improve system effectiveness, efficiency, and through-put.

The geriatric day hospital (GDH) is an innovative program designed to provide diagnostic, therapeutic, and rehabilitative services that clinicians can use to manage frail elderly patients on an ambulatory basis. GDH programs include patient needs assessment, comprehensive and coordinated patient care by a multidisciplinary team, extensive retraining assisting patients to adapt their activities of daily living to the constraints of their functional limitations, opportunities for social interactions with staff and other patients, and some respite care for patient informal caregivers.

Although well-established in the United Kingdom, GDHs have only recently been introduced into North America. Published studies evaluating GDH effectiveness and efficiency are methodologically suspect, compare different alternatives, and report mixed findings (see Eagle et al, 1987 for a comprehensive appraisal of this literature). One scientific study reported improved physical and emotional patient functioning following management in a GDH (Tucker, Davison, and Ogle, 1984), while other studies (Cummings et al, 1985; Weissert et al, 1980) reported no significant differences in patient outcomes. All three of these studies reported substantially greater costs for patients treated in GDHs. Furthermore, it is not clear that these findings can be generalized to the context of the Ontario healthcare system. Therefore, to provide decision-makers with valid evidence applicable to the Ontario healthcare system, the effectiveness and efficiency of patient treatment in the Chedoke-McMaster Hospitals GDH compared to usual care (UC) available in the Hamilton-Wentworth region were examined using incremental analysis – i.e., comparing the differences in costs and consequences between alternative programs.

METHODS

Effectiveness and efficiency were evaluated in a randomized controlled trial. Patients were defined as "day hospital eligible" if they: 1) were 65 years of age or older, 2) had impairment of function to the extent that independence in their present living arrangement was threatened, 3) had a positive prognosis for long-term improvement, 4) lived at home or in a home for the aged, 5) resided in the Hamilton-Wentworth region, and 6) were referred to the consultant geriatricians (CP, IT). Individuals were excluded if their life expectancy was less than six months or their illness/disability required 24-hour monitoring. Following assessment by a consultant geriatrician, "day hospital eligible" patients were randomly allocated (using a randomized block design with a blocking factor of 4) to receive care in the GDH or to receive the UC provided prior to the advent of the GDH. Patient costs of care and clinical outcomes were monitored over the one-year period following randomization.

Effectiveness was estimated by incrementally comparing average clinical outcome scores per group (experimental minus control) over four assessment points (baseline and 3, 6, and 12 months). Clinical outcomes were measured using several instruments assessing patient functional status and health-related quality-of-life. Repeated measures of ANOVA using baseline data as a covariate were used to separate treatment and time effects.

Efficiency was estimated using cost-effectiveness analysis (CEA), cost-utility analysis (CUA), and cost-minimization analysis (CMA) to compare the estimated incremental costs to the measured incremental clinical outcomes (see Drummond, Stoddart, and Torrance, 1987 for a detailed discussion of economic evaluation methods). The between-group cost differences were estimated by incrementally comparing average costs per group (experimental minus control) measured over the one-year period following randomization. In Figure 1, the incremental costs appear in the numerator of all three analytical formulations, and the denominators of the CEA and CUA formulations express the difference in average clinical outcomes between the alternatives; CMA assumes that there are no differences in clinical outcome (i.e., the alternatives are equally effective). The CEA denominator is the incremental change in a single-dimension measure of patient health-related quality-of-life (i.e., a measure of morbidity or mortality); the CUA denominator is the incremental change in quality-adjusted life-years (QALY) (a multi-dimension index of patient health-related quality-of-life combining morbidity and mortality).

Costs are estimated from the perspectives of the Ontario Ministry of Health, patients and informal caregivers, and society. Societal costs is a comprehensive measure that includes the costs to the Ontario Ministry of Health, patients and informal caregivers, and other public and private agencies (e.g., community agencies and private insurance firms).

ECONOMIC EVALUATION ANALYTICAL FORMULATIONS

$$CMA = C \qquad (\$ \text{ per patient})$$

$$CEA = C / E \qquad (\$ \text{ per clinical effect gained})$$

$$CUA = C / U \qquad (\$ \text{ per QALY gained})$$

Where: C is the incremental (experimental minus control) between-group difference in average direct costs per patient measured using 1987 Canadian dollars.

E is the incremental between-group difference in clinical outcome measured by a single-dimension index of patient health-related quality-of-life.

U is the incremental between-group difference in clinical outcome measured by the time-tradeoff (TTO) method and converted into quality-adjusted life-years gained.

Figure 1

PROGRAM DESCRIPTIONS

Patients randomized to the experimental group attended the GDH every Tuesday and Thursday for approximately four hours per visit until they were judged capable of managing their day-to-day activities and of functioning relatively independently in their own home environment. To ensure continuity of care, discharge planning usually involved relatives and community caregivers. The GDH, established in 1984 by Chedoke-McMaster Hospitals (a secondary and tertiary care teaching hospital providing care to the Hamilton-Wentworth Region), included facilities for physical and occupational retraining, areas for patients to practice activities of daily living, examining rooms, and workshops and crafts rooms. The clinical team included: 1) a physician trained in geriatrics; 2) a full-time nursing coordinator and two registered nurses; 3) physical, occupational, speech, and nutritional therapists; 4) a social worker; and 5) a pharmacist. With the exception of the on-call pharmacist and nutritional therapist, all clinical staff were available in the GDH during its hours of operation.

Patients randomized to the control group received care in the usual manner provided prior to the advent of the GDH. Before randomization, the consultant geriatrician specified where patients would be managed if they were assigned to the control group. Control patients with complex medical problems requiring comprehensive assessment and treatment were admitted to the inpatient Geriatric Assessment Unit (GAU); of the remaining control patients, those requiring monitoring and limited rehabilitative services were followed through the ambulatory Geriatric Clinics (GC).

Patients in both the experimental and control groups received necessary care and services as required from hospitals, community agencies, and informal caregivers. Hospital care was provided through inpatient nursing units, ambulatory clinics, and emergency units. Agencies providing community health care services included the Hamilton-Wentworth Home Care Program, the Public Health Unit, community physiotherapy clinics, community visiting nursing organizations, and physicians (primary care and specialist). Patient support was provided by community agencies including the Visiting Homemaker Program, Meals-on-Wheels,

Disabled and Regional Transport Services (DARTS), and recreational programs provided by several organizations. Informal care was usually provided by a spouse or cohabitant.

CLINICAL OUTCOME MEASURES

The clinical outcomes used to estimate the effectiveness and efficiency (using CEA and CUA methods) of the GDH compared to UC were estimated using several instruments measuring functional status and health-related quality-of-life. A brief mental status questionnaire (Robertson, Rockwook, and Stolee, 1982) was administered to all patients at baseline to identify individuals who could not understand or respond meaningfully to the more complex instruments.

The instruments used in this study are fully described elsewhere (see Eagle et al, 1991), so only a brief summary is presented here.

All patients, regardless of their mental status score, were assessed for: 1) functional status as measured by the Barthel Index (BI), 2) emotional function as measured by the Rand Questionnaire (RQ), and 3) overall health state as measured by the Global Health Question (GHQ). For the GHQ, patients were asked to rank on a 7-point scale (with 7 being the best response) their answer to the following question: "Generally speaking, how has your OVERALL HEALTH been over the past two weeks?"

The condition-specific (i.e., functional limitation) BI (Mahoney and Barthel, 1965) is a valid (Granger et al, 1979), reliable (Granger et al, 1979), and responsive (Deyo, 1984; Donaldson, Wagner, and Gresham, 1973; Gresham, Phillips, and Labi, 1980; Kane and Robert, 1981) instrument measuring functional levels of self-care and mobility in the physically impaired. Although the BI does not measure the more complex activities of daily living (e.g., food preparation, shopping, housekeeping, management of personal finances), and hence is not a complete measure of the basic activities most critical for patients to remain in community settings (Applegate, Blass, and Williams, 1990), a score of 60 (out of 100) appears to predict the point at which individuals move from assisted independence to dependence on others (Fortinsky, Granger, and Seltzer, 1981; Goldberg, Bernad, and Granger, 1980; Granger, Sherwood, and Greer, 1977; Granger et al, 1979).

Patient caregivers were also asked to rate the patients using the BI, GHQ, and RQ. A patient caregiver was defined as someone who had direct daily contact with the patient for the purpose of giving care. This was usually a spouse or cohabitant who assisted the patient with daily activities over a 24-hour period. At home, the caregiver was asked to rate the patient's current performance; hospitalized or institutionalized patients too ill to respond meaningfully were rated by a health professional (usually a nurse).

Study patients with a mental status score of 7 or higher (out of 10) were administered the person-specific Geriatric Quality of Life Questionnaire (GQLQ) and the generic Time Tradeoff (TTO) instruments. The GQLQ, developed specifically for this study along established principles (Kirshner and Guyatt, 1985; Guyatt, Bombardier, and Tugwell, 1986) and validated against the BI, RQ, and GHQ instruments, contains 25 items in three dimensions: activities of daily living (ADL), symptoms, and feelings/emotions generated by the patient's health state.

Although condition- and person-specific instruments are useful for evaluating the effectiveness and efficiency of alternative health care programs that generate comparable outcomes, they do not provide comprehensive measures that are comparable across programs producing diverse outcomes (Guyatt and Jaeschke, 1990). Utility measurement is a holistic approach widely used to assess patient preferences for health states using a cardinal index ranging in value from 0 (death) to 1 (perfect health) (Torrance, 1986, 1987).

Most studies that measure the utility of health states use either the standard gamble method (von Neumann-Morgenstern) or the time tradeoff technique (TTO). Although the standard gamble has the advantage of being based directly on the fundamental axioms of von Neumann-Morgenstern utility theory, giving the results a precise interpretation, the method is somewhat complex in that it requires the understanding and use of probabilities. Given the limited cognitive capacity of many elderly subjects in this trial, we elected to use the TTO to avoid possible patient conceptual problems with probabilities. The TTO technique is easier for subjects to use than the standard gamble (Torrance, 1987) and has been shown to yield comparable results (Guyatt and Jaeschke, 1990; Torrance, 1976). Moreover, in this study, the TTO results were not to be used directly as utilities in an expected utility decision model, but were to be interpreted as comprehensive measures of quality-of-life for use as quality weights in calculating quality-adjusted life-years (QALYs). In addition, the treatment effect was estimated over time using within-person changes from baseline. Finally, the TTO method has been used successfully in several studies of older and/or cognitively diminished subjects (Churchill et al, 1987; Mohide et al, 1988).

COSTS OF CARE

Patient costs were estimated from patients' utilization of health care and other resources over the one-year period following randomization and valued using prices expressed in 1987 Canadian dollars. Because patients and informal caregivers were retired, the indirect cost of lost productivity was not estimated and only the direct costs were measured. The statistical significance of the incremental costs being genuine (i.e., non-zero) is estimated using the two-tailed t-test.

The costs of resources consumed by study patients include: 1) the costs to the Ontario Ministry of Health of patient care and services provided in hospitals, institutions, and the community; 2) the costs to public and private agencies of the services and equipment used by patients and not funded by the Ontario Ministry of Health; and 3) the out-of-pocket costs to patients and informal caregivers arising from treatment-related activities. Overall, the costs of over 50 types of care and services used by study patients were estimated. Because treatment in the GDH compared to UC could affect the subsequent quantity and mix of care and services utilized, we estimated costs over a one-year period following patient randomization. To facilitate between-group comparisons and to identify possible substitution effects (e.g., decreased institutionalization at the expense of increased utilization of community resources), the costs of patient care and services were grouped into five broad categories: 1) hospital care and services, 2) medical care and services, 3) institutional (excluding hospital) care and services, 4) community care and services, and 5) recreation and transportation.

The costs to the Ontario Ministry of Health of hospital care and services include all therapeutic and rehabilitative services provided by acute-care hospitals through inpatient, outpatient, and ambulatory programs; diagnostic services and medications provided by hospitals to inpatients and ambulatory patients are included in the following section. Because the distinction between acute- and chronic-care hospitals for the provision of long-term care is not clear, long-term care provided by acute-care hospitals to study patients is included in this category.

Although most patients were cared for in the Chedoke-McMaster Hospitals, geographical considerations and physician referral patterns also caused some patients to obtain care from other hospitals within the region. To control for the possible confounding effect of price differences between hospitals providing equivalent care and services, utilization was valued using prices estimated for the Chedoke-McMaster Hospitals. Furthermore, except for care provided in specialized inpatient nursing units (e.g., cardiac care unit) and ambulatory clinics (e.g., urology) located at the McMaster Division, the costs of all hospital care and services were estimated using Chedoke Division prices.

Episodes of hospitalization can include: 1) care provided in inpatient (e.g., medical, surgical, intensive care) and ambulatory (e.g., short-stay, urology clinic) nursing units; 2) patient services (e.g., physiotherapy, occupational therapy, dietary, central stores and receiving, pharmacy); and 3) administrative and other activities supporting the provision of patient care and services (e.g., administration, housekeeping, plant operation and maintenance, laundry and linen). The costs of the care, services, and support should reflect the operating expenses (wages and supplies) and the opportunity costs of equipment, buildings, and land. Support costs were allocated to patient care and service departments on the basis of actual charges or appropriate parameters (e.g., floor area and paid hours) using the method of simultaneous allocation to account for interactions between support departments (Drummond, Stoddart, and Torrance, 1987). The average prices of nursing care and patient services were estimated using departmental costs and the outputs produced (e.g., patient-days, clinic visits, service work-units). Patient utilization of hospital care and services was abstracted from medical records.

The costs to the Ontario Ministry of Health of medical care include physician consultations, professional (e.g., podiatrist) services, all prescribed medications, a portion of the charge for ambulance service, and diagnostic services (laboratory and radiology). The costs of services provided by primary care physicians, specialists, and GDH physicians were estimated using the 1987 Ontario fee-schedule. The costs of prescribed medications were estimated using the 1987 Ontario Formulary; the cost of medications not provided by hospitals includes the customary dispensing fee charged by local pharmacists. The costs to patients of over-the-counter medications were estimated from prevailing drugstore prices. The Ontario Ministry of Health and patients (or welfare) are each charged $22.00 per trip for ambulance services. The costs to the Ontario Ministry of Health of all diagnostic services were calculated using prices estimated for the Chedoke Division laboratory and radiology departments; the cost to the Ontario Ministry of Health of collecting and transporting specimens obtained from patients in their place of residence was included when appropriate. Utilization data were obtained from patient medical records and self-reports; whenever possible, patient self-reports were corroborated.

Institutional care and services were provided by retirement homes and nursing homes (patients in this sample did not require care provided by chronic care hospitals). Retirement homes provide residential services but no nursing care (Level 1 care); the cost to patients was estimated using prevailing charges. Nursing homes provide residential services plus limited nursing care and therapeutic services (Level 2 care); the base amount paid by the Ontario Ministry of Health and the remaining amount paid by patients (or welfare) were estimated using prevailing charges for the type of accommodation. Utilization data were obtained from institutional records; charges were estimated by the Hamilton-Wentworth Regional Placement and Coordination Services coordinator.

Study patients residing in private homes and satisfying eligibility criteria could obtain care and services from community agencies. Nursing care is available through the

Hamilton-Wentworth Home Care Program, the Public Health Unit, and private agencies; other services can be provided by the Home Care Program, physiotherapy clinics, home-maker agencies, and Meals-on-Wheels. Recreation and transportation services are excluded from this category because they are used by patients regardless of their place of residence.

Home Care Program case-managers assess patient needs and arrange for required nursing care, home-maker assistance, and therapy services (physio-, occupational-, speech-, and nutritional therapy, and social work). Home Care is fully funded by the Ministry of Health. Actual costs for the 1986-7 fiscal year were used to estimate the unit prices (including a share of support costs and the opportunity costs of the building, land, and equipment) of case-management and professional services; nursing care and home-maker services are purchased under contract from local agencies. Utilization data were obtained from Home Care records.

The Hamilton-Wentworth Public Health Unit provides visiting nursing care. Funding is provided by the Ministry of Health (75%) and the Hamilton-Wentworth region (25%). The cost per hour of nursing time provided to patients was estimated using 1986-7 fiscal year expenses (including a share of support and opportunity costs). The numbers and types of contacts (telephone monitoring, home visits to provide care) were abstracted from patient records. The time required for each type of patient contact was estimated by the Unit administrator. Physiotherapy clinics are directly reimbursed by the Ontario Ministry of Health at rates specified by the fee schedule. Patient self-reported utilization was verified against clinic records.

Paid helpers assist patients with the activities of daily living, perform home-making tasks and residential maintenance, and provide companionship. Patient self-reported costs were verified whenever possible from receipts. Self-reported expenditures by patients and informal caregivers for equipment and supplies (e.g., walkers, support bars, rails) used to adapt homes for patient functional limitations were verified whenever possible against receipts. The costs of hot meals delivered to patients' homes are largely funded through an operating grant from the Hamilton-Wentworth region, so only the costs to patients (or welfare) were estimated. The numbers of meals provided to study patients were obtained from the agency's records.

Recreational programs and transportation services are available to patients regardless of their place of residence. Recreation programs provide patients with access to leisure activities and opportunities for socialization. Utilization was estimated from self-reported expenditures. Although these programs are funded by public and private agencies, only the costs to patients (or welfare) were estimated. The costs to patients and community agencies of transportation used to access health care (primarily treatment in the GDH or GC) were estimated from patient self-reports, verified whenever possible. The Disabled and Aged Regional Transit System (DARTS) is an important source of transportation used by the study patients; other sources include private automobiles, taxis, and public transportation. Because the DARTS operating expenses are funded through direct user charges and grants, the costs to patients and informal caregivers and to public agencies were estimated. The operating costs of automobile travel include expenditures on fuel and parking; the costs of bus and taxi transportation include only the direct charges to patients or their informal caregivers.

RESULTS

Randomization was successful in that the two groups were initially comparable with respect to age, sex, presence of a caregiver living in the home, and proportion of patients with degenerative joint disease or cerebral vascular accident; depression was, however, more frequent among the control group.

Of the 113 (55 GDH, 58 UC) patients who entered the study, 12 (8 GDH, 4 UC) died within one year of randomization. Of the 101 surviving patients, 99 (47 GDH, 52 UC) were administered the BI and 84 (39 GDH, 45 UC) were administered the GHQ at the four assessment points (baseline, 3 months, 6 months, and 12 months); caregivers, on behalf of patients, also completed the BI and GHQ. Of the 76 (35 GDH, 41 UC) patients at baseline who had sufficient mental status (as determined by the mental health status questionnaire) to respond meaningfully to the complex quality-of-life instruments, 60 (28 GDH, 32 UC) completed the ADL dimension, 55 (26 GDH, 29 UC) completed the emotions dimension, and 60 (28 GDH, 32 UC) completed the symptoms dimension of the GQLQ; 67 (32 GDH, 35 UC) patients completed TTO at all four assessment points or died after three measurements (and therefore their 12-month QALY value was imputed to be 0 [i.e., the value of death as a health state]).

Although the costs of care of all the study patients were compiled for the one-year time period (or until death) following randomization (i.e., no patients were lost to follow-up), only the findings of the 57 (28 GDH, 29 UC) patients completing all four TTO measurements are reported here. Mentally lucid and comprehending patients surviving beyond the one-year follow-up period may obtain the greatest benefit from GDH treatment.

The treatment effects estimated from the between-group difference (experimental minus control) in average clinical outcomes measured by the BI, GHQ, GQLQ, and TTO instruments are reported in Table 1. For all instruments, a positive difference favours the experimental group. Although the health status of both groups decreased over time, the incremental treatment effects (adjusted for the effect of time) measured by all instruments except TTO were negative. However, all estimated treatment effects were small and, at the conventional level of statistical significance ($p = 0.05$) adjusted for multiple sample testing

Table 1

INCREMENTAL AVERAGE CLINICAL OUTCOMES

Instrument	Difference[1] in average score	95% confidence interval	Statistical significance
Barthel Index	-4.9	(-11.3, +1.6)	p = 0.18
Global Health Questionnaire	-0.50	(-0.89, -0.11)	p = 0.012
Geriatric Quality of Life Questionnaire			
Symptoms	-0.33	(-0.80, +0.14)	p = 0.17
Activities of Daily Living	-0.32	(-0.92, +0.28)	p = 0.29
Emotion	-0.63	(-1.13, -0.13)	p = 0.015
Time tradeoff	+0.056	(-0.017, +0.183)	p = 0.38

1 The difference was calculated as the average experimental group score minus the average control group score over the one-year period following randomization. In all instruments, a positive difference favours the experimental group.

(p = 0.008; see Hassard, 1991), there was no statistical evidence of any genuine between-group differences. (See Eagle et al, 1991 for a detailed discussion of these clinical findings.)

The incremental cost of the five costs categories, estimated as the between-group difference (experimental minus control) in average costs, are graphically displayed in Figures 2 - 6 by perspective. A positive cost difference indicates that the GDH program was more costly than the UC alternative; a negative cost difference means that UC was more costly than GDH treatment.

In Figure 2, there is statistical evidence (at the conventional level of significance; i.e., $p = 0.05$) that GDH treatment increased the costs to the Ontario Ministry of Health and to society of ambulatory care (AC) and therapeutic services (TS); there is no evidence that the costs of inpatient care (IC) and surgery differed. The higher AC and TS average costs estimated for the experimental group are explained by the attendance of these patients at the costly GDH nursing unit and their higher utilization of TS associated with treatment in the GDH. Although utilization of the GC by control patients was significantly higher, this increase was not sufficient to offset the costs of GDH care and therapeutic services. There were no significant cost differences in the remaining inpatient and ambulatory nursing units. Overall, hospital care and services were more costly for the experimental group.

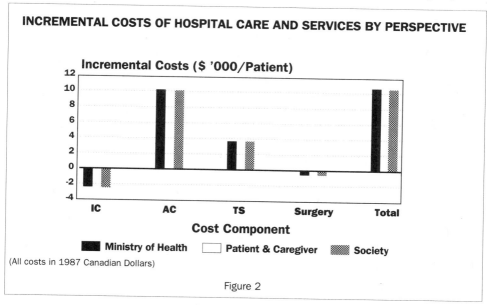

Figure 2

There is no statistical evidence that the incremental costs in Figure 3 of professional services (PS), prescription and over-the-counter medications (MEDS), ambulance transportation (AT), and diagnostic tests (DT) are different from zero. However, the significantly higher costs of physician consultations (PC) to the Ontario Ministry of Health and to society are explained by the assessments and consultations given by GDH physicians to patients receiving treatment in the GDH; no cost differences for services provided by specialists and primary care physicians were found. Overall, there is some (marginal) evidence that the costs of medical care and services were higher for patient treated in the GDH.

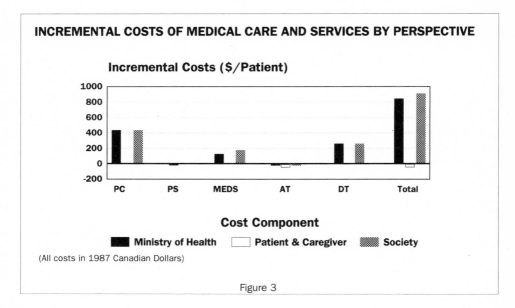

Figure 3

Although, in Figure 4, the negative incremental costs of residing in retirement homes (RH) are less than the positive incremental costs of nursing home (NH) care and services to patients (or their families), the Ontario Ministry of Health, and society, there is no statistical evidence that these differences are genuine. The finding of no significant between-group difference in nursing home costs suggests that GDH treatment may not reduce the subsequent loss of independence of living arrangements for experimental patients compared to control patients receiving UC.

Figure 5 shows that study patients residing in the community during any portion (or all)

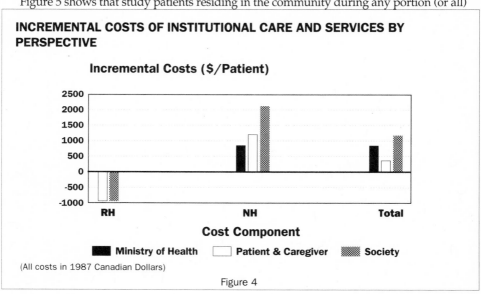

Figure 4

of the one-year period after randomization did not exhibit any statistically significant incremental costs for the care and services provided by home care (HC), public health nursing (PHN), physiotherapy clinics (PTC), paid help (PH), equipment and supplies (E/S), Meals-on-Wheels (MOW), or the overall costs of community care and services to any study perspective.

Finally, in Figure 6, the between-group difference in the costs of recreation programs

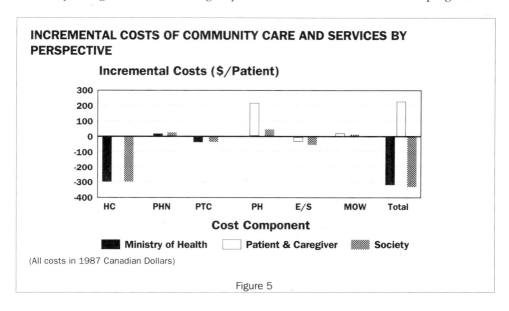

Figure 5

(RP) to patients and informal caregivers is not statistically significant. The average costs of transportation (TRANS) to both patients and informal caregivers and to society were signif-

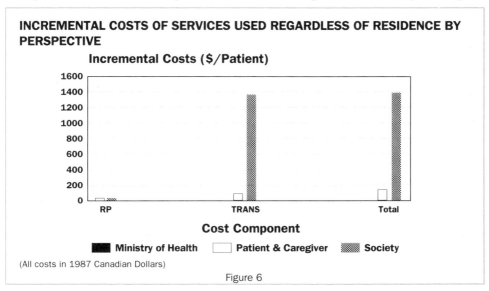

Figure 6

icantly higher for the experimental group. This higher cost to both perspectives is related to the higher usage of DARTS transportation (no differences were noted in the costs of other forms of transportation) by the experimental group to attend GDH treatment.

The incremental social costs of GDH treatment compared to UC, by perspective, for all care and services utilized by study patients over the one-year period following randomization are graphically displayed in Figure 7. The average costs of the experimental group are higher than those of the control group for all of the analytical perspectives. The positive incremental costs to the Ontario Ministry of Health (p<0.000) and to society (p<0.000) are highly significant; however, the positive incremental costs to patients and informal caregivers (p = 0.552) and to the other public and private agencies (p = 0.054) are not statistically significant.

The sensitivity of these results to the effect of a lower intensity of care and services

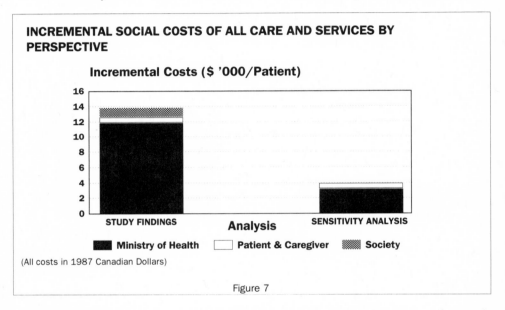

INCREMENTAL SOCIAL COSTS OF ALL CARE AND SERVICES BY PERSPECTIVE

Incremental Costs ($ '000/Patient)

STUDY FINDINGS   Analysis   SENSITIVITY ANALYSIS

■ Ministry of Health   □ Patient & Caregiver   ▧ Society

(All costs in 1987 Canadian Dollars)

Figure 7

provided to GDH patients was examined by reducing the estimated incremental costs of the following GDH-related care and services to the lower value of their respective 95% confidence intervals: 1) nursing care provided in the GDH, 2) therapeutic services provided in the GDH, 3) physician consultations provided during GDH treatment, and 4) DARTS transportation used to access the GDH. The revised incremental social costs estimated using these reduced values are also shown in Figure 7. Although the estimated incremental social costs were sensitive to these changes, GDH treatment remained more costly to all perspectives.

When, as for this study, no differences in clinical outcomes between alternative health care programs are detected, the appropriate analytical formulation is CMA (Drummond, Stoddart, and Torrance, 1987); however, for academic interest, the implications of findings from the CEA and CUA will also be discussed. The CMA finding that the incremental costs to all study perspectives are positive is clear empirical evidence that (within the limitations of this study) GDH treatment is not an efficient alternative compared to UC for providing the frail elderly with therapeutic, rehabilitative, and diagnostic care and services. Moreover, because the sources of the costs-increase appear to be directly associated with GDH-related activities (i.e., there is no statistical evidence that the costs of the remaining care and services differed between the experimental and control groups), the GDH appears to be a costly health care program neither affecting patient outcomes nor influencing the utilization of other care and services. This finding is robust with respect to a large reduction in the incremental average costs of the GDH-related activities.

Although the between-group average treatment effects are not statistically significant, all estimated clinical outcomes (other than TTO, which is used in CUA) are negative. Therefore, CEA using these effects will also be negative to all study perspectives (i.e., incremental costs to all perspective are positive). These findings indicate that GDH treatment increases the average costs of care and decreases patient average functional status or single-dimension health-related quality-of-life (the worst of all possible worlds) compared to UC.

Similarly, although a small estimated difference of 0.056 QALYs favouring GDH treatment was measured using TTO, the large incremental costs required to produce this small increase (when compared using CUA) yield a large cost per QALY-gained to all study perspectives. These findings indicate that GDH treatment is not efficient (from any perspective), compared to UC, because the opportunity cost of implementing the GDH is the lost improvement in health-related quality-of-life that could otherwise have been gained by investing in other (more cost-effective) health care programs. Such programs could produce larger improvements in patients' health-related quality-of-life using these scarce health care resources.

SUMMARY AND DISCUSSION

This analysis failed to find statistical evidence (using several instruments measuring clinical outcomes) that treatment of the frail elderly in the Chedoke-McMaster Hospitals GDH improved patient outcomes compared to UC available in the Hamilton-Wentworth region. Furthermore, the estimated average cost of care for the GDH group was significantly higher than that of the UC group to both the Ontario Ministry of Health and to society; no statistical evidence of a significant cost difference was found from the perspective of the patient and informal caregiver. Using CMA (supported by findings from CEA and CUA), the analysis found that GDH treatment was not an efficient alternative to UC.

Although the power of the study to detect real differences in clinical outcomes using the more complex instruments (GQLQ and TTO) may be compromised because patients with insufficient mental status were excluded, the finding of no treatment effect using the GHQ and BI instruments administered to all surviving patients (or, in some cases, their caregivers) indicates that, at least along these dimensions, GDH was no more effective than UC. Because functional limitation (as measured by the BI) is an important aspect of patient health status that should be affected by GDH, the failure of this study to detect any difference strongly suggests that GDH is no more effective than UC for caring for the frail elderly in the Hamilton-Wentworth region.

Given that treatment in the GDH appears to be no more effective than UC, the most appropriate analytical formulation for evaluating GDH efficiency is CMA. Because the average costs of care for the GDH group were significantly higher than those for UC, the estimated positive incremental costs (experimental group minus control group) to all study perspectives indicate that the GDH program is not an efficient use of scarce health care and other resources compared to UC. This finding is supported by the incremental comparison of costs and clinical outcomes by the CEA and CUA formulations. Although CMA is sensitive to a large reduction in the costs of GDH-related care and services, our finding that treatment in the GDH is not efficient compared to UC is robust.

The generalizability of this study is limited by the population studied and the alternatives compared. For example, GDH treatment may be effective and efficient compared to usual care available in other settings if therapeutic, rehabilitative, and diagnostic services through a GAU and GC (supported by comprehensive community care and services) are not available. In such settings, treatment in a GDH may be cost-effective compared to possibly inappropriate hospitalization or institutionalization. However, unless strong empirical evidence showing improved patient outcomes and/or lower costs of care is found, clinicians, administrators, and planners located in settings rich in programs caring for the frail elderly should consider the opportunity costs of implementing a GDH.

ACKNOWLEDGEMENTS

This study was supported by a grant from the Ontario Ministry of Health, Research and Planning Division. We are grateful to Amiram Gafni, Roberta Labelle, Greg Stoddart, and especially George Torrance for their constructive comments and advice. We thank Ron Goree (McMaster University) for providing us with the prices of care and services produced by the Chedoke-McMaster Hospitals, Judy Duncan for completing the chart audits, and Jenny Whyte, Lynne Sackett, and Ashish Kohli for data management.

REFERENCES

Applegate WB, Blass JP, Williams TF: Instruments for the functional assessment of older patients. *New England Journal of Medicine* 322:1207-1214, 1990.

Churchill DN, Torrance GW, Taylor DW, et al: Measurement of the quality of life in end-stage renal disease: the time trade-off approach. *Clinical and Investigative Medicine* 10:14-20, 1987.

Cummings V, Kerner JF, Arones S, Steinbock C: Day hospital service in rehabilitation medicine: an evaluation. *Archives of Physical Medicine and Rehabilitation* 66:86-91, 1985.

Deyo RA: Measuring functional outcomes in therapeutic trials for chronic disease. *Controlled Clinical Trials* 5:223-240, 1984.

Donaldson SW, Wagner CC, Gresham GE: A unified evaluation form. *Archives of Physical Medicine and Rehabilitation* 54:175-179, 1973.

Drummond M, Stoddart G, Torrance G: *Methods for the Economic Evaluation of Health Care Programmes.* Oxford: Oxford University Press, 1987.

Eagle DJ: *Evaluation of a Geriatric Day Hospital.* A thesis submitted to the School of Graduate Studies in partial fulfilment of the requirements for the degree of Master of Science. Hamilton, Ontario: McMaster University, 1985.

Eagle DJ, Guyatt G, Patterson CJ, Turpie I: Day hospitals' cost and effectiveness: a summary. *The Gerontologist* 27:735-740, 1987.

Eagle DJ, Guyatt GH, Patterson C, Turpie I, Sackett B, Singer J: Effectiveness of a geriatric day hospital. *Canadian Medical Association Journal* 144:699-704, 1991.

Fortinsky RH, Granger CV, Seltzer GB: The use of functional assessment in understanding home care needs. *Medical Care* 19:489-497, 1981.

Goldberg RT, Bernad M, Granger CV: Vocational status: prediction by the Barthel Index and PULSES Profile. *Archives of Physical Medicine and Rehabilitation* 61:580-583, 1980.

Granger CV, Lester SD, Nancy C, et al: Stroke rehabilitation: analysis of repeated Barthel Index measures. *Archives of Physical Medicine and Rehabilitation* 60:14-17, 1979.

Granger CV, Sherwood CC, Greer DS: Functional status measures in a comprehensive stroke care programme. *Archives of Physical Medicine and Rehabilitation* 58:555-561, 1977.

Gresham GE, Phillips TF, Labi ML: ADL status in stroke: relative merits of three standard indexes. *Archives of Physical Medicine and Rehabilitation* 61:355-358, 1980.

Guyatt G, Bombardier C, Tugwell P: Measuring disease-specific quality-of-life in clinical trials. *Canadian Medical Association Journal* 134:889-895, 1986.

Guyatt G, Jaeschke R: Measurements in clinical trials: choosing the appropriate approach. In: Spilker B (ed.): *Quality of Life Assessment in Clinical Trials.* New York: Raven Press, 1990.

Hassard TH: *Understanding Biostatistics.* St. Louis: Mosby Year Book, 1991.

Kane RA, Robert L: *Assessing the Elderly.* Toronto: Lexington Books, 1981.

Kirschner B, Guyatt GH: A methodologic framework for assessing health indices. *Journal of Chronic Diseases* 38:27-36, 1985.

Mahoney F, Barthel D: Functional evaluation: the Barthel Index. *Maryland State Medical Journal* 14:61-65, 1965.

Mohide EA, Torrance GW, Streiner DL, et al: Measuring the wellbeing of family caregivers using the time trade-off technique. *Journal of Clinical Epidemiology* 41:475-482, 1988.

Robertson D, Rockwook K, Stolee P: A short mental status questionnaire. *Canadian Journal on Aging* 1:16-20, 1982.

Torrance GW: Utility approach to measuring health-related quality of life. *Journal of Chronic Diseases* 40:593-600, 1987.

Torrance GW: Measurement of health state utilities for economic appraisal: a review article. *Journal of Health Economics* 5:1-30, 1986.

Torrance GW: Social preferences for health states: an empirical evaluation of three measurement techniques. *Socioeconomic Planning Sciences* 10:129-136, 1976.

Tucker MA, Davison JG, Ogle SJ: Day hospital rehabilitation – effectiveness and cost in the elderly – a randomized controlled trial. *British Journal of Medicine* 289:1209-1212, 1984.

Weissert WG, Wan T, Livieratos B, Katz S: Effects and costs of day care services for the chronically ill. *Medical Care* 18:567-584, 1980.

ECONOMIC COSTS OF SELF-SUFFICIENCY IN BLOOD PRODUCTS: THE CASE OF ALBUMIN

Philip Jacobs
A. Robert Turner
L. Duncan Saunders
Faculty of Medicine
University of Alberta

INTRODUCTION

Provincial ministers of health, through the policy making and financial coordination of the Canadian Blood Committee, have mandated that "national self-sufficiency for blood products", a goal espoused in a number of other countries (Morris, 1984; Gunson, 1984), is to be a goal of the Canadian blood system as well (Canadian Blood Committee, 1987). Currently, Canada is self-sufficient in blood components such as red cells, platelet concentrate, and frozen plasma – components which are prepared at the 17 regional blood centers serving the Canadian population from blood donated to the centers. However, Canada is not self-sufficient in products manufactured from plasma and lacks the manufacturing capacity to provide albumin (a volume expander), intravenous immune globulin (used in a variety of hematologic and immunologic diseases), or coagulation Factors VIII and IX (required to treat hemophiliacs). The fractionation of plasma is a sophisticated procedure carried out by commercial operators. The current cost of providing these products for Canadians is approximately $100,000,000. In 1988, Canadian source plasma covered 95% of total Canadian albumin use, but only 56% of Factor VIII use (Canadian Red Cross Society, 1989).

In the context of plasma products, the term "self-sufficiency" can have several meanings. A country may be self-sufficient in the *collection* of plasma, but can then have its plasma fractionated into albumin, Factor VIII, and other components externally. Alternatively, self-sufficiency can refer to domestic collection and fractionation. The goal of self-sufficiency in collection is more readily achieved than that of self-sufficiency in production, and most of the benefits of any sort of self-sufficiency can be achieved through self-sufficiency in collection.

The importance of this subject lies in the potential benefits of self-sufficiency. One traditional argument for self-sufficiency – the one that seems to be most relevant – lies in assuring that supply is *available.* A country may be unwilling to be vulnerable in the event that foreign sources of supply are shut off. In the case of blood products in Canada, the Canadian Red Cross, being the government-delegated provider of blood products, has a policy mandate to assure that such supplies are adequate. The argument is more compelling when the product is a "necessity". There are alternative products for albumin, but not for Factors VIII and IX, which in present times represent survival for hemophiliacs. This makes the case for self-sufficiency even more compelling. A second argument for self-sufficiency lies in the need to assure the *safety* of the blood supply. Much of the albumin purchased from the United States is commercial source plasma, and in the past the quality of commercial source plasma has been suspect. Although recent improvements in testing have reduced the likelihood of HIV infected plasma's being fractionated, there are still concerns that commercial source plasma may have higher infection rates for other (as yet undiscovered) conditions. Another argument in favor of national sufficiency relates to the importance of creating manufacturing jobs in Canada.

Whatever these arguments, the *economic* aspects cannot be ignored. Increases in self-sufficiency will be accompanied by additional costs as well as financial savings and other economic benefits. It is important to understand the economic magnitude of this endeavour to assess the policy's impact. In this paper, we conduct an analysis of the economic costs of achieving self-sufficiency in collection in Canada. Our analysis, which is a preliminary one, focuses on the product albumin, for which self-sufficiency is a more realistic short run goal. It is conducted in terms of the net change in social costs of achieving self-sufficiency, as compared with the present situation. That is, we focus on production costs and consider any potential disease costs. As such, our analysis includes the benefits of self-sufficiency as well as its additional costs. It should be pointed out that there is no single method of attaining self-sufficiency in the collection of plasma. Plasma can be obtained from processed whole blood and from pheresis. Since both are viable methods, the economic implications of obtaining self-sufficiency will be examined for both. Finally, we should point out that this is a preliminary analysis. Our recruitment cost analysis is currently getting under way, and the recruitment costs presented herein are therefore subject to change.

METHOD

In this paper, we first determine the number of litres of plasma which must be collected to achieve self-sufficiency in albumin. To do this, we estimate the number of collections of plasma that must be made to replace the volume of albumin that was imported in 1988/89. This estimate is based on the assumption that for each vial of albumin imported, 1.03 litres of plasma must be processed (Canadian Blood Committee, 1987).

Second, we determine the number of whole blood and pheresis collections that must be made to obtain the required volume of plasma. We base our analysis on the assumption that for each collection of whole blood, 200 ml. of plasma is processed at each blood center. Therefore, five collections must be made to obtain a litre of plasma. Since an average pheresis collection results in 550 ml. of plasma, 1.818 collections must be made to obtain a litre of plasma in this way.

Third, the net change in social costs of achieving self-sufficiency in collection, compared with the present situation, are estimated. Social costs of achieving self-sufficiency include "direct" and "external" (to the Red Cross) costs. Direct costs include costs of recruiting blood donors (recruitment costs), costs of collecting and processing plasma (collection costs), and costs paid to the fractionator for processing the plasma into albumin (processing costs). External costs include donor time costs and disease costs (costs resulting from infection by the product). These costs are compared with costs of purchasing the imported albumin directly from the fractionator and the disease costs resulting from the imported albumin to provide a complete picture of the net social gain (or loss) from pursuing self-sufficiency. In the case of albumin (unlike Factors VIII and IX) the cold ethanol production process appears to ensure that the product is not infected. Disease cost differences for this product are therefore likely to be negligible.

For obtaining plasma by whole blood collections, recruitment costs for plasma are estimated based on the average values per unit collected for a single blood center. Collection costs are estimated using a process costing procedure and are based on marginal, rather than average, costs. Despite the fact that plasma and red cells are joint products in this process, all relevant costs of expanding output are attributed to plasma alone (Kopetsky,

Jacobs, and Turner, 1990). For obtaining plasma by pheresis collections, recruitment and collection costs at various volumes are derived by estimating a stepwise cost function from data of one blood center based on cost accounting methods. This costing procedure recognizes the capacity levels of the various semi-variable inputs, labor and equipment (Hart, Jacobs, and Turner, 1990). Cost accounting methods have been used in both cases because of (data) difficulties in applying standard cost equations.

Costs external to the blood donor centers include the indirect costs of foregone leisure time of the donors and the disease costs associated with the greater infection rates for undetected disease in U.S. commercial source products. We have not included the donor time costs in this study. For the reasons mentioned above, calculation of disease cost differentials between domestic and imported blood, which would pose a special problem for Factors VIII and IX, does not pose a problem in the case of albumin.

RESULTS
IMPORTED UNITS AND NATIONAL REPLACEMENT NEEDS

In Canada in 1988/89, 237,000 vials of albumin were shipped to hospitals; 211,000 of these vials came from Canadian source plasma. Since 26,000 were produced from foreign source plasma, this is the number of vials that would need to be replaced to achieve national self-sufficiency in collection.

COLLECTION NEEDS

The most recent data (1987) indicate a yield factor of 1.03 vials per litre of plasma. To meet the 26,000 vial deficiency, 25,240 litres of plasma must therefore be collected. If the plasma is obtained by collecting and processing whole blood, and assuming each whole blood collection results in a yield of 200 ml. of plasma, five whole blood collections would be needed to obtain a litre of plasma. If, on the other hand, the plasma is obtained with the pheresis procedure, and assuming each collection results in 550 ml. of plasma, 1.818 collections must be made for each litre of plasma.

BLOOD DONOR CENTER (DIRECT) COSTS

Our preliminary cost per *whole blood donor* recruitment is $7. Based on our analysis of the whole blood collection and production process, collection costs are $28 per collection and $140 per litre. Recruitment and collection costs for *pheresis* are $69 per collection or $129 per litre.

Although we do not have the processing fee for Canadian albumin and the cost of importing a unit of commercial albumin, we do know that the U.S. source albumin costs $11 more than the processing fee. It should be noted that this $11 does not represent the net price differential of plasma, because plasma yields at least four products. The net price differential of the American to Canadian plasma must take into account all four products.

OVERALL COSTS

The overall cost picture is shown in Table 1. In this table we show the different costs – recruitment, collection, and net difference between the purchase cost and replacement fee. This allows us to compare the status quo (i.e., continuing to import the 26,000 vials) with two alternatives: collecting enough plasma to replace the 26,000 imported vials by either

(1) whole blood collection or (2) pheresis methods. Focusing only on direct costs, we estimate that if the imported units were replaced by internally collected units, the additional cost would be $3.967 million if all the plasma were collected with whole blood and $2.995 million if it were collected by pheresis.

Table 1
NET COSTS OF ACHIEVING SELF-SUFFICIENCY FOR ALBUMIN

	Self-sufficiency with whole blood collections vs. current	Self-sufficiency with pheresis collections vs. current
Cost category		
Recruitment and collection	$4,237,000	$3,265,000
Purchase of commercial less processing fee for domestic (net difference)	($270,000)	($270,000)
Net cost of self-sufficiency	**$3,967,000**	**$2,995,000**

DISCUSSION

We would like to stress first that the feasibility of an expanded recruitment effort is essential to our final analysis. This subject is currently under study, so we cannot yet present final estimates. However, it is important to gain some notion of the relative magnitude of collections needed in relation to current quantities collected. In Canada, in 1988/89, there were 1.14 million units of whole blood collected, and 68,000 units of plasma collected by apheresis. Given the additional national requirements to achieve self-sufficiency of 26,000 vials of albumin, if the additional plasma were collected from whole blood, 126,200 extra collections would have to be made. This would mean an 11% increase in collections. If collections were done solely by pheresis, 45,900 extra collections would have to be made. This would mean an increase in pheresis collections of 72%. As a result, we have more confidence in our whole blood estimate than in our pheresis estimate.

In fact, the additional plasma would likely be collected from both sources. With our current estimates, the net cost would be in between the two estimates (for whole blood and plasma). A ballpark figure would be $3.5 million extra to achieve self-sufficiency in collection for albumin.

Not mentioned in this analysis was the role of demand. Self-sufficiency can also be achieved in part by reductions in overall demand. This may be more feasible for albumin than other products.

Economic measurement provides summaries of the quantifiable factors, but by itself it is not sufficient to reach a conclusion. Intangible factors must also be taken into account before a decision is reached. Some of the intangible factors in the decision to achieve self-sufficiency include an increase in the security of supply and the maintenance or development of national expertise in blood products. With regard to *security of supply*, reliance on foreign sources places one at risk in the event that some event in the foreign country causes the supply of the product to dry up. If Canadian producers can provide a more reliable source of plasma, then the risk is reduced and, although difficult to quantify, certainly is of some relevance to the decision. With regard to *maintaining local expertise,* the existence of a local industry might conceivably help in the development of the blood services in Canada and thus, in the long run, might result in higher quality services. Finally, one might argue that, in producing its own plasma supply, Canada is acting as a *good citizen of the world* in not draining supplies from poorer regions and countries.

Mention should also be made of the fact that we have focused solely on self-sufficiency in collection for albumin. If anything, the arguments for self-sufficiency in the other products, Factors VIII and IX, are even more compelling. Canada is more dependent on foreign sources for these supplies. And unlike the case of albumin, the safety of these products is much less assured, since their production processes differ. As a result, disease costs may play a significant role in enumerating social costs for these products. This would be especially true if Canadian plasma is less prone to disease than foreign plasma.

Additionally, we should point out that if Canada becomes self-sufficient in these other products as well, the recruitment and collection costs for those units considered would not have to be duplicated, since the other products can be made with additional processing of the same plasma. There may, additionally, be savings in disease costs which would be very difficult to estimate. These topics are currently under study.

ACKNOWLEDGEMENTS

We thank Dr. Roger Perrault, Steven Vick, and Sean McGuire of the Canadian National Red Cross, Ottawa for suggestions and data.

REFERENCES

Canadian Blood Committee/Canadian Red Cross Society: Plasma Fractionation Seminar (mimeo). Ottawa, October 15, 1987.

Canadian Red Cross Society: *Blood Services Statistical Report 1988-1989.* Ottawa: Canadian Red Cross Society, 1989.

Gunson HH: The needed volume of plasma. *Vox Sang* 46(suppl. 1):66-71, 1984.

Hart S, Jacobs P, Turner AR: A Cost Accounting Methodology for Plasmapheresis Program Expansion (mimeo). Edmonton: University of Alberta, Faculty of Medicine, 1990.

Kopetsky D, Jacobs P, Turner AR: Joint costs in health care: the case of blood component production. *Journal of Ambulatory Care Management* (in press).

Morris JP: National self-sufficiency in blood components and plasma fractions. *Vox Sang* 46(suppl. 1): 7-9, 1984.

DISCUSSION
Chair: Jack Boan
University of Regina

Raisa Deber (University of Toronto)

The question I have is for Phil Jacobs. I was just wondering what you think the effect of recombinant drugs is going to be. You could certainly project the possibility that rather than take anything from a blood supply, where one bad unit could kill a lot of people, you might want just to use recombinant techniques to produce what you need. Is the entire blood collection enterprise going to become largely obsolete?

Philip Jacobs (University of Alberta)

I'll let my co-author, Bob Turner, answer that. Bob is a hematologist.

A. Robert Turner (CRCS Blood Transfusion Service/University of Alberta)

This certainly has been the subject of a lot of speculation, and indeed it is within the realm of possibility now to replace Factor VIII with recombinantly engineered products. But I would caution all of you who are interested in economics not to expect any savings. Look at what TpA costs or what erythropoeitin has cost on introduction. The other difficulty with Factor VIII at the present time is that in trying to scale up to the needs of the world's hemophiliacs, difficulties have been encountered so that, at least in the short term, we are going to require human plasma to produce Factor VIII. I think I can say this relatively confidently: There will not be substitution of albumin with an engineered product. Albumin is so cheap that it is not economical to make it from a microbiological point of view. And for the other products, it is really up in the air.

Larry Wiser (Manitoba Ministry of Health)

Question to Peter Coyte. We've heard off and on during this conference that we've got too many doctors and it's costing us an arm and a leg. We've heard about supplier-induced demand. Well, let's talk about lawyers, then, as far as malpractice. The Prichard Report, that you worked on with Rob Prichard – who's now president of this university, I understand – he quotes in his study that the rate of malpractice is 5 to 10 times higher in California than in Canada. Now in California, you have 10 times as many lawyers per capita. The question that I had is, is this just coincidence? Does anything in your study support the idea of supplier-induced demand in malpractice, referring to the number of lawyers?

Peter Coyte (University of Toronto)

No, we looked at that particular question, and the figures that Rob Prichard provides are the figures that came out of our study. We looked at the supply of lawyers – lawyers per capita – over the period in question to see whether it was related to the frequency with which people sued physicians. And there was no relationship whatsoever that was found – no statistically significant relationship. Lawyers appear not to be related to malpractice litigation, at least the prevalence of lawyers. Other factors seem to be more important than lawyers. And studies in the U.S., when they control for urbanization, also come to the similar conclusion that lawyers are not chasing ambulances as much as the press and other people might have otherwise thought. So the lawyers are innocent. So you not only heard it from Rob Prichard, who's a lawyer, but...

Wayne Sullivan (Nova Scotia Department of Health and Fitness)

A question for Dr. Jacobs. Federal law requires that all blood donated in Canada should be tested for syphilis, hepatitis C, HTLV I, HIV, and hepatitis B. Why did you not include that data in your cost of albumin? And secondarily, how cheap is it to buy albumin on the open market compared to being self-sufficient?

Philip Jacobs

We did include all the testing costs – they are in the collection costs. All of these tests that you mentioned – the lab costs are included in our estimates. Unfortunately, in 12 minutes it is hard to summarize them all. But we have several papers, which we would be glad to let people look at, and these costs are included. The differential of purchasing albumin vs. collecting it and sending it out is $11 per 25% unit.

Don MacNaught (Health and Welfare Canada)

Question for Mr. Jacobs. First of all, you define self-sufficiency in relation to albumin. You didn't define it in relation to Factor VIII and Factor IX, which has essentially been the policy debate for 20 years in Canada. Why did you choose albumin?

Philip Jacobs

Oh, it's only a beginning for our study. We chose to define self-sufficiency for all the products, but this is a pilot. The next step is to look at these other products as well. These or other products have significant disease costs associated with them, but we just chose – because of the pilot – to do it for one product. And as we get the data, we plan to do the other products. That's what we're going to be doing during the coming year. But I recognize that the other products, especially Factors VIII and IX – I think it's got to be stressed, and I tried to stress it – these other products are especially significant. And this is where the goal of self-sufficiency is going to become important. Ignoring the recruitment costs, I should stress that the cost of self-sufficiency will come down, I think, when you bring in these other products. The total cost of self-sufficiency will come down.

Participant

I thought the question that Wayne was trying to get at was the question of the regulation of private vs. public blood supply, to some extent. There are external costs associated with regulating blood supplies. And the second thing is the issue of the relative cost of manufacturing – U.S., south of the border, vs. cutting, making, and producing in Canada. And your study is not seeming to address that question.

Philip Jacobs

No, the study didn't look at the alternative of producing in Canada. We could look at that alternative, but we chose to look at the two most immediate alternatives. But certainly producing in Canada is something that – I don't say it's financially viable, but it's certainly something that could be considered and put into a study.

Jack Boan (University of Regina)

I have a question, perhaps facetious, but it's about the gentleman that was reported in the *Medical Post*, who was suing the hospital for not letting him die. Apparently, he had a heart attack and they rushed him to the hospital, and he was stable but he asked them if got a recurrence to let him go, and it was written on his chart. Well, he went into cardiac arrest, the nurse came in, she didn't look at the chart and she pulled all the stops, and they rescued him and they brought him back to life, except that a few days later he had a very severe stroke and it paralyzed him on one side, and he decided to sue the hospital for not letting him die. So I'll ask Peter Coyte, from his vantage point of malpractice, whether he thinks that the chap has much of a chance of success.

Peter Coyte

I'm not a lawyer.

MARKETING CHANGE: HOW CAN WE GET ANYWHERE FROM HERE?

MARKETING CHANGE – HOW CAN WE GET ANYWHERE FROM HERE?

Maureen Dixon
Institute of Health Services Management, U.K.

The three themes for the conference were laid out for us in the opening remarks:
- What should be the goals, the direction for changes in the Canadian health care system?
- What are the likely consequences of pursuing different routes to achieve these goals?
- How do we get there? What are the necessary prerequisites for *implementation?*

THE GOALS

In the Canadian system as elsewhere, there is a high degree of consensus about the goals in terms of changed patterns of service delivery and funding. These goals include less stress on acute/hospital care, more stress on outcomes and quality, the need to contain and where possible to reduce costs, emphasis on health promotion and quality of life rather than on aggressive, interventionist approaches to medical care, and so on. Not only are these goals common across a wide variety of (national) health care systems, but they have also been the prevailing wisdom for many years.

Our relatively slow progress towards achieving these goals is explicable at least in part by the intractability of certain underlying political realities. In political terms, the primary goals which must be recognised and accommodated are:
- how to ration health care;
- how to make the rationing process acceptable to the electorate, or how to 'market' the necessary changes;
- how to ensure reasonable value for money once the priorities are decided.

CONSEQUENCES OF CHANGE

Consideration of the likely consequences of change can become a justification for inaction and often turns out to be irrelevant, or at least ignored, when real decisions about change are taken. There are some important pragmatic reasons for this continuing to be the character of political decision-making in health care.

First, politicians in a representative democracy inevitably work on a much shorter time scale than that involved in redirecting and redesigning a health care system. After allowing for pre- and post-election 'noise', there is effectively only a one- to two-year period during which significant, long-term policy initiatives can be pursued.

Secondly, as illustrated by the recent White Paper reforms of the NHS in the United Kingdom, ideology has become an increasingly powerful driving force in social change. Major changes to the British NHS are to be introduced in the complete absence of evidence about the likely effects – a classic example of a solution in search of the problems.

A further difficulty in predicting the likely consequences of change is the fallibility of research evidence or pilot projects. Even if the evidence is reasonably valid and reliable, the 'not invented here' syndrome tends to lead to rejection of findings that do not fit local preconceptions.

Furthermore, however accurate our assessments of the cost-effectiveness of particular programs of care, the decision to continue or develop a program will still be taken either on pragmatic political grounds or because it is what we 'ought' to do, even if it costs more. The American and Canadian accounts of home care provision earlier in the conference demonstrated this well – we feel home care is the right way to go from a social policy point of view, even though it can be more expensive than other forms of care.

A final reason for not agonising too much over the possible consequences of change in the system is the innate resilience and adaptability of human beings. They seem to survive in spite of the health care system!

IMPLEMENTATION

So if you can accept my propositions that there is sufficient consensus about goals, and that the consequences of change are largely predicated on political and social values rather than scientific evidence, we come to the most difficult task of all, implementation. The lack of a public consensus about the need for change is one of the reasons often given for retaining the status quo. But that public perception is largely a function of what the politicians and providers of health care tell the public. As such, it is amenable to adaptation, and indeed it is often the public voice which challenges the professionals' conventional wisdom. Politicians' concerns about the next election and the providers' concerns to stay in business are much more powerful forces for inertia than the so-called public view.

We have to find somehow a way of empowering our elected representatives to take hard decisions, to be a step ahead of the conventional wisdom, to be the community's alter ego. Three steps would help to switch into this implementation mode.

To escape analysis paralysis, send all the health service researchers and management consultants overseas for two years! We do not need to know more about the possible effects of actions; we need to get more action.

To escape consultation paralysis, disband all commissions, task forces, etc.! Have the politicians decide the top priorities for change and mandate implementation throughout the system. The decisions about how to achieve change need to be as decentralised as possible, but the drive for change must come from the top.

Concentrate on the management of the system and the training and development of skilled managers at all levels in the organisations. Recent moves towards involving physicians more in the management of clinical services and resources are all to the good. But the complementary demand on managers is to become both more sophisticated and more practical in mediating the relationship between clinicians and limited budgets.

In conclusion, it is worth remarking on the excellent relative position of the Canadian health system. There is lots of money in the system, services are of high quality and generally accessible. If Canadians cannot get anywhere from here, the rest of us have little chance.

THE
EMPIRE
STRIKES
BACK

HOSPITAL COMPETITION IN THE U.K.: A (POSSIBLY) USEFUL FRAMEWORK FOR THE FUTURE

A.J. Culyer
University of York, England

THE BACKGROUND

Three White Papers (together with associated "Working Papers") form the policy background to the current wave of radical reform of the National Health Service. They are *Promoting Better Health* (Department of Health and Social Security, 1987), *Working for Patients* (Department of Health, 1989a) and *Caring for People: Community Care in the Next Decade* (Department of Health, 1989b). The first two will be substantially implemented by April 1991, and the arrangements proposed in the third will be phased over several years. The three interrelated sets of proposals cover general practice, hospital and community health services, and Local Authority social services. Formally, GPs are currently organised within local Family Practitioner Committees (FPCs), now Family Health Services Authorities; hospital and community health services (such as community nursing) are organised under District Health Authorities (DHAs); and related social services, including homes for the elderly and most domiciliary services, fall under the aegis of the elected Local Authorities and their Social Services Departments (though services may be provided by voluntary and private agencies, and private residential accommodation for the elderly is often financed by the Department of Social Security).

In this paper, I shall focus on the hospital and community health services. *Working for Patients* contains myriad details that, although important, are not central; its main proposals are the following:

1. "Purchaser" and "provider" roles are separated. Purchasers are of two main kinds: DHAs and Fund-holding General Practices (FGPs). DHAs receive budgets from Regional Health Authorities (RHAs) to purchase the services they require for their client populations from providers with whom contracts or "agreements" can be made. The providers contracted need not be from within the DHA's geographical boundary nor, indeed, even within the U.K., nor need they be publicly owned institutions. Fundholding practices (of more than a minimum size) receive budgets from the RHA to purchase hospital diagnostic services, outpatient care, and a range of elective surgical procedures.

2. DHAs are charged with the assessment of their local populations' health care needs and the determination of the best pattern of services to be purchased to meet them. Within the service availabilities thus set, physicians – both GPs and hospital doctors – will make their clinical decisions.

3. Within the NHS, there are two forms of provider: (1) Directly Managed Units (DMUs) whose control remains directly under the DHA but at arm's length, with separate management lines corresponding to the "purchasing" and "providing" roles, and with agreements analogous to contracts between them and (2) Self-Governing Hospital Trusts (SGHTs) (though community units are also eligible for self-governing status), which are managed independently of the local DHA and are directly accountable to the Secretary of State. They are also able to set their own wage and salary levels via local pay bargaining (compared to the national bargaining that continues to characterise the rest of the NHS).

The public discussion in the U.K. has concentrated largely on the first and third of these aspects. To my mind, however, it is the second that is of greatest significance for the future of the NHS, as I shall try to show.

There has been considerable opposition to the reforms. Organised medicine has resisted the GP proposals, which increased the element of capitation in GP incomes (to encourage competition between practices), specified "core" services to be provided, and set targets to be achieved (e.g., particular rates of inoculation). The proposals for the hospital and community health services, however, are far more complex and it will take several years of experience before satisfactory arrangements in respect of details are fully operational (some of which, like the allocation and finance of capital investment, are of central importance). A lot of the opposition probably arises from the idea that health care is not a "commodity" to be marketed by quasi-commercial principles and a feeling that economic realities should not be too directly confronted in clinical practice, even at the budget setting or general performance monitoring levels. There is also a suspicion that the proposals are the product of a "hidden agenda" whose true purpose is to prepare the way for a wholesale privatisation of health care provision and health insurance in the U.K.

These doubts may arise in part because the White Papers in general, and *Working for Patients* in particular, have lacked what one might call a general conceptual framework in terms of which the policy aims and actual implementation might be assessed and monitored. In this paper, I shall attempt to provide such a framework.

ONLY THE END CAN JUSTIFY THE MEANS

Let us assume, without too much discussion (even though it is plainly contentious), that the objective of health services is to promote health and to do so, moreover, in such a fashion as to maximise the impact on the nation's health of whatever resources are made available to that end, while satisfying various equity constraints to do with geographical availability and individual terms of access. Although what "health" means in this context is plainly a major issue, I do not want to get bogged down in problems of definition and measurement for present purposes. Imagine, if you like, a battery of health indicators ranging from SMRs, data on disease incidence and prevalence, and extending even to QALYs. For managerial purposes, it is plainly an important task to develop usable outcome measures that can assist the planning of collective demands for care, and it is also crucial for the purchasing authorities to be well-informed about the epidemiological and clinical evidence on the effectiveness of medicine. But if you accept this general premise as a properly moral point of departure, then without all the details that will need subsequent addressing, a number of major implications still flow from it that affect the general character of the health service:

1. The health service should be as *efficient* as it can be made (we should not be namby-pamby about this – efficiency is not only important, it is highly *moral*, given the objective for the NHS that I have posited).

2. We need better information on health needs and health outcomes than we currently have (more important, perhaps, we need to create the environment in which there is an effective demand for such information from those who run the system).

3. Competition among financing (viz. insurance) agencies is inconsistent with these aims.

4. Provider competition may be the most effective means of attaining the efficiency objective.

5. Provider competition need pose no threat to the traditional equity objectives of the NHS.

The rest of the paper seeks to explain these inferences. It is worth emphasising at the outset, however, that the fundamental touchstone relates to the meeting of the health needs of individuals. It is in terms of this end that means such as the separation of purchaser and provider, and provider competition, are to be evaluated. It is in this sense that means are to be justified (or not, as the case may be) by the ends. Indeed, it is hard to see what, other than ends, could ever possibly justify any means. This is not, of course, to say that *any* means can be justified by reference to an end. It is all too easy to imagine some means so awful that no end could possibly justify them. It is also easy to imagine some ends that are themselves so awful that we would immediately reject all means of attaining them. But if we agree on a morally acceptable end (or ends), then the question becomes one of selecting the most appropriate means of achieving it (or them). In this sense, it is only the end(s) that can justify the means – if anything can. I hope, therefore, that we can for present purposes accept the ends I have postulated (and, at least for the time being, bear with their ill-definition) and discuss the separation of function and provider competition in internal – or even wider – markets in terms of its appropriateness as a means.

THE MORALITY OF EFFICIENCY

I have emphasised ends because the pursuit of efficiency is a moral pursuit only in so far as the end sought is also moral. Both governments and the economics profession have done a rather poor job of explaining to the general public and the professionals working within the health services that efficiency is a highly moral notion. Since the papers of a meeting like this may fall into the hands of such, I make no apology for an elementary homily on the subject. Efficiency (they need to be told) has three moral meanings, each of which embraces the previous ones(s).

1. NOT USING MORE RESOURCES THAN ARE NECESSARY TO ACHIEVE AN END

This is sometimes referred to as *efficacy* or *effectiveness*. It enjoins us not to squander resources. Given an objective, such as returning the patient in need to normal functioning as speedily as possible, one should therefore seek those combinations of diagnostic procedures, medicines, surgical procedures, inpatient and outpatient care, health and social services, family caring, and the patient's own time that are most effective in promoting health. To use *more* of any of these resources than is necessary is wasteful and inconsistent with the objective of maximising the impact of resources on health in the community. For if more than is necessary is used, the excess could have been used at no cost to the patients in question to further the health of some other patients. Overall community health is therefore lower than it need be. Overall community SMRs may also be higher than they need be.

Although this definition seems fine to me – so far as it goes – it does not really go terribly far, for it enjoins us to do no more than sit on, rather than float above, the relevant isoquant (or, if you prefer, iso-QALY curve). There is of course usually more than one combination of resources represented in more than one method of case management that satisfies the definition. There are substitutions between drugs, between medicine and surgery, between institutional and community care, and so on, which can be made. This can give rise to the great variety of practice that can be observed within and between health districts and across national boundaries. Although some of these variations may represent inefficiency, many of them may be equally efficient in the sense of effective (or ineffective). We therefore need a tighter definition. The second meaning of efficiency meets this requirement.

2. NOT INCURRING A HIGHER COST THAN IS NECESSARY TO ACHIEVE AN END

This is usually termed *cost-effectiveness*. It requires the selection from among the effective modes of case management of the one judged to be least costly: tangency of an iso-QALY curve (if QALYs gained are an acceptable outcome measure) with an iso-social cost line. To incur a higher cost than is necessary is again wasteful and inconsistent with the objective of maximising the impact of resources on health in the community. If a higher cost than is necessary is incurred, the excess could have been used at no cost to the patients in question to further the health of some other patients. Overall community health is therefore lower than it need be.

The trouble with this definition is that, although it affords a clear criterion for evaluating the efficiency of whatever it is that one is doing so that, for a given expected outcome and other patient-oriented attributes of the procedure the cost is minimised, it does not tell us whether the procedure is actually *worth* what it costs. In particular, it does not tell us whether there are not other programmes of care whose health payoffs may be higher at the margin (given the resources currently committed to them) than those of the programme whose cost-effectiveness is being considered.

We need constantly to remind the rest of the world that the notion of "cost" that we employ is the economist's standard notion, but that it is no simple financial concept. If benefit is to be seen in terms of health outcomes obtained (or expected), then cost is the benefit (similarly defined) that could have been obtained had the resources in question been applied in the most beneficial alternative way. In market transactions, prices tend not to signal the value of these lost benefits for a variety of reasons of market failure, and second-best shadow prices are in general needed – though they are rarely estimated in most economic studies of health care. Without a market – for example, within a hospital – *direct* judgments have to be made about such opportunity costs, which should again, if they are to be consistent with the objective, be couched in terms of benefit to the patient.

The concept of opportunity cost may be quite consistent with my point of departure, but the second meaning of efficiency is still deficient because of its failure to address questions to do with the *value* of health, the worthwhileness of any particular activity, and its ideal rate of implementation. We need a still tighter definition and, of course, we have one to offer. The third meaning of efficiency meets this requirement and is:

3. NOT INCURRING A HIGHER COST THAN IS NECESSARY TO ACHIEVE AN END PLUS ATTAINING AN APPROPRIATE RATE OF THROUGHPUT OR OUTPUT

This meaning requires not only cost-effectiveness but also an appropriate workload, which may be higher, lower, or the same as the current rate. Policy makers, managers, and clinicians need constant reminding (or telling) that the judgment needing to be made here is usually a *marginal* one: Is the gain to be had in the form, say, of added community health from a cost-effective programme (or what is very often lost sight of – even by skilled economists – from particular *parts* of such programmes) worth the additional cost or, in the case of a possibly reduced scale of activity, is the value placed upon the lost health smaller, larger, or the same as the costs thereby saved? The general idea here is that a fully efficient (first best) health care system will have sufficient resources devoted to it such that, at the margin, the gain in health is judged to be of equal value to the additional costs incurred, and that the resources within the health care system are so distributed that their payoff per additional pound of cost is equalised across all programmes of care (Culyer, 1976).

The morality of this definition of efficiency is again clear: If the condition is not met, then either resources used elsewhere would be better employed in health care or resources used in health care would be better employed elsewhere. The "elsewhere" may, of course, be in programmes that affect health but that are not themselves health services. Economists will recognise that there will be some nice judgments to be made of a second – and third – best sort.

HEALTH NEEDS AND HEALTH OUTCOMES

The NHS, like all health care systems, has been handicapped in its pursuit of both efficiency and equity by a desperate shortage of information about needs and outcomes. On the efficiency side, it is only recently that it has become possible to make approximate assessments of the health payoffs from alternative packages of care. The main reason for this has been the absence of quantitative measures of even an approximate type that would permit more subtle comparisons than can be made by means of relative mortality or survival rates. In the U.K., one such new instrument that has proved useful in such fields as the care of the elderly and clinical practice is the Quality Adjusted Life Year (or QALY). The QALY has the great merit of highlighting the value content inherent in *any* outcome measure. Although it is pretty obvious that there are important value questions embodied in the notions of both benefit and cost discussed earlier, it is less obvious *precisely* what the crucial judgments are that need to be made and who should be making them. The QALY sets this agenda out very clearly. It also indicates that there are quite substantial variations in the average costs per QALY across programmes. Although these are not the marginal costs one would ideally prefer, data of the sort indicated in Table 1 suggest pretty strongly that current resource allocations are not making their maximal impact on need and they also suggest the general directions in which it may be sensible to try to redistribute resources.

Developments of this kind can also afford ministers an enhanced bargaining power with the Treasury in the competition for public resources, as *evidence* for the expected payoff of judiciously targeted additional public expenditure. They also offer – at least in my judgment – the most satisfactory means of reaching a view on that very vexed question of whether the NHS is underfunded.

Given my starting point, consumer demand is replaced by need and, at the macro level, this is to be determined collectively by health authorities. A need for health care exists when a patient has the capacity to benefit from the consumption of health services (Culyer, 1976; Culyer, Lavers, and Williams, 1971; Culyer, 1989c). If the care is not effective, it cannot be said to be needed. If the technology that would improve someone's health for the better does not currently exist, current services cannot be said to be needed (though it may well be that *research* is needed). In deciding what needs shall be met, however, it is essential to be able to form a judgment about the likely *size* of the benefit (in terms of enhanced health), and this is also true if needs are to be *fairly* met (for example, equal treatment for equal need) as well as efficiently met. It is also worth noting that the

Table 1
COST PER QALY FOR SELECTED PROCEDURES, U.K. (1983-4 PRICES)

Intervention	Present value of cost per QALY (£)
GP advice to stop smoking	170
Benign intracranial tumours	240
Subarachnoid haemorrhage	310
Pacemaker implantation for heart block	700
Hip replacement	750
CABG for severe angina LMD	1,040
GP control of total serum cholesterol	1,700
CABG for severe angina with 2VD	2,280
Kidney transplantation (cadaver)	3,000
Breast cancer screening	3,500
Heart transplantation	5,000
Metastatic tumours in central nervous system	11,000
CABG for mild angina 2VD	12,600
Hospital haemodialysis	14,000
Malignant brain tumour	69,000

CABG Coronary artery bypass graft
LMD Left main vessel disease
2VD Two vessel disease

Adapted from Williams A: Economics of coronary artery bypass grafting, *British Medical Journal*, 291:326-329, 1985; and Pickard JD et al: Steps towards cost-benefit analysis of regional neurosurgical care, *British Medical Journal*, 301, 629-635, 1990.

important thing about capacity to benefit is that it must be seen in terms of *changes* in health status. An absolutely or relatively high mortality or morbidity rate does not in itself indicate a high need: that depends on whether there is a capacity for the rate to be *reduced* sufficiently by the application of the relevant resources for it to command a priority relative to other needs. Moreover, it is the contribution of health care to the potential health improvement that is important. Many conditions are, for example, self-limiting, so one is concerned with the *faster* recovery that health care permits rather than the probability of recovery itself. In other cases one may not actually expect a payoff in terms of better health *than before,* but rather in terms of better health than would otherwise have been the case – amelioration rather than cure, reduction rather than elimination of disability, slowing rather than stopping of deterioration.

The interpretation and local measurement of need is the job of the new authorities and requires them (and especially Directors of Public Health) to have a good grasp of local demography and epidemiology and of trends. It also requires them to have a thorough understanding of the effectiveness of specific health care procedures – both those embodied in current technologies and those expected (by those at the "leading edges" of their subjects who are in the best position to know) to be available over a relevant contract period. Just think what a purchasing authority, armed with this kind of information and largely insulated from improper provider interests, might achieve by the selective placing of contracts. If there is a prospective revolution in health care in the U.K., it arises more from this aspect of the reforms than any other. Moreover, these are possibilities that should be heartily welcomed by the political left as well as the right.

There may also be a "big tradeoff" (to use Arthur Okun's phrase) (Okun, 1975; see also Culyer, 1988a, 1989a) between efficiency and equity. For example, in remote areas where the population is thinly distributed, the cost per unit of effectiveness may be relatively high, implying that on efficiency grounds alone community health could be increased by redistributing resources away from such localities towards those where population density is greater and cost per case lower. This is, however, likely to offend against any equity principle that requires approximately equal geographical accessibility. If such is the case, it is natural to allocate general resources (say, in the form of regional or district budgets) on a capitation basis, with the pursuit of efficiency in the meeting of local needs being conducted within the constraints that the equity rule imposes, and accepting that the ultimate cost of equity may be higher overall mortality and morbidity than it actually lay within our power to attain (Culyer, 1971a, 1971b, 1982).

Time and space prohibit my indulging in the details of health and needs measurement – fascinating though such an indulgence would be. Moreover, I am well aware that "health" is not the only product of health services. I do not wish it to be thought that I think the NHS should neglect important dimensions of performance like the supply of "reassurance" or comfort, courtesy and respect for individual dignity, or the hotel dimensions of institutional care whose neglect the NHS has frequently been taken to task for in the past. Indeed, it is clear that such dimensions of performance are regarded as very important by the authors of the White Paper. If I have focussed on health status in all this talk about efficiency, equity, and need, it is because this is the *prime* business of the NHS (I make no apology for asserting that) and because it is only relatively recently that it has become possible to assess effectiveness – and cost-effectiveness – in such a fashion that decision-makers like doctors and purchasing authorities are going to be able to use these ideas alongside some real evidence to evaluate their practice and to frame the terms of contracts. It can scarcely be doubted that the reforms of *Working for Patients* also lend a renewed urgency to the further development of operationally and managerially sensible measures of need and outcome. Fortunately, there is now lots on which people can build.

THE NHS AS A DEMAND-SIDE ORGANISATION

The traditional arguments for why health care is "different" from other goods and services are almost exclusively demand-side arguments (Culyer, 1971a, 1971b, 1982). They argue in particular for a low or zero user-price, for low-cost subsidised insurance, and for preserving so far as possible the integrity of the "agency" role of the physician – in particular for helping the doctor, whether in general or hospital practice, to form professional judgments about the principal's (patient's) needs and how best they might be met out of available resources, without being contaminated by other professional (provider) interests (especially those that determine the doctor's pay) (Evans, 1974).

In my view, these arguments amount to a pretty unassailable case for a health service having the following characteristics:

1. The insurance function is monopolised by the state rather than by competitive private insurers, thereby avoiding premium-loading through failure to secure scale economies on the finance side, the possibility of monopoly premium-setting, extensive billing and fraud-checking administrative and legal costs, adverse selection through community premium-setting, inequity through experience premium-setting, a host of gaps in coverage arising from employment status and inability to pay, and publicly unaccountable methods of controlling the moral hazards that all insurance systems throw up (and which otherwise might be met by such mechanisms as indemnity limits, deductibles, co-insurance, and privately determined quantity limits on the supply side) (for a review, see Culyer, Donaldson, and Gerard, 1988).

2. Access to care is determined by need rather than (for example) willingness to pay, insurance status, income, social or ethnic group, or any other nonhealth related factor.

3. The bargaining and regulatory power of the state is used to countervail the monopoly professional and supplier organisations and to enforce standards of safety and quality determined in publicly accountable procedures.

4. Professionals are rewarded adequately, but primarily by salary and capitation rather than by fee-for-service.

It is striking that, while these desiderata all require the partial rejection of free market solutions, they do so for demand-side reasons and for the most part involve a heavy rejection of market-determined resource allocations only on the demand side. The relevance of the *collective* expression of demand lies in its ability to specify and regulate need. It is appropriate therefore that health authorities, for example, should specify a demand for the care of their client populations. But none of these traditional arguments for health care's being "different" requires the public ownership of the means of production (viz. doctors' practices or institutional care providers). Not least among the benefits of *Working for Patients*, therefore, is the clear distinction between purchaser and provider which it has introduced into public discussion. I contend that *all* of the major ideological strengths of the NHS relate to characteristics of demand. The job of the supply side is simply (!) to be cost-effective at meeting whatever demands are placed upon it by the demand side. Its ownership and structure ought to be whatever pattern of ownership and structural features prove as a practical matter to be cost-effective and responsive in the way just described – nothing less than this, but also nothing more. What matters is what works. What matters is what means are best suited to the ends determined by the collective demanders. The supply side is not judged by ideological but by practical criteria. Whether directly managed units, or trusts, or private organisations (for-profit or non-profit) best satisfy the requirements of NHS demanders is something to be determined by experience and judgment. It is not an *a priori* matter. The NHS is essentially a demand-side organisation – or so it should be. Muddling supply-side features inside the public NHS not only begs the question as to the most effective means of delivering what is needed, it also exposes it to the serious hazard of domination by supplier interests that are independent of, and may be inconsistent with, the true objectives of the patient-oriented demand side.

PROVIDER COMPETITION

If competition between providers of finance has scarcely any redeeming features, the same cannot be said for competition between providers of care. The particular attraction of competition on the health care provider side is that it provides the very *systematic* (Culyer, 1988b) incentives for efficiency and innovation that are so conspicuously lacking in the NHS and dispenses with the need for the periodic sledgehammer strategy of financial squeeze (which has penalised the efficient and the inefficient rather indiscriminately).

There are two forms of competition that can be exploited, though *Working for Patients* emphasises only the first of these:

1. competition **within** a market, and
2. competition **for** a market

The first of these is competition between existing or incumbent providers (public or private, SGHTs, or DMUs) for various contracts offered by purchasing authorities, fundholding GPs, other GPs, local authorities, private demanders, and overseas demanders (increasingly, one may expect, from the rest of the European Community). The second is competition between incumbents and potential new entrants to the market for the *right to provide service*. It is contestability: a competition for franchises (Baumol, Panzar, and Willig, 1988).

I wish to fasten on to three aspects of provider competition as worthy of particular attention: the rather poor performance of competition in the U.S.A.; the problems arising from possible monopoly behaviour by providers and the attendant need (though this is not unequivocal) for some form of price, quantity, and quality regulation; and the problems that may arise from having multiple demanders under the arrangements in *Working for Patients.* Let me address each of these briefly.

THE U.S. EXPERIENCE

Competition between providers in the U.S.A. has led not to greater efficiency and lower costs, but to duplication of services, excess capacity, higher costs (and hospital cost inflation persistently above general inflation), and (though the evidence is somewhat ambiguous here) inferior clinical outcomes. I conjecture that these adverse results are less the result of provider competition *per se* than of the particular market environment in which U.S. providers operate. One factor is that insurance (which is far from comprehensive or complete in the world's richest economy, as witnessed by the 50 million U.S. citizens without – or with inadequate – coverage) reduces the incentive for demanders, whether patients or physicians, to select providers on the basis of quality balanced by cost and generates pressures on providers to compete on a nonprice basis. Any consequential upward pressure on premiums has a muted effect on demand (though it may be significant for equity) because it depends on income effects and there is no direct substitution effect. In the NHS, by contrast, purchasers are effectively expenditure capped and are to make contracts in the interests of an entire resident district population or an entire GP's list. Demand is at one level expressed in a collective fashion that sets the availability of resources into which the individual decisions of (mostly) doctors at a lower level have to fit (and which is to be planned in conjunction with the expected demands of GPs).

Moreover, in the U.S. the retrospective cost-based reimbursement system has historically enabled most providers to bill the insurer for whatever costs are implied by the services it has been decided (e.g., by physicians and hospitals) to provide, usually on a fee-for-service and per diem basis. Third party reimbursement plus retrospective compensation at a rate determined by providers confronts demanders with an effectively open-ended budget constraint which, to the visitor, is apparent in the spectacular atriums and lavish parklands that greet one on entering a hospital's precincts. (For a fuller review of U.S. experience, see Culyer and Posnett, 1990.) The prospective arrangements in *Working for Patients* substantially immunise the NHS from such problems and also protect patients in need.

MONOPOLY

Resource misallocation through monopoly most likely took the form in the pre-reform NHS of a higher rate of use of some inputs than was necessary (especially highly skilled human ones and the technical equipment that every able technician can never get enough of) or of shirking. These sources of on-the-job (or on-the-golf-course) utility can easily be passed off to the innocent public as better quality. The question is altogether begged, of course, as to whether the extra costs incurred actually benefit patients or, even if they do, whether the benefit is large enough to justify the cost. Under the White Paper's arrangements, there is also the possibility that pricing and output decisions may be set monopolistically (as well as some rents continuing to be taken in the form of cost-raising X-inefficiency).

The policy response can be of two kinds. The first seeks to *suppress* the operation of the market via centrally determined price schedules (e.g., based on DRGs) and other controls. The second seeks to *enhance* the effective operation of the market by disseminating appropriate information (e.g., about historical patterns of cost locally and elsewhere, DRGs, performance indicators of various kinds, and prices struck elsewhere in the system between purchasers and providers which may be judged by the bargainers to be relevant to their case) and by exposing incumbent providers (especially those with a monopoly) to the threat of entry of new providers by making markets more contestable. I lean strongly towards the second of these two responses for several reasons: (1) any suppression of the market will tend to destroy its beneficial and adverse effects alike (especially evident with central price schedules imposed on all alike); (2) such regulation is costly and may come, through customary political processes, to be dominated by provider interests; and (3) a strategy aimed at making the market work more effectively is more likely to deliver cost-effective contracts, especially if there were a greater emphasis on contestability, which theory tells us can even be a complete answer to a monopoly problem posed by one or a few incumbent providers. I am not, however, at all hopeful that we are going to see either contestability or real competition in the NHS – I think the providers may have already seen to that!

Indeed, politicians may well connive at this, and not merely because of the routine operation of the "Establishment". Contestability, selective contracting, openness about costing and prices and outcomes accomplished, can all impose awkward dilemmas for politicians. These politicians may not be able to escape a residual responsibility for poor performance as it becomes easier to identify and may come under intense political pressure to prevent some incumbents from going out of business – even if they offer no service that anyone wants or that purchasers are able to purchase satisfactorily elsewhere with no net loss of either employment or service for their client populations. The government clearly attaches great significance to provider competition. I doubt whether there is really a great deal of X-inefficiency to be squeezed out of the NHS, though there is doubtless some. The efficiency gains from competition alone are likely to be far smaller than those to be had from clearer definition of need and the use of the contracting process to eliminate ineffective (and cost-ineffective) medicine.

MULTIPLE DEMANDERS

Under the new arrangements, a collective demand is not expressed solely (as would in my judgment have been preferable) by a single purchasing agency acting for its population catchment area; purchasing from a wide variety of potential providers (or as wide as it judges useful) including voluntary agencies and local authority social services; and able to exert considerable monopsony power to hold down prices for maximum throughput of contracted caseloads with contracted arrangements for quality assurance and the ability to stipulate the providers to whom GPs would normally be able to refer. What we have instead is the clear possibility of different local judgments of need being reached by health authorities, FPCs, GPs of both kinds, and local authorities, which may be difficult to reconcile and impossible, even if agreed at some stage, to enforce as the funding scene for each changes. With competition between GPs (particularly nonfundholding ones), moreover, there is the danger that they will be under greater pressure than hitherto to refer to non-contracted providers offering relatively attractive packages of services but whose cost consequences the health authority has little power to control. It is not possible to assess the likely practical significance of this at the present time but there is clearly the possibility that some of the adverse features of the U.S. may arise in the U.K. via this route, since the demand decision and the bearing of financial consequences are effectively separated.

The ability of health authorities to make appropriate deals with FPCs, fundholders, other GPs, and local authorities remains to be tested. At present, it is an area of considerable uncertainty. As the number of GP fundholders increases, the problem will in one sense become less, because the demand and its financial consequences will become increasingly localised on the same decision-making unit. By the same token, however, the bargaining power of health authorities will also be strangled as this process takes place and their recurrent funding becomes increasingly topsliced on behalf of fundholders when RHAs set the budgets for DHAs and GPs. As the principal agencies responsible for assessing a district's needs and determining the most cost-effective means of meeting them, health authorities may find themselves increasingly unable to implement the strategies that would seem most appropriate. These problems will be the more pressing in a world in which local authorities feel their budgets to be under great pressure and may decide to allocate resources to nonhealth priority areas.

EQUITY

Provider competition and the separation of purchasers and providers pose in themselves no particular impediment to the attainment of whatever equity objectives are set. Indeed, if the effect is to increase cost-effectiveness and better matches of case-mix, workload, and quality to population needs, equity (at least in the sense of equal treatment for equal need) is likely to be enhanced. The revision of RAWP (a weighted population means of allocating regional recurrent budgets) is not an inherent part of the competition strategy, but budget allocations within regions can clearly depart from the stricter capitation basis towards which the system is now moving if regional needs assessments suggest that this would be more equitable in the vertical sense. Regional initiatives in clarifying and implementing local notions of equity will, of course, be need- rather than supply-based. If district *funding* is need-based, decisions at that level about the *place of treatment* of patients will need to weigh the advantages of treatment close to patients' homes against the possibly lower costs, and/or higher quality and/or shorter waiting times, that may be available elsewhere. This partly involves equity judgments (both horizontal and vertical), but it also involves judgments of effectiveness and efficiency in matters like the integration of community, GP, and institutionally-based care that it would seem entirely appropriate to make at local levels within the general equity constraints set by government and region.

It will be important for purchasers to bear equity issues in mind when formulating and placing contracts. For example, the horizontal equity notion of equal treatment for equal need has implications for hospitals' admissions policies that will need to be made explicit in contracts – and be monitored and enforced.

The development of much better information about community health and health care needs and the most cost-effective means of meeting them is one of the more promising (though sadly much down-played) aspects of *Working for Patients* and should eventually enable much more explicit judgments to be made at all levels about both efficiency and equity. It can also be expected that, within the regions and districts, not all will reach the same view of equity, how best to implement strategies designed to improve it, and the way tradeoffs between it and efficiency should be made when the two conflict. Perhaps this is as it should be for, if the meanings of efficiency and effectiveness are reasonably clear – at least in principle – the same cannot be said for equity, for which many different criteria vie for supremacy (see, e.g., Mooney, 1986). It may therefore be neither surprising nor undesirable if different criteria and different judgments in their application emerge in different places.

CONCLUSIONS

The strategy of *Working for Patients* seems to me to be one that can be welcomed in principle by all who care about the NHS, though for reasons that may not be immediately apparent. It does not prejudice the equity objectives of the NHS and it offers considerable scope for enhancing its efficiency – particularly its *efficiency at meeting need*. This is highly acceptable morally because inefficiency implies that some patients necessarily go without the effective care that a more efficient system would, with the same resource base, have provided. It also promises to be a more responsive service: more responsive, that is, both to the collective expression of need by authorities (which, if they are bold enough, can simply decline to contract for those services whose effectiveness – let alone cost-effectiveness – is in serious doubt) and probably also to the individual preferences of patients, especially in matters of hotel facilities in hospitals and the convenience of admission dates. The NHS is, however, already cost-effective at "normal medicine" and probably performs fewer needless operations than most other systems (Culyer, 1989b) (though the variance across districts is very high). So whether the new strategy will generate sufficient cost savings and sufficiently substantial resource reallocations between activities according to the best evidence of effectiveness so as markedly to improve the impact of the NHS's resources on the nation's health remains to be seen. Nor has there been any real appreciation of the potentially enormous costliness of operating markets – even of the relatively limited sort envisaged in the reforms. However, at the very least what has hitherto been extremely opaque will, over time, become more clear – the link (at the margin) between resources and outcome, for whatever else happens, the demand for relevant information about needs and effectiveness is going to be huge and it is only to be expected that the supply side will respond to this demand too. I believe that this better evidence of the productivity of health care (as it increasingly becomes available) will also have the effect of assisting ministers in their battle for resources in the annual ministerial bargaining round with the Treasury.

Any major changes of this sort are bound to bring major uncertainty and worry. I have alluded to my worries about the fragmented demand side. The pace is also frenetic. Indeed, the biggest threat to the strategy's success is probably that insufficient time will have been allowed to ensure that the early stages operate smoothly and without imposing delay on patients and their doctors in the prompt matching of need and care.

Although I was once (in 1987/88) an advocate of regional experiments, I have come to the view that such experiments could all too easily have served, as ministers have claimed, to postpone or sabotage any real change. But even were that not so, such major experiments are quite extraordinarily difficult to evaluate independently of the vast array of incidental pressures and changes that accompany them. It is also always necessary to compromise in the design of any experiment based on only a *part* of the system but intended to model the workings of the whole (for example, by omitting regional interactions or failing to include professional reactions of a national kind that may be exogenous in a small experiment but endogenous to the system). So we are in for an all-or-none experiment.

But the all-or-none game implies that we (and here I think especially of the research community) will have to monitor carefully what goes on, and the government should be prepared to invest substantially in such monitoring of the system's behaviour. Policy makers at *every* level must be adaptable so as to close off avenues that are destructive of the ends of the strategy and to open up new avenues that might be helpful. I expect that there will have to be lots of "cleaning up", particularly on the demand side.

I conjecture, however, that the separation of purchaser and provider is going to be a reasonably assured success. The adverse effects of competition as seen in the U.S. are unlikely to emerge in the U.K. (with a caveat regarding the GP sector). The strategy has much to commend it in principle (though the payoffs to competition *per se* are likely to be relatively small) and, even if the strategy is less than perfectly consistent on the demand side, we shall have time enough to monitor progress and make the required changes.

A final area of uncertainty lies with the politicians. The opacity of the present system protects them from true accountability in a way that will increasingly be less available. The ruthless judgment of the market on poor provider performance will test them in particular. If they prove chicken, or are effectively captured by provider interests, or fail to insist that the health authorities discharge their estimation of needs and effectiveness boldly and diligently, the politicians' ability to compromise the good that the reforms can generate is, of course, limitless. There are signs that these chickens have already given much away. It could be that we have simply swapped one mess of pottage for another. But, although compromises are inevitable, there remain grounds for optimism (so long as we do not make the perfect the enemy of the merely good). Moreover, there are reasons, which I have tried to bring out, that some aspects of the reforms which have commanded relatively little attention can be welcomed by both sides of the political spectrum. So it may be that the Conservative reforms of 1990/91 will turn out to be the best thing yet for health care in the U.K. since 1948.

REFERENCES

Baumol WS, Panzar C, Willig RD: *Contestable Markets and the Theory of Industrial Structure.* New York: Harcourt Brace, 1988.

Culyer AJ: Medical care and the economics of giving. *Economica:* 38:295-303, 1971a.

Culyer AJ: The nature of the commodity "health care" and its efficient allocation. *Oxford Economic Papers* 23:1889, 1971b.

Culyer AJ: *Need and the National Health Service.* London: Martin Robertson, 1976.

Culyer AJ: The NHS and the market: images and realities. In: McLachlan GM, Maynard A (eds.): *The Public/Private Mix for Health.* London: Nuffield Provincial Hospitals' Trust, 1982, 25-55.

Culyer AJ: Inequality of health services is, in general, desirable. In: Greed D (ed.): *Acceptable Inequalities.* London: Institute of Economic Affairs, 1988a, 31-47.

Culyer AJ: The radical reforms the NHS needs – and doesn't. *Minutes of Evidence Taken before the Social Services Committee.* London: HMSO, 1988b, 238-242.

Culyer AJ: Commodities, characteristics of commodities, characteristics of people, utilities and the quality of life. In: Baldwin S, Godfrey C, Propper C (eds.): *The Quality of Life: Perspectives and Policies.* London: Routledge, 1989a, 9-27.

Culyer AJ: Cost-containment in Europe. *Health Care Financing Review,* Annual Suppl. 21-32, 1989b.

Culyer AJ: The normative economics of health care finance and provision. *Oxford Review of Economic Policy* 5:34-58, 1989c.

Culyer AJ, Donaldson C, Gerard K: *Financial Aspects of Services: Drawing on Experience.* London: Institute of Health Services Management, 1988.

Culyer AJ, Lavers RJ, Williams A: Social indicators: health. *Social Trends* 2:31-42, 1971.

Culyer AJ, Posnett J: Hospital behaviour and competition. In: Culyer AJ, Maynard AK, Posnett J (eds.): *Competition in Health Care: Reforming the NHS.* London: Macmillan, 1990, 12-47.

Department of Health and Social Security: *Promoting Better Health.* London: HMSO, 1987.

Department of Health: *Working for Patients.* London: HMSO, 1989a.

Department of Health: *Caring for People: Community Care in the Next Decade.* London: HMSO, 1989b.

Evans RG: Supplier-induced demand: some empirical evidence and implications. In: Perlman M (ed.): *The Economics of Health and Medical Care.* London: Macmillan, 1974, 162-173.

Mooney G: *Economics, Medicine and Health Care.* Brighton: Wheatsheaf, 1986, ch. 8.

Okun AM: *Equity and Efficiency: The Big Tradeoff.* Washington DC: Brookings Institution, 1975.

HOSPITAL COMPETITION IN THE U.K.: A PROSPECTIVE
Discussant: W. Vickery Stoughton
The Toronto Hospital

"Will competition between health care providers work to solve a number of the problems of the British health care system?" is the issue that has been addressed by Professor Culyer and is the issue that I will attempt to address.

At the outset I must point out that I have very limited direct knowledge of the British health care system. For a number of years The Toronto Hospital has had an exchange program for managers with the Cambridge District Health Authority and more specifically the Addenbrook Hospital in Cambridge, England. This was set up at my initiative and that of the CEO of Addenbrook.

Once we had agreed that it would be a useful opportunity for both institutions, it received Board approval after about 15 minutes and District Health Authority approval after about two years. If issues as simple as this take two years to decide, then I am amazed that such fundamental structural reform has been initiated and predict that it will create havoc because it will require much more decentralization and much quicker decision making than the system seems to be able to demonstrate given what I repeat is, at the best, my highly limited perspective.

A more fundamental issue is whether competition will work in helping to achieve improved health status and reasonable health costs while maintaining equity and improving access. Professor Culyer in his paper seems to be giving competition the benefit of the doubt, with some skepticism admittedly.

I personally postulate a much less ambiguous opinion. Competition will not solve the problems that are identified, but it will take sufficient time to figure this out that all those associated with this approach will be long gone and off the hook.

Now, to get myself into additional hot water I am going to add my two cents about the folly of the application of economic theory to health care. Competition and consumer choice are fundamental principles of market place supply and demand. Quality, cost, and supply theoretically are influenced by demand associated with consumer choice. But social services and their related structures have consistently demonstrated that they march to different and much less perfect economic principles. Specifically, health care choices are seldom made by those who receive the services but rather by those who benefit financially.

Furthermore, there is evidence that limiting professional income structures to salary and capitation approaches will in the long term have negative effects on productivity. On the other hand, fee-for-service, while improving productivity, has no beneficial impact on appropriate utilization.

A number of years ago, Barbara W. Tuchman wrote a book entitled *March of Folly; From Troy to Vietnam*. The book has four chapters on the folly of positions taken by ruling parties. Applying economic principles to health services delivery presents a unique future opportunity to add a fifth chapter.

I personally am an advocate of a multiplicity of structural approaches such that various structures and models can be used to demonstrate to other structures and models greater effectiveness and efficiency.

If nothing else, the United States has demonstrated that market-based competition between institutions has resulted in unnecessary duplications of technologies and services. Even in the more laissez-faire environment of the United States, those who can afford health services will not tolerate lower quality and lack of access.

Does the British government really believe that health care quality, access, cost, and equity can be turned over to the market place with no political fallout? In a system which will continue to be supported by tax dollars distributed to payers/providers, will the British government be able to avoid political heat? I seriously doubt it. Providers in a government-sponsored system are not allowed to go out of business because the one who has-failed, as seen by the public, is not the provider but the funder. Will the new approaches change this political reality? I doubt it.

As in any politicized service, the public perception of the success of the system is directly related to staying in office. And if health care costs too much, as it will in any quasi-competitive approach, i.e., one that does not allow closures attributable to financial failure, then the effect of the competitive approach will simply be to expand the resources of the system. Whether this is good or bad can be argued from many points of view.

I suspect that the current British approach was directly related to the policies and philosophy of the Thatcher government concerning the market place and less government involvement. It is almost a reflection of government desires to let local agencies (District and Regional Health Authorities) take the heat.

Finally, it is likely a tool to delay facing the real problem with British health and that is the public perception, because of long waiting times, that not enough money is spent. These changes will slow down having to face this problem for a while longer. But in all likelihood, when it is ultimately faced it will be in a more expensive and less responsive system than currently exists. Having said all this, perhaps Professor Culyer is correct, the system will be more responsive and then we would have to admit finally that the beloved Brits are truly the smarter fellows. But by the time the evidence is in we will be too old to understand the data.

In conclusion, I suspect that if I were part of the British health system facing the introduction of this new approach I would adopt an optimistic attitude about the benefits it will bring to resolving problems. Hence, I can understand Professor Culyer's cautious optimism.

However, as an outsider who has worked in two less restrictive systems – the United States and Canada – I can sit back and predict that these approaches will not solve access, curtail costs, or be as responsive to health needs and status because health service delivery does not function in a perfect market – for reasons I mentioned – as well as many others which add enormous complexity to the issue.

DISCUSSION
Chair: Orvill Adams
Curry Adams and Associates

Peter Ruderman (Toronto)

I hate to do this every day, but I would like to ask Professor Culyer one thing. How do you reconcile your reference to the monopsony power of the state with what Canadians would consider to be the fundamental flaw in the design of the NHS more than 40 years ago, and that was to permit a parallel insured private sector?

Anthony Culyer (University of York, England)

Well, I think – the private sector in Britain still remains pretty small. It has grown very slightly; it's actually in decline at the moment. But I don't perceive any inconsistency between the exercise of monopsony power in the NHS itself and the co-existence of private health care, sometimes operated within a National Health Service institution and sometimes within private institutions. I think I may be missing the point of your question, but in the context of what's going to happen now, I think there is a major risk of the break up and the diminution of the monopsony power of the NHS through the system of trusts which will have their own local bargaining authority. Aside from that, it seems to me, although quantitative evidence on this is very difficult to get, that arguably one of the principal reasons the proportion of GDP in Britain spent on health care is still only around about 6% and rising very slowly relatively to GDP, compared to most other countries, is precisely because of this powerful monopsony pressure. Whether you think it's inconsistent with private medicine probably reflects more your attitude to private medicine than the problem about inconsistency. You don't have to interpret monopsony (or, come to that, monopoly) *too* literally. The NHS has been close enough to a monopsony for all purposes.

Michael Rachlis (Toronto)

Tony, I gather that different Regional Health Authorities – and tell me if I am wrong – but I gather that they have been establishing objectives – health status objectives.

Anthony Culyer

That's correct.

Michael Rachlis

And I'm just wondering how much those are going to be used as solid benchmarks for assessing success or failure? That's the first question. And the follow-up is, what technological and epidemiological and economic expertise is being used in the strategic planning process?

Anthony Culyer

I don't know the answer to the first either. It's a healthy sign that people are making mission statements that are fairly precise and by and large good, I think. I mean, they are good statements. At least, they are consistent with the sorts of objectives that I've been trying to describe. The use that purchasing authorities will make of epidemiological, etc. information is hard to predict, since they don't yet exist. I think at present everybody's too obsessed with actually getting the organizational structure sorted out and these rather broad statements of objectives established, and trying to get a commitment to those as well. I mean, there's a lot of effort going into getting genuine commitment by managers, in particular, to these sorts of things. But in the longer run, your second question is one we are going to have to address very seriously. And indeed if we don't, then all my optimism will vanish. My own priority is to get the Directors of Public Health on the purchasing authorities better trained.

Michael Rachlis

To follow up on that quickly, I think that that may be the way the Premiers' Councils and provincial health councils, etc. in Canada, which are designing overall health status objectives, may fail, because they have not appreciated the need for that kind of expertise in their planning and therefore are not using – and are not developing – accurate targets and a full fledged strategy for achieving those targets.

Anthony Culyer

Yes. I think in our system it puts the Director of Public Health in a key position, and many of them are ill equipped for it. Maureen [Dixon] would probably say they're all ill equipped for it, grotesquely ill equipped for it. And I'm not sure that we're doing enough, quick enough, to remedy them.

Richard Plain (University of Alberta)

Tony, you've spoken about local bargaining authorities. And not being terribly familiar with the British system, I was trying to understand – whom would they bargain with? Have the unions decided that they will enter into bargains with individual units, and somehow that will differ from what in our case would be a provincial province-wide bargaining with nurses, physicians, and the rest, and somehow the sisterhood or the brotherhood would compete against each other and not have any cohesive power on its side? I don't know, I'm trying to visualize what would happen.

Anthony Culyer

Let me give you a quick answer. The way you're thinking is exactly the way the managers of – Maureen, correct me – is exactly the way prescient managers are thinking. And so far as I know, all of them, so far, all of those managers in prospective trusts who have enunciated their views on this matter, say they are going to follow the national wage agreements.

Maureen Dixon (Institute of Health Services Management, U.K.)

My understanding is that what we are likely to get in the final analysis is retaining central bargaining with the major unions, but with local flexibility in how those agreements are applied, much more extensively. We are already getting the phenomenon of potential trusts having price fixing cartels in terms of the rates they are going to pay locally in any one region or any one district, to make sure that they are not doing each other out of business. Interesting phenomenon.

Raisa Deber (University of Toronto)

I am trying to put some of the pieces together. I found the presentations interesting, but a little opposite to the direction that we've heard in Canada, where there is the talk about the need for more regional planning, in the sense of less competition among institutions and more designation of who's going to be doing what. This is also the direction in terms of a lot of the commissions. And I'm wondering if there's been attention to that, and how, for example, particularly for specialized services, competition can be real unless you have multiple excess capacity, which you then decide you are going to use or not use? For things where there are volume-outcome relationships, where you don't want a whole lot of diffusion, for expensive things – what's the sense about how competition is supposed to work under those circumstances?

Anthony Culyer

I think that, particularly in the short run, it's crucially dependent upon the existence of excess capacity, of which there is very little or, alternatively, on the ability of capital and relevant human capital as well to be able to move in or out quickly, neither of which is the case in the U.K. So those are very very major constraints which were, I think, in the similar debate which took place in New Zealand, critical in the rejection of the competitive solution there. As to regionalization: the regions will still continue, of course, and regional and subregional hospital specialties will doubtless also continue. What I predict will be new is that purchasers will often amalgamate and emerge in general as having larger populations than the previous DHAs.

HOSPITALS
REVISITED

HOSPITAL RESOURCES IN METROPOLITAN TORONTO: THE REALITY VERSUS THE MYTH

Paul A.W. Gamble
Hospital Council of Metropolitan Toronto

In Metropolitan Toronto, the provision of inpatient services is encountering realities never before envisioned by the policy and program designers of the health care system. As we enter into the 1990s, predictions abound as to the circumstances and trends that will emerge in the next decade. Forecasts include both good and bad economic times, with ever-rising health care costs, an aging population, labour shortages, technological growth, and expanded interest in health promotion and disease prevention. With respect to urban hospital resources, we are presented with numerous predictions for changes in the mix of inpatient beds, reduced occupancy levels, and fewer inpatient services. At the same time, we are rarely presented with an accurate picture of the current institutional situation and the challenges and realities being faced. The purpose of this paper is to use the databank and resources of the Hospital Council of Metropolitan Toronto (HCMT) to outline current realities faced by the institutional health care sector versus the perceptions and myths.

THE HOSPITAL COUNCIL OF METROPOLITAN TORONTO

The Hospital Council of Metropolitan Toronto (HCMT) is a voluntary association with a mandate to serve the diverse needs of the hospital community in the Greater Metropolitan Toronto region. Its members are the University of Toronto Health Sciences Division and 42 acute care, rehabilitation, convalescent, chronic, and specialty hospitals within Metropolitan Toronto. In addition, eight hospitals within the surrounding urban communities hold associate membership. The municipalities served by HCMT include the Cities of Etobicoke, York, North York, Toronto, and Scarborough; the Borough of East York; and the surrounding regional municipalities of York, Durham, and Peel.

The member institutions of HCMT comprise approximately 23% of the hospitals in Ontario and historically have accounted for over 35% of the provincial hospital bed total. From a budgetary perspective, the HCMT constituency represents approximately $2.7 billion in operating allocations, which equates to almost 40% of the $6.5 billion of the provincial health transfer payments allocated to hospitals.

CURRENT SITUATION AND CHALLENGES

As in most metropolitan areas, the challenges facing the Metropolitan Toronto hospital industry are both diverse and numerous. When addressing the evolution of our health care system, a priority for both health care providers and planners will be to separate myth from reality as it applies to the resources and utilization of the hospital based services.

To date in Metropolitan Toronto, occupancy rates related to inpatient hospital care have continued to grow, with no indication of any slowdown or decrease. During the period from February 1, 1990 to July 31, 1990, across the acute care institutions in Metropolitan Toronto, the average occupancy of beds in service was 91%. Table 1 provides a more detailed breakdown of the data, by clinical specialty, for this period.

This table also illustrates a number of other significant facts regarding acute care hospital bed utilization in Metropolitan Toronto. There is an inventory of approximately 15,000

Table 1

AVERAGE DAILY BED REPORT FOR HOSPITALS BY SERVICE GROUP

(February 1, 1990 – July 31, 1990)

Service group	Average allocated	Average in-service	In-service as % of allocated	Average occupied	Occupied as % of in-service
Chronic	1,374	1,282	93	1,253	98
Critical care	595	508	85	404	80
Medical	4,183	3,606	86	3,559	99
Obstetric	1,012	954	94	782	82
Paediatric	1,062	983	93	639	65
Psychiatric	1,947	1,793	92	1,671	93
Rehabilitation	335	284	85	259	91
Specialty	35	14	40	13	93
Surgical	4,507	3,813	85	3,424	90
Total	*15,050*	*13,237*	*88*	*12,004*	*91*

beds in the HCMT hospitals which are currently on the HCMT electronic database (the Central Resource Registry). Of that total some 11,394, or 76%, are categorized as "acute care" beds. However, only 13,237 of the total allocated beds are actually staffed and "in service", indicating that the remaining 1,813 beds are out-of-service. Further complicating this picture, however, is the fact that according to the Metropolitan Toronto District Health Council, the local voluntary advisory health planning agency, some 13.9% of the local acute care beds are occupied by "inappropriately placed patients"– patients who would be more appropriately served by a resource other than an acute care bed, if these resources were made available to these patients.

During periods of traditional decrease in service demand (e.g., summer), the bed inventory and availability picture can be even more dramatic. Table 2 gives the "out-of-service" numbers that were projected for the summer months of 1990. In fact, by August 15, 1990 the total number of "out-of-service" beds had peaked at 2,868 and was slightly in excess of the projected maximum number of closures.

Even this information does not convey the entire picture. The institutional sector in Metropolitan Toronto is currently facing major manpower, recruitment, and retention problems. In 1988, in response to growing concerns on staffing issues, HCMT undertook a study of nurse staffing in Metropolitan Toronto and identified 27 major recommendations for consideration by hospital administrators. The vacancy problems, however, continue.

In October 1989, the Ontario Ministry of Health undertook a Nursing Vacancy Survey. Subsequent analysis by HCMT indicated that Metropolitan Toronto is experiencing an FTE (Full Time Equivalent) vacancy rate over twice that of the rest of the province – 9.7% versus 4.5%. Table 3 illustrates the percentage of FTE vacancies, and Table 4 illustrates the "hard to fill" or "real" vacancy rates, i.e., the rates remaining after including the use of temporary staff.

These tables clearly illustrate that the vacancy rate is most severe in the tertiary care teaching facilities and the 1-400 bed community hospitals. Although these data refer specifically to nursing staff, there are similar concerns with vacancy rates in the allied health professions (e.g., occupational therapy, physiotherapy) and domiciliary workers (e.g., housekeeping, dietary aides).

Table 2

PROJECTED BED CLOSURES: SUMMER 1990

Service group	Prior to June 1	June 15-June 30	July 01-July 15	July 16-July 30	Aug 01-Aug 15	Aug 15-Aug 31	Post Aug 31
Critical	71	112	113	113	113	113	108
Medical	603	849	983	983	1,011	1,011	896
Obstetric	51	85	90	90	90	90	66
Psychiatric	141	176	205	205	205	205	171
Surgical	448	847	877	917	949	919	823
Chronic	142	147	147	155	155	155	155
Paediatric	76	75	92	92	126	126	78
Other	98	134	169	169	169	169	121
Total	*1,630*	*2,425*	*2,676*	*2,724*	*2,818*	*2,788*	*2,418*

Table 3

TOTAL REPORTED STAFF RN OCTOBER 1989 METRO TORONTO FTE VACANCIES
by Institution Type

Hospital type & size	Critical care	Acute care	Psych care	Long-term care	All others	Total FTE vacancies	% of total FTE vacancies
Teaching	243.2	317.5	17.0	41.0	6.0	624.7	10.0%
400 + beds	71.0	94.0	18.0	13.0	2.0	198.0	5.8%
1-399 beds	104.5	120.4	10.3	8.5	6.0	249.7	14.6%
Rehab/chronic	4.4	0.0	5.1	98.5	19.7	127.7	11.0%
Psychiatric	0.0	0.0	18.5	0.0	0.0	18.5	5.1%
Other	1.0	4.0	0.0	0.0	50.0	55.0	15.7%
Total	424.1	535.9	68.9	161.0	83.7	1,273.6	9.7%
% of total FTE vacancies	13.5%	7.9%	8.4%	12.7%	7.3%	9.7%	-

Table 4

"REAL" STAFF RN OCTOBER 1989 METRO TORONTO VACANCY RATES
(includes temporary and agency staffing)

Hospital type & size	Critical care	Acute care	Psych care	Long-term care	All others	Total vacancies	% of total vacancies
Teaching	141.2	184.3	12.0	17.7	2.0	357.2	5.7%
400 + beds	14.0	24.5	3.5	0.0	0.0	42.0	1.2%
1-399 beds	37.3	40.9	2.0	4.7	3.0	87.9	5.1%
Rehab/chronic	0.0	0.0	.1	18.1	3.4	21.6	1.9%
Psychiatric	0.0	0.0	6.0	0.0	0.0	6.0	1.7%
Other	0.0	2.0	0.0	0.0	0.0	2.0	0.6%
Total	192.5	251.7	23.6	40.5	8.4	516.7	3.9%
% of total vacancies	6.1%	3.7%	2.9%	3.2%	0.7%	3.9%	-

Obvious to all managers and supervisors is that at least part of the reason for these ongoing recruitment and retention difficulties can be traced to the economic realities of living and working in Metropolitan Toronto, where the rate of inflation consistently outpaces the rate for the rest of the province.

Another major concern of the Metropolitan Toronto hospitals is the availability of capital funds. On November 29, 1989 the Treasurer of Ontario announced that a total of $250 million in capital funds would be provided to the institutional sector, with fully 1/3 of that amount going towards the cost of the expansion of specialty programs such as cancer, cardiovascular, emergency, critical care, dialysis, and care for mothers and the newborn.

This allocation must be contrasted against capital requirements of the Metropolitan Toronto hospitals alone. In a survey undertaken by HCMT, the membership identified a current level of capital need of approximately $500 million with a projection for that figure to increase to $1.75 billion by 1995. These capital funds are required to replace as well as update and renovate physical plants, not only to provide efficient care but also to meet regulatory standards (e.g., fire codes, environmental controls, occupational health and safety standards).

This enormous difference between the identified capital needs of the industry and the availability of capital funds from the provincial government has led to intense competition between hospitals and has resulted in massive capital fundraising campaigns. These activities are not only time consuming but also reduce the likelihood of co-operative service provisions or the regionalization of services.

How then is access to institutional care, particularly acute care, viewed by the public? Contrary to opinion often expressed in the popular press, on the whole the public seems to remain relatively satisfied with the current system. According to an Environics research study commissioned by the Ontario Hospital Association, almost 75% of the Metropolitan Toronto population are satisfied with the quality of health care available, and 77% are satisfied specifically with the quality of care provided by hospitals. At the same time, while 95% of the population did not support a reduction in available hospital beds, 90% supported the idea of an increase in the capacity for diagnosing and treating hospital patients on an outpatient basis.

SCANNING THE FUTURE: TRENDS OF THE 1990s

From the above description, it appears obvious that the hospital resources of Metropolitan Toronto are changing. There are significant number of beds "out-of-service", occupancy rates remain high, there are staffing and retention problems, and physical plants face huge capital retooling costs. Nevertheless, the public still remains fairly satisfied.

What, then, does the future hold?

It is predicted that there will be a change in the mix of inpatient beds. Mergers such as the one between Toronto General Hospital and Toronto Western Hospital and the one under way between St. Joseph's Health Centre and St. Michael's Hospital may well be justified in terms of removing excess inpatient bed capacity from the system and increasing efficiencies.

The 1990s should see more mixed use facilities which provide a more humane environment, with linkages and interaction for the elderly and other groups within the community. A renewed emphasis on home care and hospitals reaching out to their communities is also advocated by the provincial government.

In recent months the Ontario government has unveiled a "New Vision" for the Ontario health care system. This vision involves the development of social and health policy advisory bodies such as the Premier's Council on Health Strategy and a multitude of governmental discussion papers and legislative changes. During the last session of the Ontario Legislature, the Ontario Hospital Association identified the introduction of 16 separate pieces of legislation which will impact the health care system. Among the most relevant are the:

(a) *Development Charge Act*
(b) *Employer Health Tax Act*
(c) *Evidence Amendment Act*
(d) *Independent Health Facilities Act*
(e) *Occupational Health and Safety Law Amendments*
(f) *Workers' Compensation Amendment Act*
(g) *Health Professions Legislation Review*

In addition, the new role described for District Health Councils, the piloting of Comprehensive Health Organizations, and hospital investigations by Legislative Officers such as the Public Trustee and Provincial Auditor have all contributed by modifying the way hospitals operate.

Of particular concern to the institutions in Metropolitan Toronto will be the impact of the changing demographics of Metropolitan Toronto (e.g., aging population, increasing population projections, ethnic diversity) and the impact of new technology.

CHANGING DEMOGRAPHICS
The Aging Population

Age is the most powerful factor determining the use of health care. The very old, those 85 and over, make up the fastest growing age group in Canada. The number of people over 75 is expected to grow almost 35% by the year 2000. This group tends to use health care services 5 to 7 times more frequently than the average population.

In 1986, the median age of the population in Canada was 31.5 years; in 2001 it will be 37.7 years. The numbers of people in their forties will grow at 4 to 5 times the average national rate as baby boomers enter middle age. Since the demand for diagnostic medicine begins to rise dramatically after age 40, it is expected that the demand for outpatient services will also explode.

Elderly persons in the 1990s will be more sophisticated consumers of health care services. They will deal with health care providers as professionals and not as high priests. They will expect a greater role in medical decision making and will be instrumental in making new health care delivery systems operational.

The numbers of 15- to 24-year-olds in North America are on the decline and are expected to continue to decline over the next 6-7 years. This decrease in the number of young people entering the labour force will have an impact on shortages of nursing and other personnel.

Metropolitan Toronto Population Projections

In 1987, the Metro Toronto hospitals' referral population was 2,859,091. This is projected to increase 3% to 2,946,226 by 1992. The 15-44 age group is now the largest Metro Toronto hospital referral group, with 1,375,205 persons, but this cohort is expected to decline to 1,359,545 by 1992.

In the next five years, the 65 and over group is expected to experience the greatest percentage increase, 16%, from 302,795 to 351,626 persons.

Cultural and Ethnic Diversity

At the end of the 1960s, Canada abandoned its preference system and opened its doors to people of all nationalities. Whereas previously 80% of immigrants had come from the British Isles or countries of European heritage, in the last three years 70% came from Africa, Asia, the Caribbean, or Latin America, and only 24% from Europe.

Between 1976 and 1986, 90% of all immigrants settled in the eight largest metropolitan areas in Canada. The result has been that Metropolitan Toronto now has the heaviest concentration of non-British, non-French, and visible minority segments of the Canadian population. In 1986, approximately 40% of City of Toronto residents reported a native language other than English. The Portuguese are the largest non-English speaking group at 7%, followed by the Chinese at 5% and Italians at 4.1%. Scarborough, Mississauga, and Etobicoke are popular places for new immigrants to settle, resulting in an ongoing shift in ethnic mix from Italian and Greek to Chinese, Caribbean, and Indo-Pakistani.

The increasing diversity of this population presents a real challenge to the Toronto institutional sector to provide adequate channels of communication between patients and providers and to ensure that practitioners have an understanding of this broad mix of cultural backgrounds.

IMPACT OF NEW TECHNOLOGY AND FUTURE DIRECTIONS

By the year 2000, medical technology will radically reconfigure the way health care is delivered, particularly in urban centres such as Metropolitan Toronto. Dramatic breakthroughs are anticipated in diagnostics, pharmaceuticals, therapeutics, biotherapeutics, communications, and information systems.

The introduction of complex, expensive new technology will present tough choices as to who gains access to these technologies, where they are located, and who pays for them. These types of decisions are presently being experienced by the Metropolitan Toronto hospitals with respect to the introduction and/or expansion of both lithotripsy and nuclear magnetic imaging.

It has been predicted that up to 90% of diagnostic procedures and 70% of therapeutic services will be provided outside the hospital. Technological advances and new practice patterns will make the custodial care of the past decades even less of a necessity during the 1990s. Measuring performance by means of current yardsticks such as the inpatient census or bed utilization will become almost meaningless.

Inpatient medical care will likely range from the most critical and serious (i.e., trauma and multi-organ failures) to the highly technical (i.e., prosthetics and joint replacement). Such care will be both high-tech and high-cost. A 20% to 40% increase in overall hospital costs is forecast with the adoption of new medical technologies. This cost will have to be judged and justified not only in economic terms, but also in terms of both ethical and quality of life considerations.

In Ontario it is probable that the smaller and more remote facilities will tend towards outpatient care and limited inpatient holding capacity, while larger urban facilities are expected to maintain the sophisticated high tech services.

Chronic care will require day treatment facilities, accessible ambulatory services, and an ability to reach into the home by caregivers and electronic monitoring.

The balance of services will be home based. Home care, self-care, and the pharmaceutical industry are expected to see strong growth in the next decade. The shift towards diagnosis and health management from later stage treatment of illness will require taking services out to patients. Services will become more decentralized. If hospitals are to survive, they must be prepared to reach out into homes and residential communities as much as they now depend on the sick coming through their doors for help.

A renewed collaboration with physicians will be required to expand ambulatory care systems and decentralize service networks successfully. As technology advances, making ambulatory surgery, diagnostics, and therapeutic care less dependent on the hospital environment, physicians may in fact regain some of the autonomy they have lost over the last decade. Physicians must also become key players in the necessary developments of utilization review and quality assurance.

Residents of local communities will be urged to become more familiar and supportive of at-home and outreach services offered by their hospitals. It has been argued that "going corporate" may have cut off many hospitals from their local constituents, losing the interest of those constituents and thus making hospitals more vulnerable to control at regional and national levels. According to the Ontario Deputy Minister of Health, Dr. M. Barkin:

> We believe in the concept of voluntary governance. The kind of governance that characterizes a self-governing profession; the kind of governance that characterizes a community; the kind of governance that characterizes our public hospital system. We believe also that the instrument of accountability is vested in that governance and that governance must know for what and to whom it is accountable.

It is this concept of governance responsibility and control which is at the centre of the current debate with respect to revisions to Ontario's *Public Hospitals Act.*

From the institutional perspective, success in bringing the above issues back to the local community is considered critical in determining the way the health care delivery system will evolve.

CONCLUSION

The changes in the way care is delivered will require the redefinition and refocusing of each facility's service offerings to meet the demands of the changing health care environment.

In Metropolitan Toronto, hospitals must begin to carve out their own niche both to provide useful services to their communities and to survive as viable entities in the next decade and beyond.

How can this be done?

The following are some of the conclusions reached at a recent conference of the Metropolitan Toronto hospitals convened to examine the future of their institutions. It was felt that there was a need to:

- implement an assessment of needs, including public needs;
- plan, especially in the areas of strategic and human resources, in the most effective collaborative manner;
- explore opportunities for collaborations with other service providers;
- strengthen the leadership role of hospitals;
- create incentives for hospitals to carry out needed changes;
- allocate financial resources in hospitals, where appropriate, for development and implementation of community based initiatives;
- focus on effective and efficient health services delivery;
- collaborate with the District Health Councils;
- change the values and measures associated with outcomes and success to be congruent with needed changes; and
- educate the consumer, especially about costs and the effects of demand.

The challenges are many. The guarantees are few. However, it is hoped that the future of the Metropolitan Toronto hospital-based resources will be guided more by reality than by myth.

REFERENCES

Amara R: Health care tomorrow. *The Futurist,* November-December 1988.

Barkin M: Remarks to The Institute of Law and Medicine on the Public Hospitals Act. Toronto, December 4, 1989.

Foster JT, Griffith JR: Hospitals in the twenty-first century: an evolutionary portrait. *Frontiers of Health Services Management* 6(2), Winter 1989.

Godet M, Barre R: Into the next decade: major trends and uncertainties of the 1990s. *Futures,* June 1988.

Goldsmith J: A radical prescription for hospitals. *Harvard Business Review,* May-June 1989.

Health Care in the 1990s: Forecasts by top hospitals. *Hospitals,* July 20, 1989.

Hospital Council of Metropolitan Toronto: *Central Resource Registry Monthly Bed Reports,* November 1989.

Hospital Council of Metropolitan Toronto: *Report of the Salaries Committee.* December 13, 1989.

Hospital Council of Metropolitan Toronto: *Scanning the Future – Trends of the 1990s.* November 1989.

Kucway C: Reaching consumers where they live. *Metropolitan Toronto Business Journal,* October 1988.

Mann G: Beyond the hospital. *The Futurist,* January-February, 1987.

Metropolitan Toronto District Health Council: *Long Term Care Bed Needs in Metropolitan Toronto.* February 1984.

Michigan Hospitals: *Technology 2000: A Window to the Future.* July 1989.

Ontario Hospital Association: *Focus Ontario: Attitudes Towards Ontario's Hospitals.* October 1989.

Ontario Hospital Association: *Hospitals in the Future: The Future Role of Hospitals Providing Care.* October 1989.

Ontario Ministry of Health: *Deciding the Future of Our Health Care.* Toronto: Ontario Ministry of Health, 1989.

Ontario Ministry of Health: *Nursing Vacancy Survey.* Toronto: Ontario Ministry of Health, 1989.

Ontario Ministry of Health: *Ontario's Health Care System, Some Facts and Figures.* Toronto: Ontario Ministry of Health, 1989.

Osberg L: The future of work in Canada. *Perception* 12(3), 1989.

Outlook 1989. *The Futurist,* November-December 1988.

Parekh N: Cultural and racial diversity in Canada. *Perception* 13(3), 1989.

Premier's Council on Health Strategy: *A Vision of Health Goals for Ontario.* Toronto, 1989.

Premier's Council on Health Strategy: *From Vision to Action, Report of the Health Care System Committee.* Toronto, 1989.

Provincial Bed Situation 1987 - 1982. Information Resources and Services Branch, 1988.

Provincial report – Ontario. *Perception* 13(2).

REDIRECTING INCENTIVES IN THE BRITISH COLUMBIA HEALTH SYSTEM: CREATING A CONSEQUENCE

Frances Caruth
British Columbia Cancer Agency

This is a tale from the trenches. The perspective is that of a middle manager who was given the mandate to implement a more effective management system in one section of a large teaching hospital.

The presentation is entitled "Redirecting Incentives in the B.C. Health System", but the issues and ideas I will discuss can apply equally to other settings.

"Creating a Consequence" is not meant in any way to convey a punitive attitude. A consequence is simply an effect or outcome resulting from a given set of circumstances. This concept of consequence is central to this presentation.

CLINICAL SERVICE MANAGEMENT IN OPHTHALMOLOGY

Vancouver General Hospital (VGH) is a large tertiary teaching hospital. It has over 1,200 beds in more than 20 separate buildings spread over eight city blocks. As part of the hospital, there is a freestanding Eye Care Centre which incorporates two daycare surgical suites and two floors of ambulatory care ophthalmological diagnostic and treatment facilities. Within the main hospital, there is a 22-bed Ophthalmology ward. These are the service areas that were incorporated into the clinical service management pilot project that has been running at the hospital for the past two years. The project was based on a traditional matrix model, customised to fit the needs of the organization. The literature related to matrix management, also called program management or clinical service management, is extensive and readily available (Fottler and Repasky, 1988; Harber and Eni, 1989; Leatt and Fried, 1985; Stuart and Sherrard, 1987). Many writers have found that the matrix model can provide a good administrative arrangement for large, technologically sophisticated organizations.

During the project at VGH, a myriad of issues and experiences have been encountered. In describing the opportunities and the incentives of the project, I am focusing on issues that need to be understood in the larger health care environment if the system wishes to take advantage of grassroots skills, energy, and resourcefulness.

PROJECT FORMAT

The structural support provided for the project was the creation of a multidisciplinary management group which reported to a steering committee made up of the hospital's vice presidents. The management group met with the steering group quarterly. A financial and workload statement was required for each of these meetings.

The management group was given the mandate to manage the resources currently being used in Ophthalmology as efficiently and as effectively as possible.

The project was provided with a facilitator/manager and technical support for data management.

Being the first clinical service in the hospital to be given such an opportunity, the group was in a position to show leadership and demonstrate the benefits of a management system that they had for some time been eager to try.

INCENTIVES

There are both incentives and disincentives in the health care system. At the same time, there is often a lack of incentives. The goal is to have incentives that encourage all participants to focus on the same goals. Success and achievement are major incentives. When organizational goals are diffuse, non-specific, or too difficult to achieve, success at the corporate level will be elusive and individuals will seek rewards through achieving their personal and professional goals. The system developed to support this clinical service management pilot offered incentives and set goals that offered an opportunity for success. Further, the achievement of the program's goals would in turn provide greater opportunity for the achievement of personal and professional goals. It is much easier to be a leader in your chosen subspecialty when those around you are also working to promote that service.

The new incentives provided to the Ophthalmology service were primarily financial. Direct cost items associated with the service were identified. Then, based on the previous year's figures, a budget incorporating both revenues and expenses was set. The Ophthalmology service generated significant revenues from the diagnostic services it provided. As with any other group in the hospital, the service was able to petition for additional funds for new or expanded programs. The budget, however, was to be adjusted downward only if the whole hospital was subject to a "squeeze"; a surplus in one year would not create the risk of a smaller budget the following year. This generated a greater feeling of control and less need to spend everything before March 31.

A set of budget transfer policies were developed to describe the way finances would be managed. The net direct program cost, a figure generated by subtracting program revenues from direct program costs, was the bottom line against which the team had to manage. This provided flexibility – decreasing costs or increasing revenues provided a surplus for which the team could develop business plans. At the same time, of course, there was the potential for a deficit, so on a quarterly basis the group was required to report its financial status to the steering committee together with its operating goals for the coming quarter. To date, the management group has had to deal only with surpluses.

A very significant incentive given to the team was the ability to carry forward surpluses into the next financial year provided an approved business plan accompanied the request. This gave the team the ability to plan for new projects, but not simply to accumulate funds. Along with this, the new policies also allowed for the submission of project proposals requiring the use of operating surpluses for capital projects. The team had the incentive to plan their service actively and to set realistic goals and objectives, because the new rules for financial management gave them a very good chance of success.

DID IT WORK?

For the clinical service management group, the pilot has been a significant success.

It was a tremendous learning experience, particularly for the physicians; many of them previously had had very little understanding of where or how the resources were allocated and used. They have even begun to discuss such issues as marginal and relative benefits from different services.

There was a real sense of optimism in terms of the potential for self determination; suddenly, the development of goals and objectives was not a required exercise, but an activity that received heartfelt attention.

It really brought out existing entrepreneurial spirits and started to kindle others; for example, the head of the eye bank quickly developed a proposal for an expanded program that could be expected to be self sustaining, based on the government reimbursement rate, in three years. On the other hand, the development of options for optimizing the benefits from the two ambulatory care surgical suites was much more difficult because the nursing personnel, who have the major role in the management of this area, were unaccustomed to exploring creative administrative opportunities. In this situation, the facilitator assumed a major role as teacher and guide.

There was an increasing sense of team amongst a group that had started off as very strongly aligned within their professions and somewhat reticent about sharing operational information with others. Part way through the pilot, in response to a request from a physician for more information about the revenues and expenses of one particular cost centre, the manager of that cost centre openly expressed concern that, with the information, the physician might then try to tell her how to run her department. The physician of course denied any such intent, simply stating that if he knew more about the cost centre he would have a better understanding of what the manager had to deal with. Bit by bit, that fear of lost control through the sharing of information is receding.

The problems that arose in the interface between the clinical service management team and the organization were significant and really served to underscore the importance of the senior administration role in optimizing the contributions of the service providers.

There was not good alignment of goals between the clinical service management group and the organization, which did not have a well organized and publicly declared set of goals. Suddenly there was a group whose goals were not motherhood statements that looked good on paper; they were intentions to act! Unfortunately, in one of their first endeavours, which was to install a centralized scheduling system, the team was well along in their planning, with the staff executive's blessing, before anyone realized that the Ophthalmology computer plans did not mesh with the corporate plans for a new ADT system. Each plan had its merits, but it has been very distressing for the clinical service group to learn that they might not be able to realize one of their first dreams because the corporate plan took precedence. Obviously, in future when the team present their goals and objectives, they will want a more seriously considered response from the executive. This in turn requires that the parent organization has enunciated quite clearly its goals and objectives.

The organization's financial and information systems were unable to provide appropriate, accurate, and timely data; large portions of technical time were spent auditing accounts. The management group became extremely careful about checking accounts. This led to the identification of anomalies in the accounting system as well as straightforward errors. The dilemma was that the only people who really cared were the management group, because only for them was there any consequence. Under our current system of management, there is little or no incentive to worry about the assignment of costs or revenues to the wrong cost centres.

Although the new set of policies sponsored decentralized decision making, several of the managers had difficulty dealing with the reality. At the start of the project, one divisional director simply never attended meetings – it was "not one of her priorities". I believe that her response was a reflection of the significance she attributed to the team's function. A second director attempted to impose her priorities and goals on her manager without reference to the common goals accepted by the Ophthalmology team. Over time there has been a change in these directors' relationship with the team but, cynically, I would suggest that the greatest impact on their perspective came when the Ophthalmology team identified a surplus and began developing plans for its use.

The organization's response time to requests from the team was slow, and team members became frustrated by the delays and a perceived lack of support from the organization; quite simply, they hit the bureaucratic wall. Clinicians are accustomed to operating in "real" time. They make an assessment, decide on a course of action, and then move on to the next problem. In administration, the time frames are much longer; the larger the system, the longer the lead time required for such things as planning and budgeting. This particular problem needed an increased level of understanding on both sides of the relationship.

From the perspective of this project as a pilot to assess the feasibility of introducing this system into other areas of the organization, there are a couple of issues that need to be addressed. If this decentralized system of management were to be introduced to many programs or clinical services, spending rights to surpluses would be totally decentralized. Without some compensating changes in the planning and budgeting process, this could threaten the central administration's leadership role, both perceived and actual. Secondly, caveats may have to be placed upon the operating to capital conversions if the hospital is to meet the Ministry's requirement for minimal levels of working capital.

CREATING A NEW ENVIRONMENT

The lessons learned from this experience can be applied not just at the level I have described, namely the clinical service/hospital interface, but also at other levels, such as hospital interfaces with the Ministries of Health.

There must be a planned environment. Subsets of the whole cannot align themselves and contribute towards the achievement of the total system if they do not know the ulti-- mate goals of the parent organization. This means starting with a better enunciation of the goals of the health ministry and health care spending.

There has to be some contract between the program or service and the parent organization. Whether a service provider's budget is $1 million or $200 million, the providers must know what is it that is required of them, how they will know when they have achieved those goals, and what sort of rewards and benefits there are for success. All this can be, and must be, incorporated into an *active* budgeting process. Last year's performance and money, plus or minus a few percent, will never inspire creative management.

The delegation of authority should be no threat if there are well specified requirements and standards and a reporting system that allows all groups to assess performance at regular intervals, coupled with pre-specified contingency plans for when performance standards are not met. In a large, complicated organization, delegation of management authority and responsibility must take place if that organization is to benefit from the skills and experiences of the service providers.

Finally, management must mean something more than financial control, more than simply "staying out of trouble", if the health care system is to realize its potential. Management must be an active process right through from planning to year end reconciliation. Administration must not be regarded as simply an unspecified add-on function to staff's primary professional responsibilities. Good management is a skill. It has to be learned, but more than that it has to be demanded and rewarded, if the functions of the system are to be optimized at all levels.

REFERENCES

Fottler M, Repasky L: Attitudes of hospital executives toward product line management. *Health Care Management Review* 13(3):15-22, 1988.

Harber B, Eni G: Issues for consideration in the establishment of a program management structure. *Healthcare Management Forum*, Fall:6-14, 1989.

Leatt P, Fried B: Organizational designs and CEOs. *Health Management Forum* Summer:65-79, 1985.

Stuart N, Sherrard H: Managing hospitals from a program perspective. *Health Management Forum* 8:53-63, 1987.

COLLABORATIVE ARRANGEMENTS FOR SERVICE DELIVERY: THE EXAMPLE OF TWO NEW BRUNSWICK HOSPITALS

Sheila A. Brown
Mount Allison University

Neil Ritchie
Sackville Memorial Hospital

INTRODUCTION

Many health care facilities are finding interdependence and collaboration preferable to independence and self-sufficiency. This paper discusses a literature review and case study of institutional collaboration between two New Brunswick health care facilities. This collaboration is further evidence of the trend toward multi-institutional arrangements which is transforming relationships among institutions, a trend which has been particularly noticeable in the United States, but is becoming increasingly common in Canada.

Changes in health care, including rapid advances in technology and increased specialization, have greatly extended the range of services available in large health care institutions compared to smaller facilities. Provincial Health Ministries across Canada have been promoting integration and rationalization of services among large and smaller facilities, but a number of factors at the local institutional level may limit or hinder the balancing of these services between large and small hospitals. Since 82% of Canadian non-teaching public hospitals have fewer than 100 beds, and these hospitals collectively account for nearly 40% of all non-teaching public hospital beds (Statistics Canada, 1988), it is important to examine ways in which smaller hospitals can collaborate with larger facilities and thereby offer better services to their user population.

The present study involved the Sackville Memorial Hospital and the Moncton Hospital. The Sackville Memorial Hospital is a 55 bed, primary care facility located in the Town of Sackville, in southeastern New Brunswick. The hospital has existed for 42 years and in 1988 moved to new premises on a site adjacent to its original location. The Moncton Hospital is a 515 bed regional hospital located 50 kilometres northeast of Sackville. There has long been a relationship between the Sackville Hospital and the Moncton Hospital, the closest hospital to Sackville offering services beyond the level offered locally. Many Sackville area patients have therefore been referred to and received treatment from the Moncton Hospital. In the past few years, this relationship has changed as collaborative arrangements between the two hospitals have steadily developed.

OBJECTIVES AND RESEARCH METHODS

The purpose of this study was to describe and evaluate the collaborative arrangements between the Sackville Memorial Hospital and the Moncton Hospital – their origins, their current status, and their future prospects.

The study had a number of specific objectives. Those reported on in this paper were:

(1) to document the extent of collaboration between the two hospitals, including the departments, individuals, services, and functions involved;

(2) to identify the institutional factors that facilitated collaboration;

(3) to document the barriers encountered in establishing collaboration; and

(4) to assess the benefits of the collaborative efforts to both institutions as well as to the individuals affected.

A critical review of the literature on multi-institutional arrangements provided guidance for the research questions to be addressed in the case study and a context for considering the findings.

LITERATURE REVIEW

The health care sector has responded in a number of ways to an increasingly complex and difficult external environment. One response is the development of multi-institutional arrangements (Fried and Gelmon, 1987; Gelmon and Fried, 1987; McKinley and Stoeckle, 1988). Jaeger, Kaluzny, and Magruder-Habib (1987), among others, have examined the various adaptations, or transformations, by which multi-institutional systems respond to the environment. These systems involve a variety of strategies to integrate, consolidate, and stabilize health-care services (Chenoy, 1987; Devries, 1978; Longest, 1980). Devries has outlined a 7-point continuum of multi-institutional systems, ranging from formal affiliation to merger.

One type of multi-institutional arrangement is shared or cooperative services, whereby an agreement is made between institutions to share medical, patient, or administrative services (Devries, 1978). The arrangements between the Sackville and Moncton hospitals involve several services.

The literature on multi-institutional arrangements identifies factors that have facilitated or impeded such collaboration and documents the benefits of collaboration for the institutions involved, their staff, and their patients. Much of the literature describes the experience of the United States, where cost containment and profit maximization for competitive advantage have been important reasons for collaboration. Shared services have tended to involve more administrative than clinical services (Moreton, 1985). Collaborative arrangements documented in Canada to date have arisen because of the need to live within cost constraints and optimize the use of limited resources to reduce competition and duplication of services, and because of the opportunity to provide new or better services to patients (Fried and Gelmon, 1987; Gelmon and Marotta, 1986). Some of the multi-institutional arrangements that have developed in Canada have resulted from legislated amalgamations.

A number of factors can work for or against the success of collaborative arrangements. Facilitating factors include:
- careful planning;
- realistic assessment of possible difficulties;
- broad view of community health needs;
- open and extensive communication;
- mechanisms for staff involvement and expression of staff concern;
- administrative responsiveness to concerns;
- management insight, commitment, and competence; and
- monitoring of progress, successes, and failures.

(Begin and Demers, 1986; Ellis, 1987; Fried and Gelmon, 1987; Gelmon and Fried, 1987; Stoughton, 1987.)

The lack of any of these factors can serve as a barrier to implementation of collaborative arrangements. Inappropriately timed financial cutbacks and staff reductions which may be seen, perhaps incorrectly, as a result of the development of multi-institutional arrangements (Fyke, 1986); fear of loss of autonomy (Fried and Gelmon, 1987; Gillock, Smith, and Pilland, 1986); or lack of staff support (Kooi, White, and Smith, 1988) have also been identified as potential impediments.

If such arrangements are successfully implemented, however, a number of benefits may be expected. These may include:

- economies of scale;
- stronger political influence;
- reduction in service duplication;
- cost effectiveness;
- better regional integration/increased efficiency;
- acquisition of new services and expertise;
- possibilities for future expansion;
- greater organizational effectiveness;
- outreach to neighbouring institutions;
- improved quality of care;
- increased patient population;
- improved human and financial resource planning;
- elimination of competition; and
- enhanced levels of community and professional satisfaction.

(Begin and Demers, 1986; Fried and Gelmon, 1987; Gelmon and Marotta, 1986; Howard and Alidina, 1987; Longest, 1980; Moreton, 1985; Stoughton, 1987; White, Migliaccio, and Smith, 1988; Zalot and Shack, 1987.)

CASE STUDY

The case study used the survey method to collect information from those involved in, or affected by, collaborative arrangements. A total of 43 interviews were conducted with trustees, administrators, and medical and other staff at the two hospitals, and a questionnaire survey was administered to patients at Sackville. Questions posed were designed to assess the particular factors that have facilitated or impeded collaboration in the Sackville-Moncton case and to identify the benefits perceived to date. Some questions were close-ended, listing factors drawn from the literature. These were followed by open-ended questions to determine whether and how the Sackville-Moncton experience differed from other cases.

ORIGINS AND DEVELOPMENT OF COLLABORATIVE ARRANGEMENTS

A key example of collaborative efforts between the Sackville and Moncton Hospitals is a day surgery program at the Sackville Hospital which involves visiting specialists from the Moncton Hospital. Development of this program was the result of a special set of circumstances. In the early to mid 1970s, when plans were being drawn up for a new Sackville Memorial Hospital, the hospital was designed and subsequently built with operating room facilities. This provision perhaps reflects the fact that Sackville had, at that time, a resident general surgeon and this situation was expected to continue. Unfortunately, in the mid 1980s the general surgeon died suddenly and over the subsequent years, despite considerable efforts, the Sackville Hospital was unsuccessful in attracting a replacement.

Contemporaneous with these developments was the origin of a number of visiting specialty clinics – for example, orthopedics, obstetrics, gynecology, and general surgery – which grew out of deliberate contacts between the medical staff and administration of the Sackville Memorial Hospital and a variety of departments at the Moncton Hospital.

During this period, operating room time at the Moncton Hospital also became quite scarce. An approach to the Sackville Hospital resulted in its operating room facilities being used to offset this shortage. Since the services of an anesthetist were available in Sackville, a day surgery program was initiated which provided for a number of low risk surgical procedures, done under either local or general anesthesia, to be carried out in Sackville. The anesthetist, chief of medical staff, and administrator at Sackville all played key roles in developing this program.

Other collaborative efforts developed in addition to the visiting specialty clinics and the day surgery program, as shown in Table 1.

Table 1

AREAS OF COLLABORATION BETWEEN SACKVILLE MEMORIAL HOSPITAL AND THE MONCTON HOSPITAL

Medical Surgical Services	**Patient Services**	**Administrative Services**
Visiting Specialty Clinics		
Internal medicine	Lab services	Computer services
General surgery	Computerized ECG	Purchasing
Orthopedic surgery	Holter monitoring	Staff education
Respiratory medicine	Pharmacy	Management consultation
Pediatrics	Rehabilitation services	Waste disposal
Geriatric medicine		Biomedical engineering
Endocrinology		
Psychiatry		
Day Surgery		
Orthopedic surgery		
Obstetrics/gynecology		
Plastic surgery		
Dental surgery		
Medical Consultation		
Telephone consultation		
Departmental reviews		

FACTORS FACILITATING COLLABORATION

A number of factors were identified from the literature as facilitating collaboration. The results of the case study confirm the importance of some of these factors (see Table 2). In particular, both the literature review and case study indicate that it is imperative that leaders within the hospital have a commitment to and involvement in the development of collaborative services. The initiative of the Sackville Memorial Hospital administrator, the rapport between administrators at the two hospitals, the movement of a key nursing staff member from the Moncton Hospital to the Sackville Hospital, and the rapport between staff at the two hospitals in general all played key roles in bringing about collaborations.

Table 2

FACTORS FACILITATING COLLABORATION

Facilitating Factor	Major Facilitator		Minor Facilitator		Unimportant	
	S	M	S	M	S	M
Hospital management	25	12	1	2	0	0
Availability of new or enlarged facilities	23	6	3	5	0	3
Good communication between institutions	25	11	1	2	0	1
Support by the institution's physicians and other health care professionals	21	11	5	3	0	0
Support of efforts to establish collaborative arrangements by the institution's governing body•	15	4	10	6	1	3
Involvement of those affected by collaboration during planning and development through consultation	20	10	6	3	0	1
Adequate planning	22	9	4	3	0	2
Other factors	6	0	0	0	0	0

S = Sackville respondents, N=26

M = Moncton Respondents, N=14, •Moncton respondents, N-13 for this item

A related facilitating factor identified in the literature is good communication and the importance of keeping staff informed of and involved in developments (Ellis, 1987; Gelmon and Marotta, 1986; Stoughton, 1987). Surprisingly, relatively few respondents in the current survey indicated that they had an extensive knowledge of existing arrangements, and few said that they had learned of these arrangements through formal processes of staff information. Nevertheless, there was no indication of resistance to the trend towards collaboration. Joint planning and commitment to the project were other facilitating elements which were identified in the present study.

An additional facilitating factor outlined in the literature is involvement and support of the medical staff and a sensitivity to the results of reorganization on them (Burchell et al, 1988; McFall, Shortell, and Manheim, 1988). An interesting finding in the current study was that, because Sackville Memorial Hospital was the principal beneficiary of collaborative arrangements, the medical staff did not appear to feel threatened by the arrangements or to fear loss of autonomy. Rather, they and other staff believed that providing additional services through collaborative arrangements contributed to the Sackville Memorial Hospital's role as an acute care institution and counteracted any perception of it as primarily a chronic care institution, which some staff regarded as less desirable for them as professionals. One factor in facilitating collaboration which received some mention in the literature is the importance of the availability of up-to-date facilities. Clearly, in the present case, the new Sackville Memorial Hospital was a major factor in permitting developments to take place in the area of surgery and is, in many ways, inseparable from the other facilitating factors.

A key point which emerged from the literature was the importance of monitoring and evaluating the process of developing multi-institutional arrangements (Kooi, White, and Smith, 1988). The study reported on in this paper has been an important element for the hospitals concerned in evaluating the successes and failures of what has been attempted to date and in identifying possible future areas for collaboration.

BARRIERS TO COLLABORATION

A major factor identified in the literature as a barrier to multi-institutional arrangements was the fear of actual loss of autonomy for the smaller hospital and its staff (Fried and Gelmon, 1987; Gillock, Smith, and Piland, 1986). However, such concern was expressed by few of our respondents and was offset by the perceived benefits. Rather, the major concern was perceived to be inadequate incentives for specialists and physicians to participate in visiting specialty clinics and day surgery (Table 3).

Table 3
PERCEIVED BARRIERS TO COLLABORATION

Service	Insufficient demand for service		Insufficient staff/ resources		Inadequate incentives for specialists/ physicians to participate		Lack of administrative will/ interest		Other	
	S	M	S	M	S	M	S	M	S	M
Pediatrics clinic	4	0	8	2	14	3	8	3	1	5
Psychiatry clinic	3	0	8	2	15	2	6	3	2	5
Geriatric medicine clinic	3	1	9	5	11	2	7	3	1	3
Orthopedic day surgery	5	1	6	2	16	4	10	3	3	7
Plastic day surgery	4	0	7	1	16	5	9	3	3	6
Holter monitoring	8	1	9	3	2	0	4	1	3	5
Administrative computer services	5	2	9	2	1	0	9	3	3	4
Staff education	6	2	10	2	4	1	7	5	1	3
Waste disposal	8	3	1	0	0	0	2	0	7	5

S = Sackville respondents, N=26
M = Moncton respondents, N=14
Multiple responses allowed

Another potential barrier was lack of administrative will or interest. The reasons given in the present study as facilitating collaboration indicate situations that might previously have been barriers to such collaboration. The results indicated the importance of administrative interest, initiative, and commitment.

Responses to a question on which services, if any, had not lived up to expectations also indicated the kinds of barriers that prevented the successful establishment of services. Major barriers identified were lack of staff at the collaborating hospital to ensure adequate turnaround time on certain tests and insufficient allocation of time for a specialty clinic. This concern included lack of time in relation to demand for the service provided and in particular a lack of time for local physicians to consult with visiting specialists. The major barrier identified with respect to a failed surgery clinic was a lack of interest on the part of some of the participants, along with inadequate communication.

BENEFITS OF COLLABORATION

The reasons for entering into collaborative arrangements and the benefits derived from them are many and various. The clear overriding benefit identified in the present study was the improvement of services to patients of the Sackville Memorial Hospital, including greater convenience, faster scheduling of specialist appointments and surgery dates, and access to new services and expertise (Table 4).

Table 4
BENEFITS OF COLLABORATION

Benefit	Major benefit		Minor benefit		Unimportant	
	S	M	S	M	S	M
Availability of specialized medical, patient, and administrative service	26	9	0	2	0	4
Lower operating costs	16	6	7	2	3	7
Strengthened clout with government	11	9	2	4	3	2
Reduced legal liability	11	1	10	5	5	9
Enhanced attractiveness of hospital to new physicians	18	7	6	6	2	2
Improved quality of care offered at institution	26	11	0	2	0	2
Improved service delivery and availability	25	12	1	2	0	1
Enhanced prestige in eyes of patient community	19	6	7	7	0	2
Enhanced prestige in eyes of health care industry	13	6	13	8	0	1
Enhanced employee/staff morale	13	4	11	10	2	1

S = Sackville respondents, N=26
M = Moncton respondents, N=15

In particular, patients appreciated the greater convenience of receiving surgery or specialty treatments in their own community. There was less time involved because the need for a 50 km drive was eliminated and, for a number of reasons, there was also less apprehension. The highway was perceived as dangerous, particularly in the winter, and the psychological benefits of remaining in one's home community were clearly identified. The smaller scale of the Sackville Memorial Hospital created in the patients' minds a sense of intimacy and friendliness which again had psychological benefits.

From the point of view of the staff at the Sackville Hospital, this study identified a factor which has not been widely discussed in the literature: the improvement in the quality of professional and institutional life resulting from the hospital's being perceived as able to maintain or enhance its status as a facility equipped to provide acute as well as chronic care. This was seen as a professionally more challenging environment for medical and nursing staff, one which allowed them to acquire new information, learn new approaches and techniques, and have more contact with visiting specialists. There was therefore a perception of dynamism and excitement in the working environment which a number of respondents believed would otherwise have been lacking or present to a much lesser extent. This finding relates to Begin and Demers' (1986) observation that during integration efforts in the Quebec health care system, many hospitals fought to retain acute care services which were seen as an "inherent leadership symbol". Chronic care services were much less an issue. This observation applied, however, to horizontal integration efforts; issues of cooperation and complementarity characterized the vertical integration efforts.

It was also believed by a number of respondents in the present study that collaborative arrangements would secure the future of the Sackville Memorial Hospital and perhaps even lead to future growth. The hospital is indeed a fairly major facility for the size of the immediate community it serves. The availability of operating room time, which results in the scheduling of a variety of surgical procedures, draws patients from a much broader area than the immediate environment of the hospital, again helping to ensure its current and future status as an acute care facility.

The enhanced prestige which was perceived to accrue to the Sackville Hospital and its effect on enhancing and maintaining staff morale were also referred to by many respondents.

From an administrative point of view, the provision of collaborative services undoubtedly allowed for areas of cost avoidance or cost savings, a factor which was important to the administration of both hospitals as well as to the provincial government, under whose jurisdiction health care falls. However, it was difficult to quantify the level of cost savings or cost avoidance.

There is a tendency to think only of the benefits of collaboration for the smaller institution, but some benefits for the Moncton Hospital were also clearly identified, including a strong expression of the fulfillment of its outreach mission. The collaborative arrangements also allowed more effective use of the Moncton Hospital's resources. For example, scheduling low risk day surgery in Sackville decreased the pressure on the already heavily used operating room facilities at the Moncton Hospital. The opportunity to provide specialty services and surgery in another environment was undoubtedly beneficial for the visiting physicians and surgeons, increasing their patient load and enhancing their overall level of professional satisfaction.

CONCLUSION

This study provided important information to the hospitals involved on what collaborative services have been successful and why, the reasons some services have been less successful, the benefits of collaborative arrangements, and the critical variables to be considered in implementing any expansion of these arrangements. Other information can be helpful to the administrators of the hospitals in avoiding pitfalls and tackling areas which, although not problematic to date, have the potential to create problems in the future. In particular, it appeared that a greater level of communication and information flow within the Sackville Memorial Hospital might have been undertaken to inform all staff of current and planned developments.

It appears from the literature review and case study results that there are a number of advantages to health care institutions and particularly to smaller hospitals in participating in collaborative arrangements. From the smaller facilities' point of view, the range of services offered can be expanded and program effectiveness increased. From the larger facilities' point of view, service can be improved by reducing waiting lists, fulfilling the regional outreach mission, and enhancing professional satisfaction for medical staff. As well, development of a "collaborative mentality" for larger facilities can help in attracting additional resources to these facilities.

Although service *effectiveness* may be increased, it is difficult to say whether the delivery of collaborative services promotes *efficiency*. Indeed, some authors, for example Howard and Alidina (1987), have suggested that it may not. Moreover, at present, many hospitals do not have the necessary cost accounting systems to provide adequate information on this matter. One may speculate, nevertheless, that increased use of otherwise idle or under-utilized facilities in either large or smaller hospitals would result in a lower cost per unit of service, but this is clearly an area for further study.

Each hospital facility will be faced with its own special set of circumstances that will either promote or discourage collaboration. However, the findings of this study do contribute to the literature on the kinds of factors institutions should consider in implementing such arrangements and add a New Brunswick example to the list of Canadian cases of multi-institutional arrangements. As Begin and Demers (1986) have noted, each arrangement must be viewed in its provincial context.

Further research might involve case studies of similar instances of collaboration among two or more hospitals in the Maritimes and other regions of Canada. In particular, it would be helpful to have further case studies of collaboration involving hospitals of different sizes to determine the extent to which the mutual benefits perceived in the present study are typical.

With increased public expectations and decreased levels of funding for hospital services, there are increasing pressures on all facilities to find new ways to improve services without increasing costs. For some services, collaborative arrangements may provide a mechanism for accomplishing this, and the southeast New Brunswick experience offers a case in point from which other institutions might benefit.

ACKNOWLEDGEMENTS

This research was funded by a grant from the National Health Research and Development Program, Health and Welfare Canada, which is gratefully acknowledged. Appreciation is also expressed to research assistants Elizabeth Barker, Graeme Marney, and Lori Multari.

REFERENCES

Begin C, Demers L: Quebec's multi-institutional arrangements. *Health Management Forum* 7(4):31-42, 1986.

Burchell RC, White RE, Smith HL, Piland NF: Physicians and the organizational evolution of medicine. *Journal of the American Medical Association* 260(6):826-831, 1988.

Chenoy NS: St. Joseph Health System: an experiment in institutional integration. *Dimensions in Health Service* 64(2):34-36, 1987.

Devries RA: Health care delivery: strength in numbers. *Hospitals* 52(6):81-84, 1978.

Ellis DJ: Change process: a case example. *Nursing Management* 18(4):14, 16, 19, 1987.

Fried BJ, Gelmon S B: Multi-institutional arrangements: the Canadian experience. *Dimensions in Health Service* 64(2):14-19, 1987.

Fyke KJ: Creating excellence through hospital merger. *Health Management Forum* 7(2):16-23, 1986.

Gelmon SB, Fried BJ: *Multi-institutional Arrangements and the Canadian Health System.* Ottawa: Canadian Hospital Association, 1987.

Gelmon SB, Marotta JT: Hospital merger: the Toronto experience. *Health Management Forum* 7(2):24-34, 1986.

Gillock R, Smith H, Piland NF: For profit and nonprofit mergers: concerns and outcomes. *Hospital and Health Services Administration* 31(6):74-84, 1986.

Howard JW, Alidina S: Multihospital systems increase costs and quality. *Dimensions in Health Service* 64(2):20-24, 1987.

Jaeger BJ, Kaluzny AD, Magruder-Habib K: A new perspective on multi-institutional systems management. *Health Care Management Review* 12(4):9-19, 1987.

Kooi D, White RE, Smith HL: Managing organizational mergers. *Journal of Nursing Administration* 18(3):10-18, 1988.

Longest BB: A conceptual framework for understanding multihospital arrangement strategy. *Health Care Management Review* 5(1):17-24, 1980.

McFall SL, Shortell SM, Manheim LM: HCA's acquisition process: the physician's role and perspective. *Health Care Management Review* 13(2):23-24, 1988.

McKinley JB, Stoeckle JD: Corporatization and the social transformation of doctoring. *International Journal of Health Services* 18(2):191-205, 1988.

Moreton GK: Hospital integration: theory and practice. *Health Management Forum* 6(1):62-73, 1985.

Statistics Canada: *Hospital Annual Statistics 1987-88.* Catalogue 83-232, 1988.

Stoughton WV: Negotiating hospital mergers: Toronto General and Toronto Western consolidate. *Dimensions in Health Service* 64(2):25-27, 1987.

White R, Migliaccio E, Smith H: Shared medical services between the Air Force and Veterans Administration: analysis of concerns among providers. *Military Medicine* 153(3):127-133, 1988.

Zalot GN, Shack J: Sharing services: an accepted way of life. *Dimensions in Health Service* 64(2):37-38, 1987.

DISCUSSION
Chair: Carol Clemenhagen
Canadian Hospital Association

Carol Clemenhagen

The innovations that you've reported on, and the changes that are proposed, would you attribute them to being stimulated from within the system? In other words, can the institutional sector restructure itself? Or do you think they came as a result of outside forces, of specific policy directions, or provincial commissions, or just the general environment coming to bear on the hospital sector, causing it to start thinking about some new ways of doing things?

Frances Caruth (British Columbia Cancer Agency)

It's probably some of all. I don't know that you can say that it's specifically any one. If I was to take the Ophthalmology group in particular, I think it's just the result of squeeze, and people become frustrated. The reduction in resources tends to happen centrally, and people begin to be frustrated. They think they want to have some control. And so they begin to initiate ideas as to how they can get involved in that management process more actively. So I think what I described was sort of a grass roots response to a more centrally driven pressure.

Sheila Brown (Mount Allison University)

I think that's true in the case I was describing. I think the initiatives really came internally, but you can't really separate that from the external environment. I suppose it's the view that we'd better do it before somebody makes us do it. And if there is a perception that provincial directives may make this sort of arrangement a necessity, then better to take the initiative yourself and establish something that meets your needs particularly.

Paul Gamble (Hospital Council of Metropolitan Toronto)

I think here in Metro Toronto there are a large number of external influences that are affecting the hospital operations. Although the responses that we've seen, I think, are internally coordinated within the institutions and addressing their particular future and the limitations that they see, the issue, as I've tried to point out, is that we have a problem. We need to take it beyond simply that institutional level and deal with it more on the system here in Metro Toronto. The one point I didn't make was that of the hospitals in Ontario, Metro Toronto accounts for about 23-24% of the total number of institutions, but in terms of the rated bed capacity and the budget allocations, we're closer to 35-40% of provincial allocation. Because of the concentration of resources here, it's very important, and also very complicated, to try to move that system.

Participant

I have a question with regards to the presentation about the amalgamation of the hospitals in Sackville. One of the effects that you indicated was that the physicians were very pleased as a result of this because it increased their caseload. I wonder how the provincial government reconciles its constant attempts to limit the increases in health care costs and the fact that it encourages amalgamations and these cross linkages which clearly, from what you said, increase supplier-induced demand.

Sheila Brown

I'm not sure that we're quite on the same wavelength. Let me just repeat what I think I said and make sure that we are. I think for the physicians at the Sackville Hospital, who are basically general practitioners serving the immediate community, the advantage is contact with visiting specialists and the fact that they can operate within an environment where there are more professional challenges. The six or eight physicians from Moncton are a very different situation, in that they are on staff at the Moncton Hospital and in terms of their particular professional practice, there appear to be limits on it because of resource constraints, so that what they can do is schedule procedures that they would have done there, but with a much longer waiting period, in Sackville. It's conceivable that other people who had the personal resources could have sought the care elsewhere, but what is really happening is that they are able perhaps to plan their workloads better. I'm not sure that their total caseload increases if you looked at it over a period of time, but if you look cross sectionally it is clear that there is better scheduling, and it seems to me that that fits within provincial initiatives to make better use of resources.

WHERE ELSE MIGHT WE GO? ALTERNATIVE APPROACHES AND MODELS

CO-OPERATIVE HEALTH SERVICE DELIVERY IN CANADA
L.E. Apland
Canadian Co-operative Association

THE ROLE OF CO-OPERATIVES IN THE CANADIAN HEALTH SYSTEM
INTRODUCTION

Despite the reputation of the Canadian health system for providing high quality health care, Canadians are increasingly aware that this system is in need of reform; some, in fact, believe it is in a state of crisis. Although the causes of the present status of Canada's health care system are the subject of considerable debate, many of its manifestations are clear. The consumer of health services often is faced with delays before receiving treatment or needed surgery. Health service workers and professionals often are confronted with an unresponsive system that can inhibit the quality of care they are capable of delivering. Health care administrators face increased operating costs on the one hand and government restraint on the other. Governments faced with ballooning deficits find spiralling health care costs, whatever their source, an identifiable and tempting target for expenditure reduction.

Many believe that these problems are fundamental to Canada's health care system as it exists today. They are inherent in the apparent lack of accountability of its funding and financial structures, in its hierarchical organizational structure, and in its curative focus. Indeed, an increasing understanding of the positive relationship that exists between health and wealth suggests that the present system's definition of health is in itself too narrow. As the 1984 Report of the National Task Force on Co-operative Development noted, "this appears to be a time when there must be a renewed commitment to search for more effective ways to provide health care... Canadians will have to learn to do more with less".

Not-for-profit, community-based, co-operative health clinics, with member-elected and accountable boards of directors, are natural and effective means by which to address many of Canada's health care delivery problems and, indeed, "to do more with less". "Understaffing, deterioration of quality, and long hospital waiting lists", according to the Community Health Co-operative Federation in Saskatchewan (1987), "are all manifestations of attempts at controlling health costs". Advocates of community clinics, they noted, "share the concerns of governments across Canada over the rise and uncontrollability of health costs, but... do not believe the solutions to those problems lie in cutbacks, rationing, or user fees... [They] lie in basic reform and in experimentation with alternatives in planning, organizing and financing health services".

The Canadian Council on Social Development noted in its Conference Report on Community-Based Health and Social Services (1985) that "community-based services are not a substitute for hospitals or other institutions, or for the curative model of care, but they are an alternative where sophisticated and expensive institutional or professional resources are an inappropriate response to a given need". Accordingly, community-based clinics are not seen as displacing mainstream methods of health service delivery, but rather are viewed as alternatives to them in appropriate circumstances. In addition, these organizations can add an element of competition to the field of health service delivery and, hence, can create incentives for self-improvement in mainstream delivery systems; they can provide more effective and appropriate health service delivery and, at the same time, contribute to improvements in the health delivery system as a whole.

In being considered as "alternatives" to mainstream methods of health service delivery, however, it is essential that co-operative and other community-based clinics be integrated into the Canadian health system and not treated as "optional extras" that simply contribute to ever-increasing health care costs. Appropriately utilized, these organizations can deliver health services more efficiently and promote a preventive approach to health that will also result in long-term cost savings.

HEALTH CARE IN CANADA: OBJECTIVES AND SHORTCOMINGS

In November of 1986, the Federal Minister of National Health and Welfare, Jake Epp, made public the Canadian government's blueprint for the direction of health care delivery in Canada. *Achieving Health for All: A Framework for Health Promotion* (Epp, 1986) outlined a strategy for health care wholly consistent with that promoted by co-operative and other community-based clinics. Building upon the 1984 *Canada Health Act* that stressed healthy individual lifestyles in conjunction with "collective action against social, environmental and occupational causes of disease", *Achieving Health for All* sought to shift the focus of Canadian health care delivery toward health promotion through three mechanisms:

1. Self-care, or the decisions and actions individuals take in the interest of their own health;
2. Mutual aid, or the actions people take to help each other cope; and
3. Healthy environments, or the creation of conditions and surroundings conducive to health.

Of note to co-operators is the fact that the three main strategies by which the federal government proposed to implement its "Framework for Health Promotion" are founded on basic co-operative tenets. According to *Achieving Health for All*, Strategy I is to foster public participation. "Encouraging public participation," the paper notes, "means helping people to assert control over the factors which affect their health".

Strategy II involves strengthening community health services. "A health promotion and disease prevention orientation... [among other things] takes for granted that communities will become more involved in planning their own services, and that the links between communities and their services and institutions will be strengthened".

Finally, Strategy III focuses on co-ordinating healthy public policy. "Self-care, mutual aid and healthy environmental change are integral to health promotion, and... are more likely to occur when healthy public policies are in place." Fundamentally, according to the paper, "for public policies to be healthy, they must respond to the health needs of people and their communities".

Clearly, the strategies and implicit objectives of the federal government's health care direction suggest that the co-operative model may be a natural and valuable means of assisting the implementation of federal health strategies. Indeed, in some ways, the co-operative model helps to institutionalize the structural mechanisms by which implementation can be facilitated.

The democratic governance structures of co-operatively-organized clinics, for instance, help to ensure a dialogue between the members (consumers) and providers of health services, and promote member participation (Strategy I). Because member participation is institutionalized, formal lines of communication are kept open between health care consumers and health care providers and administrators. There are several results.

Members/consumers are more knowledgeable regarding their health needs and, accordingly, health care administrators and providers are more accountable to them. Members/consumers are more involved in their own health care. Administrators and providers of health services are kept more aware of and thereby have the opportunity to be more responsive to the changing health needs of consumers and the communities in which they live (Strategy II). As an important element of community health services, the formal democratic structures of co-operative health delivery models can facilitate community development based on requirements articulated by those who live in the community itself. The co-operative democratic process allows for, and promotes, personal involvement by local individuals in "policy selection, program development and executive decision-making... [and] makes it more likely that public policies and publicly-funded programs will reflect the values and priorities of the community" (Sutherland and Fulton, 1988) (Strategy III).

Finally, the personal involvement that is promoted by co-operative democracy can reduce the sense of powerlessness of health consumers and, accordingly, is a prerequisite for them to take responsibility for personal health and well-being. Indeed, this is a prerequisite for the federal government's strategy to shift the focus of health service delivery to prevention.

The shift in emphasis in health care policy toward local involvement and preventive medicine is not entirely new, nor is it exclusively a federal strategy. In the 1960s in Quebec, for instance, the Castonguay-Nepveu Commission concluded its report "with a call for two major reforms: first, it urged the province to decentralize planning; second, it called on Quebec to develop a network of primary care facilities that would offer both medical care and social services" (Rachlis and Kushner, 1989).

Today, subsequent to these recommendations, there is a network in Quebec of over 160 CLSCs (Centres locaux des services communautaires), each "run by a community board, and each... [with] salaried (not fee-for-service) staff." (Rachlis and Kushner, 1989) In February of 1988, the Quebec government's Rochon Commission pronounced "decentralization and CLSCs a qualified success... [but] said the system needed to be more explicit about its goals and priorities... and urged the system to refocus on the needs of individual consumers". (Rachlis and Kushner, 1989). The CLSC model was Quebec policy-makers' specific response to a perceived set of health care issues in that province. In the present context, however, it is more important to note that the co-operative model is quite naturally structured for, and geared toward, addressing these same concerns and objectives.

In Ontario, the Premier's Council on Health Strategy outlined the provincial government's interest in shifting the emphasis of health care to "health promotion and disease prevention" and in helping individuals to become more involved in, and responsible for, their own health (Premier's Council on Health Strategy, 1989). This was reiterated by the Honourable Elinor Caplan, Ontario Minister of Health, in her remarks to the Ontario Hospital Association Conference on Comprehensive Health Organizations. She noted that the Ontario government recognized Comprehensive Health Organizations (CHOs) as a means to provide a "workable mechanism for shifting resources from illness response to health promotion and community care" and to promote "responsive planning through community participation in the management of services" (Caplan, 1989).

The co-operative model is decentralized and community-sponsored. In addition, because it promotes membership as active participation and involvement in the organization, the co-operative model encourages members to be responsible for their own good health without directing the blame for ill health to those who are its victims (as a campaign simply promoting individual responsibility might well do). Furthermore, with a co-operative control structure, communication about individual needs is easily and formally maintained. Democratic lines of responsibility and the accountability to the membership of properly elected directors help to ensure that members' individual needs are addressed.

Critics of health care policy and government alike are well aware of many of the changes required to set Canada's health care system aright. After their extensive critique of the Canadian health system, for instance, Michael Rachlis, a founding member of the Medical Reform Group, and Carol Kushner, a researcher of public policy, proposed their "blueprint for health care reform" based on six guiding principles:

1. **Patients come first.** Patients need to understand, and be involved in, the decisions that affect them. Only then can they become responsible for the decisions they make about their health.

2. **Planning, administration, and delivery of health care should be decentralized.** The Canadian health care system will not "be responsive to local needs until communities are put in charge of their own health... because needs are bound to differ from place to place".

3. **Quality assurance mechanisms must be developed and implemented.** This can be facilitated through continuing education, "non-threatening, constructive processes for peer review", and "more doctors practising in groups". As well, more appropriate and better use should be made of the knowledge and skills of nurses, practitioners, and other health care workers.

4. **The number of doctors entering our system must be immediately reduced.**

5. **The financial and professional incentives must be changed to encourage efficiency and quality.** Methods of payment other than fee-for-service (e.g., salary, capitation) ought to be encouraged. Patients should be encouraged to be discerning consumers.

6. **The system needs to be community based.** Community programs "developed by, and for, the community... will mean a relative shrinkage in hospital-based services and a dramatic expansion in community services" (Rachlis and Kushner, 1989).

Although perhaps not explicitly stated, some of the concerns and recommendations of governments are similar to or overlap those expressed by Rachlis and Kushner. In concluding her address on Comprehensive Health Organizations, Elinor Caplan echoed their approach when she indicated several ways CHOs could contribute to resolving immediate and fundamental issues facing Canada's health system. In addition to a stronger emphasis on prevention and community participation, Caplan noted that CHOs:

- provide an "opportunity to develop an alternative practice model for physicians";
- encourage "a team approach to health care and... [foster] the appropriate use of health manpower";
- integrate "health services in a true continuum of care and support";
- facilitate "the measurement of effectiveness and progress toward health goals";
- offer "the promise of reductions in the demand for hospital beds"; and
- "will make health care costs more predictable" (Caplan, 1989).

The point to be noted is that, in addition to a common understanding of many of the issues facing Canada's health system, there also appears to be reasonable consensus on the means by which they ought to be addressed. Both the issues raised and the characteristics of the generally-proposed means of dealing with them are elements upon which co-operatively-organized health clinics are naturally predicated. Virtually all of the concerns and recommendations, except for the one on the reduction of the number of doctors entering the system (which is not an objective of community-based clinics), could be addressed by the co-operative model. On a broader scale, co-operatively-based community clinics might also be useful as a means for injecting change into a complex system that, for a range of reasons, has had difficulty adapting to it.

CO-OPERATION AND COMMUNITY-BASED CLINICS

Most co-operative advocates will be familiar with the six principles of co-operation adopted by the International Co-operative Alliance in 1966:

1. Open and voluntary membership;
2. Democratic control;
3. Limited interest on shares;
4. Return of surplus to members;
5. Co-operative education; and
6. Co-operation among co-operatives.

These principles are founded on the basic values of equity, equality, and mutual self-help that Canadian co-operators have adopted to pursue their vision (Chapman et al, 1986).

Equality, according to Leon Garoyan and Paul Mohn, "is a social value that recognizes that people are important because they are people. Although related to potentials, and often to opportunities, it does not imply that all people are equal in abilities, intelligence, motivations, or even innate capabilities" (Garoyan and Mohn, 1984). This value is reflected in, and is a prerequisite for, the co-operative principles of open and voluntary membership and democratic control.

Equity, as another basic value of co-operation, "takes into account human differences... [and] has its origins with the human person, while equality has its origin in justice and fairness" (Garoyan and Mohn, 1984). According to E.S. Bogardus, "equitable treatment is equal treatment according to the degree of participation in, and of contribution to, human relationships" (Bogardus, 1950). Equity, as a basic value of co-operation, is reflected in the co-operative principles of limited interest on shares and returns of surplus to members, or "operations at cost" in the case of service-oriented co-operatives. In the case of health care co-operatives, the principles of limited interest on shares and the return of surplus to members simply mean that the organization operates on a non-profit basis and that any surplus is used in the co-operative to enhance the quality and variety of services.

Finally, mutual self-help as a co-operative value, "identifies the conceptual attitudes of thrift and self-reliance, coupled with mutual associations with others to achieve what one alone could not. To some, it implies working with others rather than against them..." (Bogardus, 1950). Mutual self-help is implicit in the principles of co-operative education and co-operation among co-operatives.

These co-operative principles are nothing new or profound to co-operators. They illustrate, however, that although some of the ICA principles may seem more economically oriented, and not explicitly applicable to the field of health care, their underlying values mesh very well with modern community-based approaches to health service delivery.

The Conference Report on Community-Based Health and Social Services, for instance, notes that whereas "traditional [health] services are characterized by centralization, hierarchies and specialization, and are oriented toward curing physical and social ills, community-based services are predicated on decentralized decision-making, public participation, team approaches, and self-help oriented toward prevention and health promotion" (Canadian Council on Social Development, 1985). Although it is not the purpose of this paper to provide a detailed account of all the varieties of community-based health clinics, it is important to recognize that the co-operative model is entirely consistent with their characteristics and values. Indeed, the co-operative model has the formal structure to address the concerns of modern critics of Canada's health care system and to accommodate and meet the objectives of community-based clinics and provincial and national health care schemes.

It should be noted as well that regardless of the legislation under which they are incorporated, and regardless of the name by which they are called, co-operative health clinics are characterized by their organizational structure and by their objectives. They are democratically structured health service organizations whose object is to provide not-for-profit health services.

CO-OPERATIVE STRUCTURES AND HEALTH CARE DELIVERY

Some of the oldest and most successful community-based health centres in Canada are organized on a co-operative basis. Among the first to implement the co-operative model of health service delivery were the Community Health Services Associations that arose out of the Medicare crisis in Saskatchewan in 1962. The general principles upon which this co-operative model was founded remain essentially unchanged:

1. Community-based organization and control;
2. Emphasis on prevention and education in provision of direct health services and by way of specialized programming;
3. Remuneration of health service professionals by way of salary or other alternatives, rather than fee-for-service payments;
4. Provision of a variety of health services in one location; and
5. Group practice as the basis of medical service (Community Health Co-operative Federation, 1987).

Because co-operative health clinics are community-based and democratically controlled by the community in which they operate, they tend to be more innovative and responsive to the requirements of the people they serve. Accordingly, their services can be more appropriate to local needs and, as a result, more effective and cost efficient.

The innovativeness of these organizations was illustrated when the Saskatoon Community Health Services Association, "out of concern over the high cost of prescription drugs, pioneered a pharmacy program where first quality medications could be obtained at cost plus a small dispensing fee. In the mid-1970s, this formulary approach was adopted as the basis for the Saskatchewan Prescription Drug Plan" (Community Health Co-operative Federation, 1987). As well, health concerns and issues raised by members at the Association's Annual General Meeting have resulted in the undertaking of a range of programs and the hiring of health personnel to accommodate members' health needs. For example, the Saskatoon Association hired a Native Health Worker to assist with the health needs of the substantial native population that uses the Association's Westside Clinic. At the Association's 1987 Annual General Meeting, during discussions aimed at instituting a PAP test recall program, it became apparent that a substantial number of members were concerned about other women's health issues as well. The result was the production and distribution of *Staying Healthy: A Preventive Health Maintenance Package for Women 45 to 64 Years*. The pamphlet contains information on risk factors for and detection of cervical, breast, and colon cancer; information on osteoporosis, influenza, blood cholesterol, and blood pressure; and a file card on which the patient can keep her own health record in respect to each of these conditions. Further discussion among clinic staff, however, resulted in recognition that the *Staying Healthy* program, on its own, was unlikely to reach women of lower socio-economic status, who are more at risk of being afflicted with health problems generally. Accordingly the Association applied for, and received, financial assistance from the federal government to hire a Community Development Women's Health Worker, who is responsible for the program's outreach.

This situation illustrates both the Association's responsiveness to the health needs of its membership and how that responsiveness has translated into health education and a shift toward preventive medicine. It is not simply coincidence that members of the Saskatoon Community Health Services Association were interested in health information and preventive services and hence used the co-operative's democratic processes to get it. As indicated by a former Saskatchewan government representative on the 1960 Thompson Advisory Committee on Medical Care, Dr. Vincent Matthews, if patients accept "good health as something which is... [their] responsibility and not entirely that of the doctor... [they are] more apt to be interested in acting to prevent visits to the doctor and stays in hospital. When patients are actively involved in their own health and in changing habits which influence it, the emphasis on preventive services, counselling and rehabilitation becomes more important." (in Gruending, 1979).

The democratic processes used by co-operatives encourage people to be informed, active, and responsible with respect to their health needs. The co-operative structure encourages and facilitates a natural emphasis on health education and preventive medicine. This is a direct result of co-operative health care clinics' being controlled, at least in part, by member consumers rather than exclusively by the providers of health care. A study by Andy Stergachis has indicated that patient education has worked to reduce unnecessary use of health services and hence has reduced health care costs, noting that a Seattle, Washington health maintenance organization whose doctors were paid on salary found that educating patients about minor respiratory illness reduced the number of calls about flu symptoms by 20% and the number of cold prescriptions by 18% (Stergachis, 1986).

In addition to an emphasis on member participation and health education that can lead to reduced health care costs, the methods of remuneration philosophically advocated and employed by the co-operative models in use in Saskatchewan and elsewhere can also contribute to a more effective and efficient health care system. Despite the good intentions of health professionals, remuneration on a fee-for-service basis allows a natural emphasis on medical care according to "volume and illness" (Marwick, 1985). The more patients and illnesses a physician treats, the more the physician is paid. Fee-for-service can have a tendency to lead to over-treatment of patients and can divert the focus of medical attention to treatments that are more expensive and away from preventive medicine that tends to pay less or not to be covered under fee schedules (Rachlis and Kushner, 1989). Accordingly, there is little financial incentive, and there actually can be financial disincentive, to practice preventive medicine or to educate patients. Health service co-operatives, however, as a general principle, "employ physicians on a salaried basis or mixed salaried and incentive basis. When their doctors visit a school or say no to a demanding patient", noted David Schreck, formerly of C.U. and C. Health Services in Vancouver, "they do not suffer a loss of income. They are rewarded for practising to the best of their ability..." (Schreck et al, 1985).

Indeed, studies have indicated that payment of health professionals by salary, rather than fee-for-service, has coincided with more preventive services and less likelihood of patient hospitalization. According to information from the Association of Ontario Health Centres, enrollees at community-based Health Service Organizations, where the Ministry of Health provides funding on a capitation basis, showed almost a 30% lower hospitalization rate than fee-for-service practice for the 1987-88 fiscal year. As well, according to the Association's April 15, 1989 news release, "These centres as a group have the broadest range of non-medical services" (Association of Ontario Health Centres, 1989). Furthermore, in Health Maintenance Organizations (HMOs) in the United States, where most "doctors are paid on salary, work in groups, and are subject to peer review", research suggests that "patients cost approximately 25% less to treat than patients attended by fee-for-service doctors, and that HMO patients spent about 40% fewer days in hospital" (Luft, 1981, as cited in Rachlis and Kushner, 1989).

Co-operative clinics can also have the effect of adding some healthy competition into the health care system and, accordingly, can offset the "less desirable aspects of fee-for-service medical practice". Saskatchewan's Community Health Co-operative Federation noted, for instance, that "when extra billing was permitted in Saskatchewan, in Prince Albert, where salaried Community Clinic physicians constitute a significant proportion of the medical community, the frequency of extra billing was considerably lower than that for the province generally" (Community Health Co-operative Federation, 1987). Methods of remuneration other than fee-for-service for medical professionals also are more conducive to a team approach to health care that allows, and encourages, more appropriate use of health care professionals and translates into savings for the health care system. Alternative methods of payment, such as capitation and global budgets, "are compatible with the development of multidisciplinary teams, with an integrated... and continuous rather than episodic approach to care, and with an emphasis on promotion" (Sutherland and Fulton, 1988). At Saskatoon's Community Health Clinic, for instance, the range of services provided includes:
- General Service and Gerontological Counselling;
- Optometric;
- Laboratory and ECG;
- Nutrition Counselling;
- Occupational Therapy;
- Pharmaceutical;
- Physical Therapy;
- Radiological; and
- A medical staff that includes an ear, nose and throat specialist, four general practitioners who practice obstetrics, and a psychiatrist.

With a payment structure that is conducive to the provision of educative and preventive health services, and because other health and social services are provided at the same location, referrals to appropriate health care providers are more easily made. The co-operative clinic produces an environment in which health care providers are encouraged to work to their highest level of ability and in conjunction with one another, rather than in competition over dollars and professional territory. Furthermore, by providing a range of health and social services under one roof, and keeping an integrated record on patients, peer review and consultation is made a more natural and accepted facet of medical practice at co-operative and other community-based clinics. The result is an environment more conducive to high quality, appropriate, effective, and economical health care.

In summation, as the Community Health Co-operative Federation noted in *Saskatchewan's Community Clinics: A Quarter Century of Innovation and Reform in Health Services:*

> In the course of setting financing levels for Community Clinics, governments can set guidelines, standards and expectations for services and... [know] precisely what these services will cost. Further, remuneration of professionals by way of salary generates cost savings throughout the health system. It eliminates the incentive to over-service and over-bill, and shows up in reduced rates of hospitalization and utilization of other health services (i.e., the prescription drug plan). Finally, the provision of out-patient and support services (X-ray, laboratory, physiotherapy, day surgery, etc.) through Community Clinics is substantially less costly than provision of the same services through hospitals (Community Health Co-operative Federation, 1987).

Extensive research data on Saskatchewan's co-operative clinics tend to be somewhat scarce or difficult to obtain, but available information supports these conclusions. An analysis of 1984-85 data conducted by administrative staff at the Saskatoon Clinic, for instance, indicates a hospitalization rate for clinic patients that is 23% lower than an urban sample population. In the same analysis, a comparison of total Medical Care Insurance Commission and hospital costs indicated that costs for community clinic patients were 77% of those for the urban sample. The trend in these figures is supported by the results of a study of two Saskatchewan co-operative community clinics, commissioned by the provincial New Democratic Party government in 1980. Although the report was completed in 1982, a newly-elected Conservative government blocked its release. Only after considerable political pressure was the report made public in 1989. Louise Simard, NDP health critic at that time, suggested that reasons for not releasing it may have been related to the "history of community clinics dating back to the start of medicare in 1962" (Community Health Co-operative Federation, 1987). Although clinic costs for general practitioner and specialist services were found to be 20% higher than those of private practice, the study shows "that overall costs were 17% lower for patients attending the Saskatoon Clinic than for those treated in the fee-for-service system. The clinic's patients had 24% fewer hospital admissions, and those who were hospitalized stayed, on average, 9% fewer days. Drug costs at the clinic were 21% lower" (Policy Research and Management Services Branch, 1983). This pattern is consistent with the philosophy and practices of co-operative and community-based health service delivery: more time is spent with clients in efforts to determine root causes of problems and to avoid the unnecessary drug prescriptions and hospital admissions. Clearly, the research supports the "contention community clinics are a big part of the solution to problems in Canada's health care system" (Saskatoon *Star-Phoenix*, 1989).

As noted by the National Task Force on Co-operative Development, the co-operative model of health care delivery has much to offer:

> For the individual Canadian it provides the opportunity to share responsibility for the maintenance of his/her own health; for communities it harnesses the ingenuity, the inventiveness and flexibility of small organizers to create innovative concepts and styles of health services delivery; for minority groups of various kinds it offers the possibility, because of the elective basis upon which co-operatives would recruit their members, to provide a focus for community life, interaction and identification; for the country and for governments it provides the potential of substantially enhanced efficiency and a mechanism for allocating the resulting savings to the priority health care needs that will otherwise come to rest at the door of governments. (National Task Force on Co-operative Development, 1984).

THE DEVELOPMENT OF HEALTH CARE CO-OPERATIVES

The 1984 National Task Force on Co-operative Development identified health services as one of four areas "of national concern and where co-operatives have significant underdeveloped potential" (National Task Force on Co-operative Development, 1984). The Task Force noted that, in a broad sense, promoting health-care co-operatives as an alternative model for the delivery of health services will "further the important and operational principles inherent in the co-operative approach" (Marwick, 1985). Specifically, however, the development of these organizations is an opportunity for the established co-operative sector to act on its commitment to the principle of social progress for its members and for society as a whole. And as Tom Marwick, Executive Director of the Regina Community Clinic, has noted, "the idea of co-operatives conceived to respond to their members' economic needs working closely with co-operatives conceived to respond to their members' health and social needs is an attractive one, and the possibilities arising out of this, both social and economic, are worthy of considerably more discussion" (Marwick, 1985).

THE ROLE OF THE CO-OPERATIVE SECTOR

Although co-operative philosophy holds that new co-operatives should be the product of grassroots initiative, developing co-operatives still have a need for external assistance. As noted by the 1984 Task Force, "[m]any grassroots co-operative initiatives founder because they do not obtain technical assistance at critical moments in their development. Others never get off the ground because they cannot get a receptive hearing with government when government support is required. Though its resources [for this type of work] are not unlimited, the co-operative system can provide critical support to get new locally developed co-operatives over some startup hurdles" (National Task Force on Cooperative Development, 1984).

National and regional co-operative organizations exist that have the structure and expertise to inform and educate people about the co-operative option and to assist them in applying it to meet their health care needs. The Canadian Co-operative Association, in English Canada, and the Conseil Canadien de la Cooperation, in French Canada, particularly, are in a position to act as a liaison between health care co-operatives and governments, the public, and other sectors of the co-operative system across Canada.

These and other co-operative organizations are in an excellent position to work together with governments to support and help shape the development of health care co-operatives. Through Canada's co-operative network, health care co-operatives can be put in touch with an invaluable source of volunteers, resource personnel, and other contacts. The co-operative sector is also a structure through which current research and information on co-operatives and health care delivery can be disseminated to the developers, directors, and administrators of health care co-operatives throughout the country.

THE ROLE OF GOVERNMENTS

Health care co-operatives are an important element of the Canadian co-operative sector. Furthermore, these organizations can make an invaluable contribution to Canadian social fabric through their involvement in Canada's health care system. Their growth and development, however, can best be assured with the leadership and support of Canada's federal and provincial governments. For their part, governments will have to put into place a legislative and financial framework that is conducive to the development of health care co-operatives and consistent with the principles of Medicare.

Primarily, to facilitate the development and continued existence of these organizations, governments should ensure that legislation accommodates their philosophy and objectives and recognizes health service co-operatives (and other community-sponsored clinics) as integral components of provincial health care systems. In some provinces, it may mean using new and creative means to fund community-based health clinics. Financing arrangements need to be sensitive to the philosophical focus of health care delivery advocated by health care co-operatives and to the general objectives of these organizations stated earlier. As a case in point, the Ontario Health Insurance Plan provides payment for a routine infant "check-up" only if the examination is performed by a medical doctor. The co-operative notion of alternative, and perhaps more appropriate, uses of qualified health care professionals, such as nurses, to provide these services is effectively undermined by these regulations. Further, since health care co-operatives often have a medical focus different from that of fee-for-service practice (preventive, rather than simply curative), the different criteria by which they should be evaluated should be recognized in legislation. Indeed, advocates of co-operative and other community-based clinics want evaluative criteria for themselves, and for Canada's established health system generally, to be laid down in legislation. For community-based clinics, evaluative criteria should address not only how many people go through the health care system and are cured, but also how many people are kept healthy. For Canadians, this will help to ensure that the system becomes accountable to those it serves.

Financial support specific to the development of health care co-operatives could take the form of startup grants, interest-free loans, loan guarantees, and the like. It needs to be stressed that this does not necessarily mean that governments should inject new funds into Canada's health system. Rather, such support might take the form of a reallocation of existing funds and resources to areas of health care that are more appropriate and compatible with the co-operative model of health delivery. Governments might also consider making research funds available for exploring various questions surrounding health care co-operatives, including evaluating the effectiveness of the different governmental and administrative structures that exist within the co-operative model, as well as exploring and assessing the differing roles of health care co-operative stakeholders.

Finally, since health care co-operatives have been shown to be an effective and an efficient means of health service delivery, the development of these organizations should be seen by governments as part of their long-term strategies to meet health care objectives.

CONCLUSION

Governments have administrative and financial responsibility for Canada's health system. Generally, however, their collaboration with the Canadian co-operative sector and community-based clinics is essential to the creation of appropriate legislative and financial frameworks within which the development of community-based, co-operative health care clinics can best be facilitated. Governments would do well, as Marwick has noted, to recognize and to explore the potential of health care co-operatives "as a weapon in the fight to control health costs and to preserve and strengthen the principles of portability, comprehensiveness, accessibility, public administration and universality upon which the public health insurance program in Canada stands" (Marwick, 1985).

REFERENCES

Association of Ontario Health Centres: *Release*, April 15, 1989.

Bogardus ES: *Principles of Co-operation.* Chicago: Co-operative League of the U.S.A., 1950.

Canadian Council on Social Development: *Community-Based Health and Social Services: Conference Report.* Ottawa, 1985.

Caplan E: *Remarks to the Ontario Hospital Association Conference on Comprehensive Health Organizations,* Don Mills, Ontario, April 5, 1989.

Chapman H et al: *The Contemporary Director.* Saskatoon: The Co-operative College of Canada, 1986.

Community Health Co-operative Federation: *Saskatchewan's Community Clinics: A Quarter Century of Innovation and Reform in Health Services.* Brief to the Saskatchewan Government, April 1987.

Epp, Honourable J: *Achieving Health for All: A Framework for Health Promotion.* Ottawa: Health and Welfare Canada, 1986.

Garoyan L, Mohn P: Equity versus equality within co-operatives. *Working Paper Series, No. 3.* Bank of Ireland Centre for Co-operative Studies, June 1984.

Gruending D: *The First Ten Years.* Saskatoon: Community Clinic, 1979.

Luft H: *Health Maintenance Organizations: Dimensions of Performance.* New York: John Wiley, 1981.

Marwick TE: Co-operatives and health services. Unpublished paper, 1985.

National Task Force on Co-operative Development: *A Co-operative Development Strategy for Canada: Report of the National Task Force on Co-operative Development,* May 1984.

Policy Research and Management Services Branch: *Community Clinic Study.* Regina: Saskatchewan Health, 1983.

Premier's Council on Health Strategy: *A Vision of Health: Health Goals for Ontario.* Toronto, 1989.

Rachlis M, Kushner C: *Second Opinion: What's Wrong with Canada's Health Care System and How to Fix It.* Toronto: Collins, 1989.

Saskatoon *Star-Phoenix:* Community health clinic benefits subject of still unreleased report, July 27, 1989.

Schreck D et al: *Presentation to the National Conference on Improving the Delivery of Community-Based Health and Social Services.* Ottawa: Co-operative Union of Canada Advisory Committee on Health Care Services, November 26, 1985.

Stergachis A: Use of a controlled trial to evaluate the impact of self-care on health services utilization. *Journal of Ambulatory Care Management* 9:16, 1986.

Sutherland RW, Fulton MJ: *Health Care in Canada: A Description and Analysis of Canadian Health Services.* Ottawa: The Health Group, 1988.

THE INDEPENDENT HEALTH FACILITIES ACT: A FIRST FOR NORTH AMERICA

Robert MacMillan
Marsha Barnes
Ontario Ministry of Health

INTRODUCTION

Ontario's health care system is a dynamic environment in which accepted policies, practices, and legislation are being questioned, challenged, and updated. This province has become fertile ground for testing new strategies and new organizational models. Words like "innovative", "creative", and "landmark" have found their way into the everyday conversation of health care professionals. With increasing frequency, the old ways are being reviewed and sometimes reconfirmed, sometimes revised, and sometimes replaced.

The *Independent Health Facilities Act* (IHFA) is only one small component of a larger revolution occurring today. This new piece of legislation, which was enacted on April 23, 1990, will permit the government to license and fund freestanding ambulatory care facilities in the province. This will include approximately 1,400 diagnostic facilities (radiology, ultrasound, nuclear medicine, pulmonary function) and an estimated 25 treatment facilities.

This paper presents an analysis of the forces that drove the development of this legislation, including a discussion of how the Act fits within the existing framework and why it may signal a change in managing this province's system. The opinions and perceptions expressed are those of the authors and are not a statement of government policy.

THE WINDS OF CHANGE

Why is the IHFA needed? What problems is it designed to solve? What forces brought it about? Where does it fit in the Ontario health care system?

The IHFA is not a panacea for all of Ontario's health care problems, nor is it a single purpose piece of legislation intended to resolve a particular gap in service. The IHFA evolved out of growing concerns in a number of areas and developed into a new legislative framework to govern the care and treatment given in freestanding community clinics.

Technological advances in medicine have been miraculous. Many diagnostic, medical, and surgical procedures once considered high risk and necessarily limited to hospitals may now be performed safely and efficiently in community settings. The IHFA provides a framework to capitalize on these changes and to permit the government to become more proactive in the management of Ontario's health care system.

Ontario's health care system was not designed to accommodate such a dramatic shift from the hospital to the community. There was no mechanism to fund overhead costs and none for structured approval or quality assurance. These are significant obstacles in a national health care system because they impede the movement of services into appropriate community settings and tie up expensive hospital resources unnecessarily.

PATIENT ACCESS

This virtually unregulated area created a window of opportunity for entrepreneurs to develop services and levy charges directly to patients. In a country which prides itself on universal access, this was indeed cause for concern.

Existing Ontario legislation, the *Health Care Accessibility Act* (HCAA) and the *Health Insurance Act*, were inadequate to meet this challenge. In 1986, the *Health Care Accessibility Act* was enacted to address extra-billing. This legislation prohibits charges to patients for insured physician services. In implementation, the HCAA was found to be inadequate to prohibit the growth of freestanding facilities where patients were "jumping queues" by paying for the additional overhead costs not covered by the Ministry. These costs were not prescribed by regulation as being part of the insured physician services because they had traditionally been covered through the hospital global budget.

The result of this absence of regulation and inability to cover the costs associated with providing these services in an out-of-hospital setting was a growth in freestanding facilities with patient participation in the cost of such services. The IHFA provides a mechanism to manage the growth of these facilities and to provide funding for overhead costs.

PRIVATE SECTOR PARTICIPATION

The private sector, entrepreneurialism and, heaven forbid, U.S. style medicine, are often considered dangerous to national health insurance. Some are showing a renewed interest in the benefits of private sector involvement and a recognition that there are significant advantages to the participation of the private sector as long as there are sufficient controls to protect those elements of the system that are seen as critical to our health insurance.

Whether we like it or not, the United States provides us with a looking glass on what is to come to Canada. If something is marketable and proves profitable in the U.S., it will not be long before it will be tried in Canada. Our health care system can benefit from much of the research and development costs borne by our U.S. neighbours, and we can learn from the types of management tools and techniques that abound in the private sector.

Even with the concern about and, sometimes, fear of the entrepreneur, there exists a recognition that there is a place in our system for private enterprise. There is also a recognized concomitant duty of the government to ensure that health care services provided by the private sector meet acceptable standards and quality. This is possible only with some sort of regulative or legislative controls.

The IHFA is an attempt to put into place a regulatory scheme which will permit the development of this "mixed economy". The private for profit sector is allowed to compete for facility ownership (although a preference for non-profit ownership must be given) and to manage facilities, but it must function within the specific regulatory framework of the Act – mandated quality assurance process, controls on ownership and share transfers, restrictions on license transfer and conditions of license, and legislated reasons for revocation and suspension.

MANAGEMENT

Ontario, like most industrialized nations, has seen a significant increase in costs for health care services. These increases are the result of a variety of factors, including an aging population, expensive technology, excessive institutionalization, increased demand for services, and increasing medical manpower.

This cost escalation has focussed attention on the expensive areas of health care: hospitals and physicians. Pressure exists to examine the use of our hospital services and ensure that they are being appropriately deployed and to look to lower cost community-based alternatives. It is acknowledged by many that the fee-for-service physician payment system is open to excessive use by both patient and provider. Care is free to the patient, and the physician has access to diagnostic and treatment services without consideration of cost.

The government has traditionally taken the position of passive payer of all claims submitted and, in a time of sufficient domestic wealth, this system was acceptable. However, with health care consuming over one third of the provincial budget, provincial politicians and administrators have become more concerned about the cost of health care and more insistent upon obtaining value for the money spent. This has led to two emerging policy shifts which are embodied within the IHFA: (1) requirements for quality assurance mechanisms and outcome reviews; and (2) increased government role in management of services.

The government is facing a double-edged sword in that it is expected not only to ensure the accessibility and availability of a broad spectrum of health care services but also to ensure that the tax burden does not become prohibitive or disproportionate to other publicly financed programs. Since the government is required to be accountable for the range, quality, and cost of health care services, it is essential that it have access to the tools needed to exercise this responsibility effectively.

The existing policies and legislation do not lend themselves easily to enhancing the role of the government in the management of the system. The emerging philosophy seems to be taking the form of a movement toward a healthy tension between the roles and responsibilities of government and those of the medical profession. Through this process it is hoped that the new partnership in management and development of our health care system will evolve.

The IHFA heralds the beginning of a new era in the relationship between the government and the medical profession. This is undoubtedly a time of tension, uncertainty, and the development of new respect and trust for each partner in this rejuvenation process. It will not be a transformation that occurs overnight or easily. By bringing all parties to the table and by presenting all sides of each position (supported with appropriate and accurate information), it is possible to gain a new appreciation for the position of the other players and to begin to develop a new shared vision which will accommodate each partner's needs balanced against those of the others. The added benefit of sharing a common goal is that it can often lead to innovative solutions and agreement on directions which can then be implemented expeditiously.

ROLE OF THE HOSPITAL

Canada has a very high rate of institutionalization and institutional care. This type of care is expensive, and there has been a recent move to become more cost conscious in the funding of hospitals.

Communities are being encouraged to examine requests for capital expansion of hospitals carefully and to consider alternatives. These alternatives often include the development of community ambulatory surgery facilities, and the IHFA provides one possible avenue to permit these to be explored.

ROLE OF THE HEALTH PROFESSIONALS

Physicians have been referred to as the "gatekeepers" of the health care system and, in large part, do control patient access to specific medical services.

The Ontario government has recognized the role of other health care professionals in our health care system. This is embodied in the *Health Professions Regulation Act* (HPRA), which was introduced in the legislature in the spring of 1990. There is a general acknowledgement that the system can be made more cost effective and that it is possible to provide better quality health care by effective use of non-physician health care professionals.

There is a real need to provide opportunities for these professionals to practice in communities outside of the hospital setting. The HPRA will go a long way to allowing these professions to be recognized as self-governing and independent, and the IHFA could provide new opportunities for practice.

WHERE DOES THE IHFA FIT?

The testing of different payment mechanisms, delivery models, and management structures continues to expand and evolve in the Ontario health care system. Some are simply expansions of existing programs, others represent a change in focus and structure of existing programs, and still others represent a transplantation and adaptation to the Ontario environment of models from other systems. Included are such activities as expanding community health centres and health service organizations, developing a network of pilot projects to test the comprehensive health service organization (Ontario's version of an HMO), and developing a hospital-in-the-home concept.

How does the IHFA fit within this framework and the existing and evolving legislative structure?

The IHFA capitalizes on many of the new directions embodied in these other initiatives – community development, de-institutionalization, de-medicalization, alternative funding, and participation of the private sector.

The delicate task ahead is to mesh the IHFA with other programs and legislation regulating complementary or, in some instances, the same areas in the health care system. Included are the *Healing Arts and Radiation Protection Act* which governs all X-ray facilities, the rewriting of the *Public Hospitals Act*, the move toward capital planning reviews which encourage ambulatory care facilities, the new self regulation of professions which could practice independently under the IHFA, and the obvious links with the *Health Insurance Act* and the *Health Care Accessibility Act*. These are massive undertakings steaming with controversy, and the changes will occur gradually.

WHAT'S INNOVATIVE, CREATIVE, OR LANDMARK?

Many features of the IHFA could be said to have been used to "test the waters" for various government policy directions, and others represent the first time that oft-articulated policies have been enshrined in legislation.

There is no single component of the IHFA that can be considered landmark in and of itself. It is the combination of elements which makes this legislation unique. The Act is certainly unique in Canada, and some interest has been expressed by other provinces in a similar type of legislative base. As always, much of what evolves in the Canadian health care system finds its roots in the United States. This is also true for the IHFA.

U.S. COMPARISONS

There are few studies that address the regulation of freestanding facilities in the United States. A recent GAO study chronicles the states' quality assurance mechanisms, and this information has been supplemented with an ad hoc survey of the legislation in 19 states.

Most freestanding facilities are essentially unregulated unless the individual states impose some sort of licensing and inspection requirements. For example, of 45 states having ambulatory care centres, 10 require licenses; of 34 states having diagnostic imaging centres, three require licenses; and of 50 states having ambulatory surgical centres, 41 require licenses.

Mandatory licensing of all types of freestanding providers is required only in New York and Montana. Other states were found to vary in the types of facilities requiring licenses. Even when licensing was required, 12 states reported not implementing requirements for certain types of providers, usually because regulations were new, had not been proclaimed, or did not apply to existing providers.

Of the 19 statutes reviewed, none required a competitive bidding process for licenses, and only three required any form of outcome review. Five of the 19 states required certificate of need reviews. From this limited review, there appears to be nothing in the United States as wide ranging as the IHFA.

RELATIONSHIP WITH THE MEDICAL PROFESSION

In Canadian society, the medical profession enjoys a special standing that has traditionally set it apart from other professional groups. This special status has recently become challenged because of a number of complex factors, including diligent media which have publicized the disputes between government and organized medicine over fee negotiations and funding for health care services. With rising health care costs and increasing public taxes, there has been an increased awareness by the public of the cost of health care and of physicians' incomes. With the change in physician lifestyles and in the image of the family physician who makes housecalls and is willing to spend more than 15 minutes with each patient, there has come a concomitant fall in the physician's status. This new image of the physician as a businessperson and entrepreneur instead of a benevolent giver of health has set the stage for a new relationship between government and practitioner. This relationship has become embodied in the IHFA and is seen by many as an infringement on physicians' autonomy to practice medicine.

One element of the IHFA which can be considered to be landmark, at least in the context of Ontario's health care system, is that this is the first time that the government has actually taken the initiative to rewrite its physician Schedule of Benefits – the list of fees that the physician will be paid for providing medically necessary services to Ontario residents.

This rewriting of the Schedule (actually a regulation under the *Health Insurance Act*) was necessary to accommodate the IHFA. Services that would become facility fees under the new Act were removed, and constituent elements of insured services which, as discussed earlier, form the basis of the IHFA, had to be more clearly defined. This change is one manifestation of the government's new approach toward the profession – one of equal partner rather than simply passive payer of claims.

The Act requires that new services covered by it be developed or expanded only when there has been recognition of an identified and documented need. This is a dramatic contrast from the previous situation, where physicians were free to practice wherever they wished and to provide whichever services they felt were required as long as those services were listed in the Schedule.

The impact has been by far the greatest on the practice of radiology, whose specialists will now be limited to practicing in hospitals and licensed facilities.

QUALITY ASSURANCE

Licensed independent health facilities will be required to participate in a quality assurance and outcome measurement program. A facility's results could affect its status for licensure and could be used to revoke a license if quality became a significant concern.

Whenever there is any type of funding control, there will always be concern about the quality of care. This makes it absolutely essential that attention is given to evaluating the quality of care provided to ensure that any restraints placed on cost or utilization are measured against the impact of that care. This recognition has led to the current interest in total quality management and to the attention to assessing services based upon parameters of practice and outcome reviews. The ultimate goal is to ensure that in the greatest number of instances the care the patient receives, the caregiver who provides it, and the time and setting in which it is delivered are the most appropriate.

The rationale behind this approach cannot be faulted, but what remains to be seen is how successful it will be in improving our health care and, more importantly, our health status. At the very least, there should be no decrease in these two factors and some improvement in cost-effectiveness. The research is still continuing on finding connections and direct relationships between setting standards/parameters/guidelines and the ability to effect change resulting in more cost-effective or better quality care.

This is one area where there seems to be potential to forge a true partnership between organized medicine and health care. It is a topic almost as good as motherhood and apple pie and is virtually impossible to argue against, that is, as long as the goal is to improve quality and not to control costs or to do "utilization reviews".

The program under the IHFA is being developed by the College of Physicians and Surgeons of Ontario (CPSO). The sheer number of facilities has necessitated that the process will be based largely upon a computerized monitoring system that will check an individual facility's performance against that of its peers. Initially, it may be necessary to adjust the established parameters to reflect current practice more appropriately. The obvious disadvantage of this approach is that it is a measurement against norms and may not, in fact, represent a statement of the practice that could achieve the best results. However, over time, with diligent monitoring of results, assessment of the parameters, and some research, it should be possible to reach a consensus on most procedures. There will always be the difficult area of emerging technologies and changing techniques and practices which will have to be addressed and integrated into the established and accepted system.

PLANNING

The Act combines a mandatory competitive request for proposal (RFP) process with a policy requirement for the participation of local District Health Councils in the development of new services. The competitive RFP permits all qualified proposers to bid for a license to establish the service. This is a move away from a situation in which a license would awarded to the first to request it rather than to the "best" one. There has been criticism about this process, suggesting that it could result in "bargain basement health care", where the lowest bidder would always be awarded the license. This attitude must be refuted by ensuring that there is a balanced review process to evaluate responses to RFPs with published review criteria. Cost is only one factor which will be taken into account when evaluating responses to RFPs.

The Act also allows for the strengthening of the role of District Health Councils and takes them a step closer to realizing the enhanced mandate being proposed. For the first time, councils will take their planning function one step further to evaluate responses to RFPs and comment on requests for facility expansion. This will assist the Ministry in the delicate task of determining whether a community need is best served by calling for an RFP to establish a new facility or by expansion of an existing facility. This determination is critical to permit new operators into the otherwise closed system created by the new licensing framework and to permit the development of services closest to the community they are designed to serve.

SYSTEM MANAGEMENT

One lever often used by governments to shape or control the system is the funding lever. This legislation has the unique aspect of allowing funding of all or any services provided in an IHF – funding is not restricted to insured and facility fee services. This is a significant advantage in allowing for the funding and delivery of a comprehensive "program" of services targeted at a specific need area. Some government programs are so streamlined and limited that it is often impossible to provide funding for a comprehensive range of services.

Access to fee-for-service billing for necessary health care services has been carefully guarded by the government, in that it is seen to be open-ended and often provides inappropriate incentives to the provision of appropriate health care. The IHFA provides the opportunity to develop more appropriate funding mechanisms through a combination of arrangements.

An area of considerable controversy is that associated with "maximum allowable consideration". This is the intangible amount that is ascribed to the value of a facility on sale and is often referred to as "goodwill".

The Act provides for the development of a formula for setting a value for each grandfathered facility for "goodwill"; for all new facilities this value will automatically be zero.

This will create a temporary two class facility system, with established facilities having a market value in excess of any new facilities. Maximum allowable consideration applies to both insured and facility fee service revenue streams and must be applied on a proportionate basis to any share transfers or partnership sales. This again is seen by some as an extreme intrusion into the business relationships of the private sector and, often, of individual physicians.

The experience of the Ministry of Health had been that once a licensing and regulatory system was introduced, the value of these licensed facilities escalated and the license itself became a commodity. This was entirely the result of the now relatively "closed" system created by the licensing framework. The Act is designed to attempt to prohibit the license from becoming a commodity in itself.

What has happened in other sectors is that the system quickly moves towards a near monopoly situation, with a few large corporations owning most of the services. Is this good for our health care system?

In Canada, there is a general feeling that "big" is bad and for-profit is even worse. There exists little hard evidence to indicate that this results in increasing the cost or decreasing the quality of services. There is a sense that it may be best to have a mixed system and a balance of types of facilities and operators to maintain that healthy competitive tension.

Another management tool which has been built into the legislation is the mandatory maximum five-year term of licensure. This requirement enhances the government's power to negotiate with individual facility operators to ensure that standards and conditions of license are adhered to. Difficulties have arisen in some areas where licenses have become virtually irrevocable, and the ability of the government to mandate the provision of quality care is undermined. In a completely unregulated, or inadequately regulated, area it is possible for a business to focus on profits and to compromise quality of patient care. This and other provisions in the IHFA provide added authority to the government to prohibit such occurrences.

The limited term of licensure has also been criticized as creating too unstable an environment to encourage business investments and creating a difficult position for securing capital financing from financial institutions. Whether this does in fact become a problem will not be known until we are further into the administration and implementation of the Act.

The IHFA brings the government further into the area of setting the legislative levers to control and direct private sector involvement in health care. With the explicit control and required reporting on ownership of facilities comes the potential to monitor and manage the potential development of conflict of interest. This is an area that has been of increasing concern and difficulty in the United States as physicians venture further into the arena of entrepreneurialism.

FLEXIBILITY

One of the most striking features of the Act is the significant regulation-making power. The flexibility given through regulation is so great that the Act is often seen as a framework within which the regulations will shape the real parameters of the legislation.

The opportunity exists to allow for extending the legislation to the primary provision of services by non-physician health care professionals. This would permit the funding and licensing of birthing centres run by midwives without physician participation. This is an area where there is great potential to allow the government to manage and provide some funding for a previously unregulated sector.

There is one limitation to much of this creativeness. As written, the IHFA cannot be easily applied to existing community services and can really be used only for new services. The transitional or "grandfather" provisions of the legislation are specific to facilities that existed prior to its enactment. No provision was made for the potential to include other facilities through regulation that were not originally envisioned as being included.

The second area of difficulty with extending the ambit of the Act is that once a service or cost has been prescribed as a "facility fee", there can be no charges for this service or cost to patients unless the facility is licensed as an IHF or exempted from the legislation. The result is that although the Act is flexible in what it may cover, it cannot be applied without automatically prohibiting the same service in the free market system.

CONCLUSION

The IHFA is a unique piece of legislation. It is complex and difficult to interpret and define. The IHFA has incredible potential and is almost so flexible that it is at times difficult to determine when and how it applies. This potential must be carefully nurtured so as to allow the legislation to take its rightful place in Ontario's health care system.

There has been much speculation and accusation about the real intentions of this legislation, and it is fair to say that there are likely many different objectives that could be achieved. There can be no question that it permits a legislated funding base for the logical expansion of services into the community. Nor can it be questioned that the Act embodies the current government position on the importance of quality assurance and outcome measures – these are explicitly stated in the Act and the CPSO is named as the principal agent through which this is to be assured. As to other presumed objectives, such as control of the profession or control of the volume of services, there is certainly the potential for this to occur. The Act brings the government into the realm of health system manager, and this is a dramatic move from the role of health system funder.

MODELS FOR INTEGRATING AND COORDINATING COMMUNITY-BASED HUMAN SERVICE DELIVERY: AN ANALYSIS OF ORGANIZATIONAL AND ECONOMIC FACTORS

Kent V. Rondeau
School of Health Services Administration, Dalhousie University

Raisa B. Deber
Department of Health Administration, University of Toronto

Incomplete, inadequate, and ineffective coordination and integration of human service delivery has become a convenient touchstone for describing what ails much of our health and social service system. Increasingly, the delivery of human services is described as being fragmented, discontinuous, dispersed, inaccessible, unaccountable, and wasteful of resources (Aiken et al, 1975; Gans and Horton, 1975; Lehman, 1975; Gage, 1976).

As public entitlements and expectations have escalated in recent years, human service needs have proliferated in tandem with an expanded concept of health and social justice. The evolution of our human service system is a process that can be described, among other things, as incremental (Lindblom, 1968), disjointed (Quinn, 1980), and emergent (Mintzberg and Jorgensen, 1987). However, this "system", or non-system, has become increasingly unwieldy and expensive and is widely criticized as unresponsive to demonstrated need.

Critics often assert that much of what is wrong with our human service system can be ameliorated with greater efforts at integrating service delivery. Unfortunately, past attempts at creating integrated services have all too often fallen far short of promise, at least partially because of a number of barriers (Redburn and Stevens, 1977; Wharf, 1977; Weiss, 1981; Deber and Rondeau, 1990).

This paper will identify some of the major political, social, and economic barriers to creating truly integrated human service delivery. Five models that illustrate how such delivery systems are normatively integrated and coordinated will be described and their ability to redress impediments to better human service integration compared.

BARRIERS TO INTEGRATED HUMAN SERVICE DELIVERY

Why have we not been more successful at creating a truly integrated human service delivery structure? A number of barriers can be identified.

Organizational autonomy and sovereignty are seen as a fundamental objectives by most organizations, and organizations tend to resist attacks on this autonomy (Litwak and Hylton, 1962; Thompson, 1967). There is a significant amount of evidence indicating that organizations facing minimal resource dependence and few external threats to their survival will strive to resist integration so as maintain their autonomy (Benson, 1975; Pfeffer and Salancik, 1978). Although organizations may be induced to develop cooperative relationships, most will be less likely to do so if they are required to accept externally sanctioned goals. Organizations will thus enter into collaborative relationships with others only to the extent that it is in their interests to do so. For those interested in fostering conditions that will facilitate the formation of interorganizational linkages, there must be sufficient inducements to facilitate the formation of cooperative associations.

Overarching *system complexity* – the sheer number of organizations and agencies involved in the planning and delivery of health and social services – is a major impediment to the development of a comprehensive, integrated human service system. As the number of system components increases, the ability to integrate across structures becomes profoundly problematic.

Impaired and contrary vision provides another barrier to effective human service integration. Blocked from the "big picture" of what human services could become by the blinders of current organizational arrangements, many agencies find it difficult to conceptualize and implement anything as comprehensive as an integrated human service delivery system. Equally, it is not clear whose mandate it is to create or sponsor such a system. Does the mandate belong to the federal government, the provincial government, local municipalities, public bureaucrats, citizen groups, human service institutions and organizations, or human service professionals? Has any of these stakeholders sufficient power, authority, or expertise to create an integrated system? Nor is it clear just what an "integrated human service system" really means, since the term may mean different things to different people. Some advocate integration that operates to the benefit of clients, making it easier for them to get the help they need when they need it. Others see integration as facilitating the work of human service providers, making it easier for them to do their jobs. Still others advocate integration that works to please administrators and funding authorities by cutting costs, eliminating waste, and increasing efficiency and financial accountability. Although these are all worthy goals, they are by no means identical. Different objectives imply contradictory courses of action.

Contrary and conflictual *professional ideologies* may hinder the formation of multidisciplinary human service teams. Different professions develop dissimilar perspectives about the main problems affecting the multiple-problem client (Wharf, 1977; Wilson, 1981). Not unexpectedly, each profession perceives its own area of expertise as the critical one, often seeing other professionals as incomplete caregivers. Separated by ideological, economic, and sociological barriers, human service professionals often have great difficulty in comprehending and facilitating the labour of their "colleagues", thus greatly undermining collaborative work.

A *lack of incentives* at the administrative level also serves to undermine integrated human service planning and delivery. It has been stated that the first law of public management is program preservation and maintenance of program integrity. The same can be said for program managers, whose worth is normatively evaluated on the basis of how well the organization provides its mandated service and not on the basis of their skill in establishing interorganizational linkages. There are too few incentives available in our present system to recognize and reward organizations for seeking and securing more collaborative arrangements.

Present *funding realities* also serve to frustrate the establishment of integrated human service delivery (Hokenstad and Ritvo, 1982). A patchwork of funding sources, coupled with a host of restrictions on their use, foster conditions that inhibit organizations and agencies from coming together to deliver integrated services.

A related phenomenon is the inability of human service providers to shift resources easily from one program to another. Economists refer to these economic and social costs which cannot readily be convertibled to secure other ends as *sunk costs*. Past practices, regardless of their success, often restrict future opportunities for change and development because they tend to lock-in resources by impairing assessments that can be used to determine where those resources could be more optimally placed (Boss, 1989).

The *uneven and fragmented capability of local governments* to integrate human service delivery effectively presents yet another obstacle. Although analysts believe that system integration has to begin at the local community level, municipal and regional governments appear to be the least equipped to be able to carry it out (Hagebak, 1979), nor do they have adequate autonomy of action to be able to do so sufficiently (Woodside, 1990). In most instances, municipalities lack sufficient authority, expertise, or resources to bring about the local integration of services, a reality which is amplified in most rural communities where resources and expertise are often at a premium (Ryant, 1976; Reid and Smith, 1984). In addition, the non-congruence of human service catchment areas with established municipal boundaries presents an additional complexity that serves to obstruct efforts aimed at local service integration. Dilemmas associated with multiple entry and exit points and the movement of the client through the system and across municipalities make it profoundly difficult to design processes that can monitor the movement of patients at the local level (Manga and Muckle, 1987).

Attempts at integrating human service delivery should be seen within the *political context*. The inherent partisan nature of publicly funded health and social services has important consequences for successful integration, because it implies that each actor in the system will seek to secure advantages that promote that actor's unique agenda. The most obvious consequence is that efforts to reform the system through increased system integration can become embroiled in political controversy on several levels. When this occurs, reform programs become tools in straightforward power struggles over control of scarce resources. Individuals and groups either promote or resist integration reforms because they see these reforms as changing the status quo. Naturally, each constituency is interested in a reform package that operates to its own relative advantage. In this context, political bargaining and coalition formation will become the organizational consequences of any efforts aimed at creating a better integrated system (Daft, 1989). The politicization of human service issues therefore means that competing groups will often be loath to work together to create integrated human service delivery, a disheartening consequence and one in direct contradiction to the kind of change that gave rise to the establishment of the reforms in the first place.

SYSTEM MODELS FOR INTEGRATING AND COORDINATING HUMAN SERVICES

What organizational arrangements are available that can reduce these impediments to collaborative association? Social theorists have examined the ways that organizational units can be structured so as to create greater collaborative action (Warren, 1967; Lehman, 1975; Provan, 1983; Gray, 1985; Goering and Rogers, 1985; Ritvo, 1987). Synthesis of this work allows one to identify five arrangements for coordinating and integrating human service delivery.

Voluntary coalition, the lowest form of integration, describes the loose arrangement of organizations, agencies, and units that voluntarily come together to achieve common objectives. Although maintaining their autonomy in most matters, members of a voluntary coalition affiliate over matters that provide mutual benefit and stability. The primary purpose of this arrangement is as much economic as political. Examples include such human service activities as the delivery of joint programs, cooperative insurance arrangements, the creation of trade associations, and the formation of interlocking boards.

Mandated coalitions differ from voluntary coalitions in that the organizations have been required by a third party, usually government, to coordinate some aspect of their function and work together to achieve common action. Although the organizations have been obliged to interact, the texture of their relationship is mutually determined by the participants. The purpose of this arrangement is to secure, by third party determination, coordinated effort through a process of dialogue and action. Increasingly, many types of human service institutions are being mandated to coordinate their operations on a number of fronts; examples include activities such as joint planning and purchasing arrangements.

Coalitions, both voluntary and mandated, are most appropriate where deliberate and cooperative interdependencies occur. They tend to be issue specific: participating organizations interact only with regard to a specific program/issue and retain their autonomy in all other matters (Warren, 1967). They do not, however, bring about any reduction in many of the barriers to better integrated human service delivery, such as promoting a uniform vision or unifying disparate professional ideologies. They are quite unable to achieve unity of purpose across disciplines, programs, or organizations.

Coalitions, although effective at creating conditions that facilitate more stability and collectivity of action, while still allowing for organizational autonomy, fall far short in reducing barriers to an integrated human service delivery system. What is needed is an organizational arrangement that more clearly and purposefully specifies the role and relationship of each participant. A federation is such an arrangement. In a federation, affiliated organizations agree to relinquish control over certain activities to the federation's mandate. In return, affiliated organizations expect the federation's management to minimize the complexity inherent in the system, reduce environmental uncertainty, and provide functional legitimacy. Federations differ from coalitions on the basis of control. When an organization becomes affiliated with a federation, it relinquishes at least partial control over decisions regarding those of its activities that are managed by a supraorganizational federative administration.

Affiliates in *voluntary federations* mutually agree to relinquish control over particular activities in exchange for certain benefits. Voluntary federations can be of two types: participative federations and independent federations. In participative federations, affiliates maintain an active role in federation management. In independent federations, a central administrative agency is created and is responsible for federation management. In both types of arrangements, the determination of goals and objectives is shared between the central federation management and each affiliate. Examples of voluntary federations in our human service system include the organization of the United Way in some jurisdictions, social service exchanges, hospital consortia, and some provincial home care programs.

In the *mandated federation*, organizations are forced by law to affiliate with the central management, although they are not expressly "owned" by it. The mandated federation differs from the voluntary federation in that goals and objectives of each affiliate are established by the central agency. Unlike the two types of voluntary federations, the major role of the central agency in a mandated federation is to represent the interests of third parties. It is this third party group, most often government, that gives the central agency its mandate and its right to control and legitimize the activities of affiliates. In a mandated federation, withdrawal from the federation by affiliates is prohibited. Examples of mandated federations typically include regional planning boards and councils.

Finally, when the affiliates are directly owned by the central agency a *conglomerate* or unitary type of arrangement is created. The amount of control over individual affiliates by the central office is variable, with some affiliates acting quite independently of the central office. Examples include such structural arrangements as holding companies, a number of horizontally and vertically integrated organizations, and many divisionalized structures. Unitary arrangements, for instance, include such organizations as General Motors, as well as the organization of a regional or state university system (Hodge and Anthony, 1988).

CONCLUSION

Do these models effectively reduce any of the cited barriers to integrated human services? Evidence suggests that coalition formation, whether voluntary or mandated, is somewhat effective at addressing impediments by reducing the degree of system complexity. Coalitions, however, do not sufficiently address problems caused by organizational autonomy, nor do they eliminate the conflict inherent in problems associated with competing values and ideologies. In addition, coalitions do not allow for the provision of adequate inducements to encourage organizations to coordinate or integrate their actions (Provan, 1983).

Federative arrangements, especially independent and mandated ones, are more effective at reducing these impediments because they more clearly specify the rights and obligations of each participating affiliate, while regulating actions from a central agency. Federations, however, may not be as effective at achieving subunit optimality of response because they diminish the degree of specialization that characterizes independent organizational action and autonomy. In addition, federations, with strong central agencies, are not without significant costs. The creation of a large federation human service bureaucracy to regulate and control the action of affiliates would no doubt be expensive and might require elaborate organizational arrangements to avoid being overcome by the requirements of excessive bureaucracy. For instance, one might envisage a scenario where a series of nested and integrated federations of human service organizations function on a number of different levels. Aiken and associates (1975) suggest that such coordination and integration would have to be made on at least four levels: resources, programs and services, clients, and information. They suggest that resources are best integrated at the societal level, programs and services at the human service organizational level, clients at the service delivery level, and information at all levels.

Short of complete system fusion which, for a variety of reasons, is unlikely to occur, how might we begin to move towards a more integrated human service delivery system? Perhaps the answer lies in designing a number of complementary and interdependent structures and processes whose collective action will begin to reduce these fundamental impediments on a variety of levels. This includes the creation of sufficient inducements that both require and reward participants to act collaboratively and cooperatively, while at the same time recognizing the positive aspects of autonomous action.

Regardless of the mechanisms we choose, it is important that we make integrated human service delivery an articulated public policy. Only by acting in this way can we provide the legitimacy and impetus for the creation of truly integrated structures.

REFERENCES

Aiken M, Dewar R, DiTomaso N, Hage J, Zeitz G: *Coordinating Human Services.* San Francisco: Jossey-Bass Publishers, 1975.

Benson J: The interorganizational network as a political economy. *Administrative Science Quarterly* 20:229-249, 1975.

Boss RW: *Organization Development in Health Care.* Reading, Massachusetts: Addison-Wesley, 1989.

Daft R: *Organization Theory and Design* (third edition). St. Paul, Minnesota: West Publishing Company, 1989.

Deber RB, Rondeau KV: *Coordination and Integration of Health Policies, Programs and Services: Annotated Literature Review on Evaluation Models* (2 volumes). Report prepared for Premier's Council on Health Strategy, March 1990.

Gage RW: Integration of human services delivery systems. *Public Welfare* 34:27-32, 1976.

Gans SP, Horton GT: *Integration of Human Services: The State and Municipal Levels.* New York: Praeger Publications, 1975.

Goering P, Rogers J: A model for planning interagency coordination. *Canada's Mental Health* 5-8 (March), 1986.

Gray B: Conditions facilitating inter-organizational collaboration. *Human Relations* 38:911-936, 1985.

Hagebak BR: Local human service delivery: the integration imperative. *Public Administration Review* 575-582 (November/December), 1979.

Hodge BJ, Anthony WP: *Organization Theory* (third edition). Boston: Allyn and Bacon, 1988.

Hokenstad MC, Ritvo RA: *Linking Health Care and Social Services: International Perspectives.* Vol 5 (Social Service Delivery Systems: An International Annual). London: Sage Publications, 1982.

Lehman EW: *Coordinating Health Care: Explorations in Inter-organizational Relations.* Beverly Hills, California: Sage Publications, 1975.

Lindblom CE: *The Policy Making Process.* Englewood Cliffs, New Jersey: Prentice-Hall, 1968.

Litwak E, Hylton L: Interorganizational analysis: a hypothesis on coordinating agencies. *Administrative Sciences Quarterly* 6:395-415, 1962.

Manga P, Muckle W: *The Role of Local Government in the Provision of Health and Social Services in Canada.* Ottawa: The Canadian Council on Social Development, 1987.

Mintzberg H, Jorgensen J: Emergent strategy for public policy. *Canadian Public Administration* 30:214-229, 1987.

Pfeffer J, Salancik GR: *The External Control of Organizations: A Resource Dependence Perspective.* New York: Harper and Row, 1978.

Provan KG: The federation as an inter-organizational linkage network. *Academy of Management Review* 8:79-89, 1983.

Quinn JB: *Strategies for Change: Logical Incrementalism.* Homewood, Illinois: Irwin Publications, 1980.

Redburn F, Stevens J: On human services integration. *Public Administration Review.*37:264-269, 1977.

Reid RA, Smith HL: Integrated rural health care systems: managerial implications for design and implementation. *Journal of Ambulatory Care Management* 13-28, (May) 1984.

Ritvo RA: Coordinating in-patient and out-patient services: the need for action. *Social Work in Health Care* 13:39-50, 1987.

Ryant JC: The integration of services in rural and urban communities. *Canadian Journal of Social Work Education* 2:5-14, 1976.

Thompson JD: *Organizations in Action.* New York: McGraw-Hill, 1967.

Warren R: The interorganizational field as a focus for investigation. *Administrative Science Quarterly* 12:396-419, 1967.

Weiss J: Substance vs. symbol in administrative reform: the case of human services coordination. *Policy Analysis* 7:21-45, 1981.

Wharf B: Integrated services: myths and realities. *Canadian Journal of Social Work Education* 3:24-31, 1977.

Wilson PA: Expanding the role of social workers in coordination of health services. *Health and Social Work* 6:57-64, 1981.

Woodside K: An approach to studying local government autonomy: the Ontario experience. *Canadian Public Administration* 33:198-213, 1990.

DISCUSSION
Chair: François Champagne
University of Montreal

Glenn Brimacombe (Ontario Medical Association)

I have two questions for Dr. MacMillan. My first question is, how do you envision the timetable to negotiate the global budgets in place of the current system of billing technical fees on a fee-for-service basis? And secondly, I'm curious as to which other provinces have expressed interest in this legislation.

Robert MacMillan (Ontario Ministry of Health)

The answer to the first question is that proclamation was the 23rd of April, so by the 23rd of April, 1991, we must have in place a license for every one of the sites that was given this grandfathered status and complies with the requirements to be licensed. So there is a very heavy schedule, inasmuch as there has been a delay in sending out the type of application we want to design to get all the information with one shot. The type of funding used to be, of course, totally on a fee-for-service basis. "Do whatever you want, add new equipment, whatever type of equipment, and start sending us the bill." Of course we saw this explosion of, in particular, free-standing X-ray facilities throughout the province and now, of course, all of them will be licensed by April of next year. The funding mechanism initially might to a great extent remain traditional – billing for a professional component and billing for a technical component, possibly within some parameters within the license. But indeed we will encourage and anticipate cooperative efforts in looking at globalizing the overhead costs of the technical side, possibly retaining a component of the fee-for-service model that most physicians want to retain on the professional side.

The answer to the second question is, I'm sorry, I don't know. My staff tell me that from time to time they are on the telephone with other provinces and I've spoken to a number of senior executives who are very interested, obviously. Now whether it's totally applicable to their setting is obviously in question, but certainly the model, if it proves effective, I think will be very much watched by other provinces who have no ability now, to a great extent, to control the growth of expensive out-of-hospital technology and medical services.

Jack Boan (University of Regina)

Question for Lars [Apland]. The development of a cooperative approach to the delivery of primary health care and other services is a laudable one, and I hope that we see a great deal more of that. But let's assume we had a lot of that in place, or mainly delivered primary care in that way. Does your organization, or has your organization, given any thought to how that is integrated with the next level of tertiary care – hospitals and so on?

Lars Apland (Canadian Co-operative Association)

I believe that right now there hasn't been a lot of thought in that area. I'm not entirely sure. It seems to me right now the focus is development at a primary level. Health Care Co-operatives – or health care for the co-operative sector – has really become an issue with

the Canadian Co-operative Association only since 1984, when a national task force identified it as one of the areas of potential for development.

Larry Wiser (Manitoba Ministry of Health)

Question for Kent Rondeau. Kent, you have a very nice description and organization
structure – progressive and incremental. If Nova Scotia is having these problems, we're
having them out in Manitoba as well. And I suggest that it may be more generalizable to a
lot of places in the country. I got a little bit lost, though, in the jump – the fourth one – the
mandated federation to the conglomerate – I'm not exactly sure what you meant by a conglomerate. I think you described it as a holding company, and I don't know anything
about holding companies, so maybe you can explain?

Kent Rondeau (Dalhousie University)

Terms such as "holding company" and "conglomerate" are frequently heard in business circles. A holding company is generally a large firm which owns enough shares in
several other companies so as to control them. A conglomerate is a type of holding company that controls a number of firms in unrelated fields of business activity. The governance of this type of arrangement is assured by the holding company owning enough
shares in the subsidiary firms so as to achieve control. Unity of action between the parent
firm and the subsidiaries is thus manifested through a complex web of interlocking direc-
torates and shared resources.

Richard Plain (University of Alberta)

I have a question for Dr. MacMillan. With respect to economies of scale on the diagnostic side, there is considerable concern that in many cases we have a multiplicity in some
provinces – I don't know whether it's the case in Ontario – of small types of facilities that
are high-cost producers, locked into a fee-for-service schedule that's far over and above
what you'd get in some type of an optimal – or a large scale – design with some reasonable
feeder elements. And what I wondered about in this procedure that you've set up, and
which it seemed like the District Health Councils were looking at, was where do we get a
look at the efficiency issues, and the economic issues, in this design? Is that in each component, or how is that carried out?

And the other thing is the Colleges – in Ontario, the College of Physicians and Surgeons
and its restrictions with respect to its practitioners and its accountability. When you talk
about the licensing, who is doing the licensing, how will the College on its side deal with
that, and what about any medical restrictions with respect to price competition or payment
or other modes?

Robert MacMillan

I was afraid that there was going to be an economist hit me. I thought you were going
to ask about how we were going to use QALYs in assessing outcome and I knew I'd be
dead, but I think I can try those two questions.

First of all, I didn't go into detail with respect to your last question, which was the role
of the College. Indeed, they are very intimately involved in the whole overview of the
quality side. And in the ability of government to impose itself so heavily on the profession

and their traditions, we of course carefully recognized that it was important that the College have an important role in order to gain that professional acceptance. The College is being funded by the Ministry of Health to develop standards – or, as they are now called, parameters, of practice. They have been funded very heavily to get on with it with respect to these guidelines and, in particular, how they will apply to the 25 treatment facilities in the first instance. In addition, they are empowered by the Act to be our assessors, so if there is breach or concern about quality on the side of the bureaucrats, it is not for us to go in and determine whether that has been breached. It's for the College to march in with the legislative authority, which as most of you know they don't have now, determining whether or not they are in breach of the Act, or substandard in quality. The first year they are probably going to be funded about $650,000 to perform those two functions, and it is a real step forward, I think, in Canada.

As far as the ability for government to become more involved on the management side of the fiscal equation, of course we are holding the bag now. It's not simply, "You go out and decide on your own that you want to do more and more of this, in more and more of these sites," and as you know, some of these are cartels now, where they are to a great extent owned by non-physician private companies – resulting in this explosion. We now control the number of sites. Obviously, there will be no new sites for a while in most areas of the province. And yet we can encourage it in areas such as the North, where such services may be deficient. We also, through our licensure and our budgetary negotiations, can do what we want to achieve the government's goal of becoming more controlled with regard to that budget. So again, not just an open-ended fee-for-service system, but certainly, initially, on the technological side, the overhead side, we can certainly work out a globe [global budget] which, to an extent, will control productivity.

Richard Plain

Just one last supplementary. In some of my experience, it turned out that some components of the public sector hospital-delivered system, many would argue, seemed to be able to provide at least a lower cost, or no worse cost, in terms of the delivery. Is the public sector free to compete with the private sector in these entrepreneurial activities? Is it a level playing field across the board? Because in many cases what's been done is to stop the public sector from competing with the private sector. In some cases, of course, it wouldn't have a chance, but in many cases, some would argue, it could beat the pants off it. But the existing regulations prevent it and stop it.

Robert MacMillan

That's a good point. And in fact until this Act there was no level playing field. Hospitals across the province were crying that just as they were finished their renovations and so on in their X-ray department, lo and behold, across the street was this private company that set up, and all the doctors were part owners, and of course that really cut off the out-patient flow (through which hospitals in Ontario, you may realize, generate considerable funds, in that they're still paid fee-for-service through OHIP). So there was no level playing field before. Ironically, since the Act was proclaimed, we see a slight tipping on the other side, and if you've heard some of the discussions this morning and yesterday about the opportunities for hospitals to get in on the game, of course we've seen some hospitals in Ontario now – just since the Act is proclaimed – trying to slip in their X-ray unit across the street with their colleagues. And there are these joint ventures. So it will be a level playing field in Ontario. Any hospital contemplating such entrepreneurial activity must have an approval by the Lieutenant-Governor-in-Council under Section 4 of our *Public Hospitals Act* – a section which I might add has been totally ignored by hospitals over the last several decades. So there will be this ability to issue licenses for for-profit, for not-for-profit, and to look at that in the context of what the local community hospital might want to offer within their global budget.

CLOSING REMARKS*
Conference Chair: Raisa B. Deber

We therefore conclude the Fourth Canadian Conference on Health Economics with the nice Canadian conclusion that there should be consensus, cooperation, and planning, but also that we should "just do it" without bothering to consult anybody! This is going to be a rather neat trick, particularly in the post-Meech Lake Canada, but I am optimistic with the conclusions that we have come to and hope that the next few years will see us actually taking steps to "get there from here".

The Fifth Canadian Conference, if we go to our usual schedule, will be three years from now. So the question is, where do we go from here? What happens to CHERA in the interim? We are delighted that there are so many new members. We hope that anybody who wants to work with CHERA to promote research in health services and linkages between the people who practice and the people who do the research will write or speak to members of the CHERA executive; we have plenty of committees eager for new volunteers.

This has also been a very notable meeting for CHERA; it marks the mellowing of Robert Evans. I hope this is only a temporary effect of becoming a B.C. Commissioner and that we will see Bob in full glory again.

The main thing I want to do here is thank people, because you can't have a meeting without an awful lot of work. And the first thing is the science. To have the science, you have to have a program committee. They were:

Geoff Anderson, University of British Columbia
André-Pierre Contandriopoulos, University of Montreal
Peter Coyte, University of Toronto
Raisa Deber, University of Toronto
Michael Loyd, Michael Loyd and Associates, Manitoba
Jackie Muldoon, Trent University
Doreen Neville, Memorial University
Bill Tholl, Canadian Medical Association
Jim Tsitanidis, Manitoba Department of Health
Mark Wheeler, Health and Welfare Canada

I'd particularly like to thank the speakers, because you can have a meeting and print up a program and if the people don't come and present good work, then you do not have a conference. I'd also like to thank the chairs, who did a wonderful job of keeping people on time; you'll see their names and contributions in this volume. The CHERA executive, particularly Bill Tholl, Mark Wheeler, and Morris Barer, and the chair of the Third Canadian Conference on Health Economics, John Horne, were very helpful.

If we didn't have the seed money, we couldn't have gone ahead, so I thank those who provided financial support. The Ontario Ministry of Health was enormously helpful; the Canadian Medical Association, the Canadian Hospital Association, and the Canadian Co-operative Secretariat also sponsored individual sessions.

I'm especially grateful to the secretaries to all of the people I dealt with, because I know where the real power lies and who is really doing the work and making sure things happen, and it's not us.

Special mention should be made of all those who worked behind the scenes to organize and run this meeting. The local organizing committee was chaired by Gail Thompson, with considerable assistance from Pamela Ko, who kept things going very smoothly and did an enormous amount of work quickly and accurately, including typing the proceedings; Ann Pendleton, who gave a lot of administrative assistance; Diane Nayda and Maria LoRé, who I hope will still speak to me, because they had to handle the books; and Peggy Leatt and Tina Pichler, who lent the auspices of the Institute of Health Management at University of Toronto. Our projectionist, John Kneller, managed to keep a lot of slides focused and take a fairly inflexible lighting system and make us fairly well able to see. Thanks to the people who provided and served the food, Mary and Jerry Catalfo of Nicola's Choice Meats on Eglinton – which I can recommend as one of the best grocery stores in town – and Gina, Nella, Antonietta, and our child labour, Sarina and Jonathan. The banquet location – Bangkok Gardens – handled health economists with flair. I'd like to thank the best-educated gopher squad who ever manned a desk. In addition to Gail Thompson and Ann Pendleton, we had the volunteer labour of Marianne Lamb, Sharmila Mhatre, Eleanor Ross, Mary Wiktorowicz, and Anne Wood – past and current graduate students, who I expect will become key members of our community in the future.

Kim Etherington, Abbie Vechter, Lesia Olexandra, and Dasha Pohoral of IMS Creative Communications were reponsible for coordinating, designing, and typesetting the Conference program and proceedings, and Suzanne Rancourt of the University of Toronto Press steered us through the production of this volume.

Finally, I would like to thank the people who programmed D-Base III and Wordstar, which enabled us to pretend that we were being far more individualized than we indeed were, and Nancy Wolff, whose presentation is going to allow me to tell Morris Barer why no computerized data base can be expected to add up perfectly.

Thank you, and I hope to see you at future conferences.

NOTE
* based on edited transcript of talk

LIST OF PARTICIPANTS
FOURTH CANADIAN CONFERENCE ON HEALTH ECONOMICS
August 27-29, 1990
University of Toronto

Julia Abelson
Harvard School of Public Health
21 Beacon Street, 9D
Boston, Mass. 02108, U.S.A.

Orvill Adams
Curry Adams and Associates
1015 - 130 Albert Street
Ottawa, Ont. K2A 2L3

Owen Adams
Can. Centre for Health Information
Statistics Canada
R.H. Coats Building, 18th Floor
Ottawa, Ont. K1A 0T6

Frank Adamson
Niagara District Health Council
P.O. Box 1059
1428 Pelham Street
Fonthill, Ont. L0S 1E0

Jean-Marie Albert
Fed. des Médecins Spécialistes du Québec
C.P. 216, Succursale Desjardins
Montreal, Québec H5B 1G8

Michael Alberti
B.C. Ministry of Health
1515 Blanshard Street
Victoria, B.C. V8W 3C8

Karim Amin
Ontario Ministry of Health
Audit Branch
7 Overlea Blvd., 7th Floor
Toronto, Ont. M4H 1A8

Geoffrey Anderson
University of British Columbia
Associate Director
Health Policy Research Unit
#400 - 2194 Health Sciences Mall
Vancouver, B.C. V6T 1Z6

Douglas E. Angus
Canadian Medical Association
1867 Alta Vista Drive
Ottawa, Ont. K1G 3X6

Aslam H. Anis
Simon Fraser University
Gerontology Research Centre
555 West Hastings Street
Vancouver, B.C. V6B 5K3

Lars Apland
University of British Columbia
Centre of Health Services and Policy
#429 - 2194 Health Sciences Mall
Vancouver, B.C. V6T 1Z6

Tariq Asmi
Ontario Ministry of Health
80 Grosvenor Street, Queen's Park
Hepburn Block, 8th Floor
Toronto, Ont. M7A 1R3

Wanda Assang
Children's Hospital of Eastern Ontario
401 Smyth Road
Ottawa, Ont. K1H 8L1

Mary Bacchus
Ontario Ministry of Health
Programs and Planning Division
80 Grosvenor Street, Queen's Park
Hepburn Block, 8th Floor
Toronto, Ont. M7A 1R3

Ronald S. Baigrie
University of Toronto
Sunnybrook Health Science Centre
2075 Bayview Avenue
North York, Ont. M4N 3M5

G. Ross Baker
University of Toronto
Department of Health Administration
McMurrich Building, 2nd Floor
Toronto, Ont. M5S 1A8

Ted Ball
President, Health Concepts Consultants
1231 Yonge Street, Suite 209
Toronto, Ont. M4T 2T8

Morris L. Barer
University of British Columbia
Health Services R & D
I.R.C. Building, 4th Floor
Vancouver, B.C. V6T 1Z6

Martin Barkin
National Practice Leader
Health and Social Services
Peat Marwick Stevenson & Kellogg
2300 Yonge Street
Toronto, Ont. M4P 1G2

Marsha Barnes
Ontario Ministry of Health
Alternative Funding Unit
49 Place d'Armes, 2nd Floor
Kingston, Ont. K7L 5J3

Jan Barnsley
University of Toronto
Hospital Management Research Unit
McMurrich Building, 2nd Floor
Toronto, Ont. M5S 1A8

Blair Barons
Comp. Health System Planning Com.
272 Dundas Street, 4th Floor
London, Ont. N6B 1T6

Bill Barrable
Ontario Hospital Association
150 Ferrand Drive
Don Mills, Ont. M3C 1H6

Shawn Barry
Alberta Health
7835 - 111 Avenue
Edmonton, Alberta T5H 1L1

Elizabeth Barton
The Toronto Hospital
585 University Avenue
Bell Wing 1-647
Toronto, Ont. M5G 2A2

Renaldo N. Battista
Director
Division of Clinical Epidemiology
Montreal General Hospital
1650 Cedar Avenue
Montreal, Quebec H3G 1A4

Andrea Baumann
McMaster University
Faculty of Nursing
1200 Main Street West, Room 2J40D
Hamilton, Ont. L8N 3Z5

Lillian Bayne
Greater Vancouver Reg. Hosp. District
4330 Kingsway Avenue
Burnaby, B.C. V5N 2C3

Dave Beavis
Health and Welfare Canada
Brooke Claxton Building, Room 1268
Tunney's Pasture
Ottawa, Ont. K1A 0K9

Pierre-Paul Bellerose
Chief, Med. Care
Health and Welfare Canada
Brooke Claxton Building, Room 1360
Tunney's Pasture
Ottawa, Ont. K1A 0K9

Alex Berland
Director of Surgical Nursing
Vancouver General Hospital
855 West 12 Avenue
Vancouver, B.C. V5Z 1M9

Charlie A. Bigenwald
Ontario Ministry of Health
Programs and Planning Division
80 Grosvenor Street, Queen's Park
Hepburn Block, 8th Floor
Toronto, Ont. M7A 1R3

Susanne Bjerno
Ontario Hospital Association
150 Ferrand Drive
Don Mills, Ont. M3C 1H6

Jean-Luc Blais
Merck Frosst Canada Inc.
16711 Trans Canada Highway
Kirkland, Quebec H9R 4P8

Jack Boan
University of Regina
Department of Economics
Regina, Sask. S4S 0A2

Ronald Bodrug
President
Scarborough General Hospital
3050 Lawrence Avenue East
Scarborough, Ont. M1P 2V5

Hildo B. Bolley
University of Toronto
Hospital Management Research Unit
McMurrich Building, 2nd Floor
Toronto, Ont. M5S 1A8

Roy Bonazza
Ontario Ministry of Health
Client Services Branch
Planning and Design
49 Place d'Armes, 2nd Floor
Kingston, Ont. K7L 5J3

Hélène Bouchard
University of Toronto
Department of Health Administration
McMurrich Building, 2nd Floor
Toronto, Ont. M5S 1A8

Gill Boyde
Ontario Ministry of Health
15 Overlea Blvd., 2nd Floor
Toronto, Ont. M4H 1A9

Glenn Brimacombe
Canadian Medical Association
1867 Alta Vista Drive
Ottawa, Ont. K1G 3Y6

Paul Brochu
Ontario Ministry of Health
381 Borden Avenue
Newmarket, Ont. L3Y 5C1

Murray G. Brown
Dalhousie University
Dept. of Community Health and
Epidemiology
Halifax, N.S. B3H 4H7

Pat Brown
Ontario Ministry of Health
Hospital Planning Branch
15 Overlea Blvd., 7th Floor
Toronto, Ont. M4H 1A9

Sheila Brown
Mount Allison University
Sackville, N.B. E0A 3C0

Guy Bujold
Health and Welfare Canada
Brooke Claxton Building, Room 1400
Tunney's Pasture
Ottawa, Ont. K1A 0K9

Charlotte Burkhardt
Homewood Health Centre
150 Delhi Street
Guelph, Ont. N1E 6K9

Fay Burton
Community and Social Services
3220 Dundas Street West
Toronto, Ont. M6P 2A3

Lynda Buske
Health and Welfare Canada
Brooke Claxton Building, Room 1370
Tunney's Pasture
Ottawa, Ont. K1A 0K9

Jim Butler
Australian National University
National Ctr. for Epidemiology and
Population Health (NCEPH)
G.P.O. Box 4
Canberra, ACT 2601 Australia

Tom Butt
Agnew, Peckham and Assoc. Ltd.
1300 Yonge Street, #700
Toronto, Ont. M4T 1X3

Bradford Buxton
Patented Medicine Prices Review Board
359 Kent Street
Ottawa, Ont. K1R 7X5

François Camirand
Chef du service Evaluation -
Recouvrement de la santé
Direction de l'Evaluation
Ministère de la Santé et des Services sociaux
1075, Chemin Ste-Foy, 3e étage
Québec, Québec G1S 2M1

Frances Caruth
Dir., Planning and Development
B.C. Cancer Agency
600 West 10th Avenue
Vancouver, B.C. V5Z 4E6

François Champagne
GRIS - Universite de Montreal
C.P. 6128, STA "A"
Montreal, Québec H3C 3J7

Denis Charette
Ontario Ministry of Health
French Language Health Services
80 Grosvenor Street, Queen's Park
Hepburn Block, 7th Floor
Toronto, Ont. M7A 1R3

Y.M. Cheung
Alberta Health
Health Economics and Statistics
Box 2222
11010 - 101 Street
Edmonton, Alberta T5J 2P4

Yoka Chung
Ontario Ministry of Health
15 Overlea Blvd., 2nd Floor
Toronto, Ont. M4H 1A9

Carolyn Clancy
Medical College of Virginia
Box 254, MCV Station
Richmond, VA 23298, U.S.A.

Carol Clemenhagen
President
Canadian Hospital Association
17 York Street
Ottawa, Ont. K1N 9J6

Bruce W. Cliff
Exec. Vice President
Professional Services
Centenary Hospital
2867 Ellesmere Road
Scarborough, Ont. M1E 4B9

Marsha M. Cohen
University of Toronto
Sunnybrook Health Sciences Centre, A443
2075 Bayview Avenue
Toronto, Ont. M4N 3M5

Lynn Cook
University of Alberta Hospitals
8440 - 112th Street
Edmonton, Alberta T6G 2B7

Brian D. Copley
Asst. Dep. Minister
B.C. Ministry of Health
7-1, 1515 Blanshard Street
Victoria, B.C. V8W 3C8

Peter C. Coyte
University of Toronto
Department of Health Administration
McMurrich Building, 2nd Floor
Toronto, Ont. M5S 1A8

Lynda Cranston
Richmond General Hospital
700 Westminster Highway
Richmond, B.C. V6X 1A2

Gloria Crotin
President
York Central Hospital
10 Trench Street
Richmond Hill, Ont. L4C 4Z3

A.J. Culyer
University of York
Dept. of Economics and Related Studies
Heslington, York Y01 5DD U.K.

Lynn Curry
Curry Adams and Associates
1015 - 130 Albert Street
Ottawa, Ont. K2A 2L3

Robert Cushman
Dalhousie Health Services, Ottawa
755 Somerset Street West
Ottawa, Ont. K1R 6R1

Debora Daigle
District Health Council of Eastern Ontario
340 Pitt Street, Suite 300
Cornwall, Ont. K6J 3P9

Joanne Daniel
Mount Sinai Hospital
600 University Avenue, Room 342
Toronto, Ont. M5G 1X5

Leslie Daniels
1960 Escarpa Drive
Los Angeles, California 90041-3015, U.S.A.

Judi David
Canadian Medical Association
P.O. Box 8650
Ottawa, Ont. K1G 0G8

Sam Mathwin Davis
Queen's University
School of Public Admin.
Kingston, Ont. K7L 3N6

Heather Dawson
Ontario Hospital Association
138 Banff Road
Toronto, Ont. M4P 2P5

Frank DeFelice
Ontario Ministry of Health
Programs and Planning
Health Program Unit
80 Grosvenor Street, Queen's Park
Hepburn Block, 8th Floor
Toronto, Ont. M7A 1R3

J. Kenneth Deane
Exec. Vice President
Welland County Gen. Hospital
Third Street
Welland, Ont. L3B 4W6

Raisa B. Deber
University of Toronto
Department of Health Administration
McMurrich Building, 2nd Floor
Toronto, Ont. M5S 1A8

Gilles Y. Derome
Sandoz Canada Inc.
P.O. Box 385
Dorval, Quebec H9R 4P5

John Dicaire
Dept. Health and Community Services
P.O. Box 5100, Carleton Place
Fredericton, N.B. E3B 5G8

Maureen Dixon
Director
Institute of Health Services Management
15 Portland Place
London, W1N 4AN U.K.

Ken Doepker
B.C. Health Association
500 - 1985 West Broadway
Vancouver, B.C. V6J 4Y3

John Dorland
Queen's University
Abramsky Hall, 3rd Floor
Kingston, Ont. K7L 3N6

Cathy Dunlop
Comp. Health System Planning Comm.
272 Dundas Street, 4th Floor
London, Ont. N6B 1T6

Marilyn Dunlop
Toronto Star
1 Yonge Street
Toronto, Ont. M5E 1E5

Martine Durier-Copp
Minister of Health and Fitness
Minister's Implementation Committee
P.O. Box 488
Halifax, N.S. B3J 2R8

Richard J. Dyke
Medical Society of Nova Scotia
6080 Young Street, Suite 305
Halifax, N.S. B3K 5L2

Richard Edwards
28 Walker Avenue
Toronto, Ont. M4V 1G2

Steve Elson
Assistant Executive Director
Niagara District Health Council
P.O. Box 1059
1428 Pelham Street
Fonthill, Ont. L0S 1E0

Al Erlenbusch
Ontario Ministry of Health
Emergency Health Services
7 Overlea Blvd., 7th Floor
Toronto, Ont. M4H 1A8

Robert G. Evans
University of British Columbia
429 - 2194 Health Sciences Mall
Vancouver, B.C. V6T 1E6

Val Evans
Chedoke-McMaster Hospitals
P.O. Box 2000, Station A
Hamilton, Ont. L8N 3Z5

Jann Everard
Ontario Ministry of Health
Teaching and Specialty Hospitals Branch
15 Overlea Blvd., 7th Floor
Toronto, Ont. M4H 1A9

Michael Farnworth
McMaster University
698 Francis Road
Burlington, Ont. L7T 3X7

Trixie Fee
Hamilton Civic Hospitals
Henderson General Division
711 Concession Street
Hamilton, Ont. L8V 1C3

Rashi Fein
Harvard Medical School
643 Huntington Avenue
Boston, Mass. 02115, U.S.A.

Brian Ferguson
University of Guelph
Department of Economics
Guelph, Ont. N1G 2W1

Susan Fitzpatrick
Ontario Ministry of Health
Claims Payment Division
49 Place d'Armes, 2nd Floor
Kingston, Ont. K7L 5J3

Martha Forestell
Ontario Ministry of Health
Women's Health Bureau
880 Bay Street, Suite 215
Toronto, Ont. M5S 1Z8

Sylvie Forgues-Martel
University of Ottawa
Heart Institute
1053 Carling Avenue
Ottawa, Ont. K0A 3B0

Denis Fortin
Ontario Ministry of Health
French Language Health Services
80 Grosvenor Street, Queen's Park
Hepburn Block, 7th Floor
Toronto, Ont. M7A 1R3

Amiram Gafni
McMaster University
Dept. of Clin. Epi. and Biostat.
CHEPA, 2C 12A
Health Sciences Centre
Hamilton, Ont. L8S 3Z5

Maris Gailitis
Ontario Ministry of Health
15 Overlea Blvd., 2nd Floor
Toronto, Ont. M4H 1A9

Paul Gamble
President
Hospital Council of Metropolitan Toronto
2 Carlton Street, Suite 1511
Toronto, Ont. M5B 1J3

Mary Gauld
McMaster University
Health Sciences Centre, 2C2
1200 Main Street West
Hamilton, Ont. L8S 3Z5

Mary Lou Gignac
Ontario Ministry of Health MCSS
Community Health and Support Services
56 Wellesley Street West, 8th Floor
Toronto, Ont. M5S 2S3

Boyde Gill
Ontario Ministry of Health
Coordinator
User Support Branch
15 Overlea Blvd., 2nd Floor
Toronto, Ont. M4H 1A9

Vivek Goel
Ontario Workers' Compensation Institute
250 Bloor Street East, Suite 702
Toronto, Ont. M4W 1E6

Ron A. Goeree
McMaster University
Health Sciences Centre
1200 Main Street West
Hamilton, Ont. L8S 4K1

Sandra Golding
CLSC Lac-Saint-Louis
145 Cartier
Pointe-Claire, Quebec H9S 4R9

Janet Greb
McMaster University
Dept. of Clin. Epi. and Biostat.
Health Sciences Centre, Room 3V 43A
Hamilton, Ont. L8N 3Z5

John Greschner
B.C. Ministry of Health
1515 Blanshard Street
Victoria, B.C. V8W 3C8

Doris Grinspun
Mount Sinai Hospital
600 University Avenue
Toronto, Ont. M5G 1X5

Dominic Haazen
B.C. Ministry of Health
6-1, 1515 Blanshard Street
Victoria, B.C. V8W 3C8

Paddy Hanlon
St. Joseph's Health Centre
30 The Queensway
Toronto, Ont. M6R 1B5

Brian Hayday
Executive Director
Ontario Prevention Clearinghouse
984 Bay Street, Suite 603
Toronto, Ont. M5S 2A5

Scott J. Hebert
Asst. to the President
Victoria Hospital Corporation
800 Commissioners Road East
Executive Offices - WT
London, Ont. N6A 4G5

Georgia Henderson
Task Force on the Use and
Provision of Medical Services
700 Bay Street, 14th Floor
Toronto, Ont. M5G 1Z6

Stephen W. Herbert
Baycrest Centre for Geriatric Care
3560 Bathurst Street
North York, Ont. M6A 2E1

Lynda Hessey
Ontario Ministry of Health
15 Overlea Blvd., 6th Floor
Toronto, Ont. M4H 1A9

Vern Hicks
Manager, Research and Statistics
Maritime Medical Care Inc.
P.O. Box 2200
Halifax, N.S. B3J 3C6

John A. Higenbottam
British Columbia Mental Health Society
Riverview Hospital
500 Lougheed Highway
Port Coquitlam, B.C. V3C 4J2

Nora Ho
Ontario Ministry of Health
15 Overlea Blvd., Room 726
Toronto, Ont. M4H 1A9

John A. Hoar
N.S. Health Services and
Insurance Commission
P.O. Box 760
Halifax, N.S. B3J 2V2

Jake Hodosy
Hansen - Toronto
620 Daytona Drive
Fort Erie, Ont. L2A 4Z4

John Horne
Sen. Vice President
Corporate Planning and Development
Health Science Centre
820 Sherbrooke Street
Winnipeg, Man. R3A 1R9

Jeremiah Hurley
McMaster University
Dept. Clin. Epi. and Biostat.
Health Sciences Centre, Room 3H2
Hamilton, Ont. L8N 3Z5

Sue Hyatt
Premier's Council on Health Strategy
56 Wellesley Street West, 15th Floor
Toronto, Ont. M5S 2S3

John Iglehart
2 Wisconsin Circle, Suite 500
Chevy Chase, Maryland 20815, U.S.A.

Juan Roberto Iglesias
Ministère de la Santé et
des Services sociaux
1075, chemin Ste-Foy
Québec, Québec G1S 2M1

Susan Iles
Exec. Coordinator
Victoria Health Project
2101 Richmond Avenue
Victoria, B.C. V8R 4R7

Diane Irvine
University of Toronto
Department of Health Administration
McMurrich Building, 2nd Floor
Toronto, Ont. M5S 1A8

Philip Jacobs
University of Alberta
Faculty of Medicine
Dept. of Health Serv. Admin./Comm. Med.
Clinical Sci.Building, 13-103
Edmonton, Alberta T6B 2G3

K. Helena Jaczek
York Region Public Health Department
22 Prospect Street
Newmarket, Ont. L3Y 3S9

Ken Jaggard
B.C. Health Association
500 - 1985 West Broadway
Vancouver, B.C. V6J 4Y3

Robert Jin
40 Gerrard Street East, Suite 1203
Toronto, Ont. M5B 2E8

Naushad Jinah
Queensway General Hospital
150 Sherway Drive
Etobicoke, Ont. M9C 1A5

Peter C. Johnson
Vice President, Hamilton Civic Hospitals
Henderson General Division, C.O.O.
711 Concession Street
Hamilton, Ont. L8V 1C3

Maija Kagis
NHRDP
Health and Welfare Canada
521 Jeanne Mance Building
Tunney's Pasture
Ottawa, Ont. K1A 1B4

Liza Kallstrom
B.C. Health Association
500 - 1985 West Broadway
Vancouver, B.C. V6J 4Y3

Joyce Kalsen
Toronto East Gen. and Ortho. Hosp.
825 Coxwell Avenue
Toronto, Ont. M4C 3E7

Elizabeth Kannon
Children's Hospital of Eastern Ontario
401 Smyth Road
Ottawa, Ont. K1H 8L1

Rosamond Katz
U.S. General Accounting Office
330 C Street, S.W.
Switzer Building, Room 1115
Washington, D.C. 20201, U.S.A.

Karyn Kaufman
Ontario Ministry of Health
880 Bay Street, Suite 215
Toronto, Ont. M5S 1Z8

David Kelly
Alberta Health
10025 Jasper Avenue
Edmonton, Alberta

Merrijoy Kelner
University of Toronto
Department of Behavioural Science
McMurrich Building
Toronto, Ont. M5S 1A8

Perry Kendall
Toronto Dept. of Public Health
East Tower, City Hall, 7th Floor
100 Queen Street West
Toronto, Ont. M5H 2N2

Joan Kennedy
Ontario Ministry of Health
15 Overlea Blvd., 2nd Floor
Toronto, Ont. M4H 1A9

Catherine Knipe
Saskatchewan Health
3475 Albert Street
Regina, Sask.

Hans Krueger
Senior Health Systems Analyst
Management Support Services
Vancouver General Hospital
855 West 12th Avenue
Vancouver, B.C. V5Z 1M9

Vaibhav J. Kulkarni
University of Toronto

Carol Kushner
Health Concepts Consultants
83 Wroxeter Avenue
Toronto, Ont. M4J 1E7

Roberta Labelle
McMaster University
Dept. of Clin. Epi. and Biostat.
CHEPA, 2C10-HSC
1200 Main Street West
Hamilton, Ont. L8N 3Z5
(deceased)

Ron Labonte
President
Ontario Public Health Association
468 Queen Street East, Suite 202
Toronto, Ont. M5A 1T7

Marianne Lamb
University of Toronto
Department of Health Administration
McMurrich Building, 2nd Floor
Toronto, Ont. M5S 1A8

Eric A. Latimer
Harvard School of Public Health
677 Huntington Avenue
Kresge 309
Boston, Mass. 02115, U.S.A.

Evelyn H. Lazare
Lazare Associates Inc.
1425 Bayview Avenue, Suite 105
Toronto, Ont. M4G 3A9

A. Eugene LeBlanc
Executive Director of Corporate Policy
Ontario Ministry of Health
80 Grosvenor Street, Queen's Park
Hepburn Block, 8th Floor
Toronto, Ont. M7A 1R3

J. Arthur LeBlanc
Co-operatives Secretariat
Sir John Carling Building, 10th Floor
Ottawa, Ont. K1A 0C5

Peggy Leatt
University of Toronto
Department of Health Administration
McMurrich Building, 2nd Floor
Toronto, Ont. M5S 1A8

David W. Lee
American Medical Association
535 N. Dearborn Street
Chicago, Illinois 60610, U.S.A.

Sidney S. Lee
Harvard Medical School
Department of Social Medicine
643 Huntington Avenue
Boston, Mass. 02115, U.S.A.

Sandra Leggat
Director of Planning
Baycrest Centre for Geriatric Care
3560 Bathurst Street
North York, Ont. M6A 2E1

Patricia Lemay
Science Council of Canada
100 Metcalf Street, 17th Floor
Ottawa, Ont. K1P 5M1

Louise Lemieux-Charles
University of Toronto
Hospital Management Research Unit
McMurrich Building, 2nd Floor
Toronto, Ont. M5S 1A8

Marion Leslie
The Toronto Hospital
585 University Avenue
Bell Wing 1-649
Toronto, Ont. M5G 2A2

Karen Levenick
Executive Director
Grey-Bruce District Health Council
945 3rd Avenue East, Suite 5
Owen Sound, Ont. N4K 2K8

Bev Lever
Ontario Ministry of Health
15 Overlea Blvd., 4th Floor
Toronto, Ont. M4H 1A9

Esther Levy
9 Menin Road
Toronto, Ont. M6C 3J1

Jack Lichter
Kingston, Frontenac and Lennox and
Addington District Health Council
P.O. Box 1690
544 Princess Street
Kingston, Ont. K7L 5J6

Karen Lichter
Ontario Ministry of Health
Alternative Funding Unit
49 Place d'Armes, 2nd Floor
Kingston, Ont. K0K 3G0

Mary Catherine Lindberg
Asst. Dep. Minister
Ontario Ministry of Health
Consumer Health and Planning
80 Grosvenor Street, Queen's Park
Hepburn Block, 9th Floor
Toronto, Ont. M7A 1R3

Adam L. Linton
Ontario Medical Association
Victoria Hospital
375 South Street
London, Ont. N6A 4G5

Stan A. Lissack
Astra Pharma Inc.
1004 Middlegate Road
Mississauga, Ont. L4Y 1M4

Dorothy Loranger
Ontario Ministry of Health
Community Health Branch
15 Overlea Blvd., 6th Floor
Toronto, Ont. M4H 1A9

Michael Loyd
45 Vavasour Avenue
Winnipeg, Man. R3C 2B5

Brenda Lundman
Employment and Immigration Canada
222 Remic Avenue
Ottawa, Ont. K1E 5W5

Jeanette MacAulay
Hospital and Health Services Comm.
P.O. Box 3000
Montague, P.E.I. C0A 1R0

Anne MacDonald
St. Joseph's Health Centre
30 The Queensway
Toronto, Ont. M6R 1B5

Sue MacDonald
Toronto East Gen. and Ortho. Hosp.
825 Coxwell Avenue
Toronto, Ont. M4C 3E7

Hugh MacKay
N.S. Department of Health
24 Dundas Street, Apt. #101
Dartmouth, N.S. B2Y 42L

Judith MacKenzie
Kingston, Frontenac and Lennox and
Addington District Health Council
P.O. Box 1690
544 Princess Street
Kingston, Ont. K7L 5J6

Robert M. MacMillan
Ontario Ministry of Health
Health Ins. Div.
49 Place d'Armes, 2nd Floor
Kingston, Ont. K7L 5J3

Don MacNaught
Health and Welfare Canada
Brooke Claxton Building, Room 1330
Tunney's Pasture
Ottawa, Ont. K1A 0K9

Kathleen MacPherson
Camp Hill Medical Centre
Veterans Mem. Building, Room 2653
1763 Robie Street
Halifax, N.S. B3H 3G2

John Maher
Cancer 2000 Task Force
77 Bloor Street West, Suite 1711
Toronto, Ont. M5S 3A1

Eileen Mahood
Ontario Ministry of Health
199 Larch Street, 8th Floor
Sudbury, Ont. P3E 5R1

Patricia Malcolmson
Ontario Ministry of Health
Claims Pay. Div.
49 Place d'Armes, 2nd Floor
Kingston, Ont. K7L 5J3

Gigi Mandy
Health and Welfare Canada
Health Insurance Directorate
Jeanne Mance Building, Room 615
Tunney's Pasture
Ottawa, Ont. K1A 1R4

Frank Markel
Vice President
Planning and Development
St. Joseph's Health Centre
30 The Queensway
Toronto, Ont. M6R 1B5

John Marriott
Ontario Ministry of Health
CHO Program
49 Place D'Armes, 4th Floor
Kingston, Ont. K7L 5J3

Deborah Marshall
University Hospital
4500 Oak Street
Vancouver, B.C. V6H 3N1

Joan Marshman
64 Araman Drive
Agincourt, Ont. M1T 2P6

Thomas E. Marwick
Regina Community Clinic
3765 Sherwood Drive
Regina, Sask. S4R 4A9

Sarah Mason-Ward
St. Joseph's Health Centre, London
268 Grosvenor Street
London, Ont. N6A 2C9

Rosemarie B. Mattocks
113 - 3907 Grant Avenue
Winnipeg, Man. R3R 2W2

Michael McEwen
Ontario Ministry of Health
Health Planning Branch
15 Overlea Blvd., 6th Floor
Toronto, Ont. M4H 1A9

Maurice McGregor
Le Conseil d'évaluation des
technologies de la santé
800, Place Victoria (bureau 42.05)
Case postale 215
Montréal, Québec H4Z 1E3

Allan McIntosh
Co-operatives Secretariat
Government of Canada
930 Carling Avenue, 10th Floor
Ottawa, Ont. K1A 0C5

James L. McIntyre
Premier's Council on Health Strategy
48 Ford Street
Sault Ste. Marie, Ont. P6A 4N4

John McLachlan
Director of Psychology
Peel Memorial Hospital
20 Lynch Street
Brampton, Ont. L6W 2Z8

Sister Winifred McLoughlin
Executive Director
Sudbury General Hospital
700 Paris Street
Sudbury, Ont. P3E 3B5

Brian R. McNab
Ontario Ministry of Health
Health Insurance Division
49 Place D'Armes, 2nd Floor
Kingston, Ont. K7L 5J3

Ron McQueen
University of Toronto
Department of Health Administration
McMurrich Building, 2nd Floor
Toronto, Ont. M5S 1A8

Christopher R. Mee
Director
Ministry of Health
217 York Street, 5th Floor
London, Ont. N6A 1B7

Michael Mendelson
Deputy Secretariat of the Cabinet
Main Legislature Bldg., Room 381
Queen's Park
Toronto, Ont. M7A 1A1

Grahame Meredith
Community Hospitals Branch
Ontario Ministry of Health
15 Overlea Blvd., 5th Floor
Toronto, Ont. M4H 1A9

Yesook Merrill
U.S. General Accounting Office
441 G Street, N.W.
Washington, D.C. 20548, U.S.A.

Sharmila Mhatre
University of Toronto
Department of Health Administration
McMurrich Building, 2nd Floor
Toronto, Ont. M5S 1A8

Robert Miller
University of California - San Francisco
Institute for Health and Aging
N631, Box 0612
San Francisco, California 94143, U.S.A.

Lenore Mills
Ont. Council of Teaching Hospitals
56 Wellesley Street West, Suite 310
Toronto, Ont. M5S 2S3

Isabel Milton
The Mississauga Hospital
100 Queensway West
Mississauga, Ont. L5B 1B8

Brenda Mitchell
Ontario Ministry of Health
Health Promotion Branch
700 Bay Street, Suite 1401
Toronto, Ont. M5E 1Z6

Peter Mix
Statistics Canada
Can. Centre for Health Information
R.H. Coats Building, 18th Floor
Ottawa, Ont. K1A 0T6

Shirley Moffs
Ontario Pharmacists Assoc.
99 Avenue Road
Toronto, Ont. M5R 2G5

Peter Molnar
Ont. Ministry of Industry, Trade
and Technology
900 Bay Street
Hearst Block, 7th Floor
Toronto, Ont. M7A 2E1

Rory Molnar
Manitoba Medical Association
125 Sherbrook Street
Winnipeg, Man. R3C 2E5

David L. Mowat
Kingston, Frontenac and Lennox
and Addington Health Unit
211 Portsmouth Avenue
Kingston, Ont. K7M 1V5

Jackie Muldoon
Trent University
Department of Economics
Peterborough, Ont. K9J 7B8

Linda Murphy
Health and Welfare Canada
Extramural Research Programs - NHRDP
518 Jeanne Mance Building
Tunney's Pasture
Ottawa, Ont. K1A 1B4

Michael Murray
University of Toronto
Hospital Management Research Unit
McMurrich Building, 2nd Floor
Toronto, Ont. M5S 1A8

Mark V. Nadel
U.S. General Accounting Office
441 G Street N.W., Room 6852
Washington, D.C. 20548, U.S.A.

Katy Nau
Ontario Ministry of Health
Manager
Training and Research Branch
80 Grosvenor Street, Queen's Park
Hepburn Block, 8th Floor
Toronto, Ont. M7A 1R3

C. David Naylor
Sunnybrook Health Sciences Centre
2075 Bayview Avenue, A443
Toronto, Ont. M4N 3M5

Doreen Neville
Director of Research and Development
Waterford Hospital
Waterford Bridge Road
St. John's, Nfld. A1E 4J8

Beverley Nickoloff
University of Toronto
Department of Health Administration
McMurrich Building, 2nd Floor
Toronto, Ont. M5S 1A8

Elizabeth J. Noyes
American Academy of Pediatrics
1331 Pennsylvania Avenue N.W.
Suite 721 North
Washington, D.C. 20004-1703, U.S.A.

Linda O'Brien-Pallas
Unversity of Toronto
Faculty of Nursing
50 St. George Street
Toronto, Ont. M5S 1A1

Gerry O'Hanley
St. Joseph's Health Centre
30 The Queensway
Toronto, Ont. M6R 1B5

Jim O'Neill
Ontario Ministry of Health
CHC/HSO Program
15 Overlea Blvd., 6th Floor
Toronto, Ont. M4H 1A9

Beverly A. Olineck
St. Paul's Hospital
1702 - 20th Street West
Saskatoon, Sask. S7M 0Z9

Darrell Osbaldeston
Alberta Ministry of Health
323 Legislature Building
Edmonton, Alberta T5K 2B6

Hélène Ouellette-Kuntz
Queen's University
Department of Community Health
and Epidemiology
Abramsky Hall, 3rd Floor
Kingston, Ont. K7L 3N6

Judith Oulton
Executive Director
Canadian Nurses Association
50 The Driveway
Ottawa, Ont. K2P 1E2

Joseph L. Pater
Queen's University
Dept. of Community Health
and Epidemiology
Abramsky Hall, 3rd Floor
Kingston, Ont. K7L 3N6

Dianne Patychuk
College of Nurses of Ontario
101 Davenport Road
Toronto, Ont. M5R 3P1

David K. Peachey
Ontario Medical Association
250 Bloor Street East, Suite 600
Toronto, Ont. M4W 3P8

Marc C. Pelletier
Oshawa General Hospital
24 Alma Street
Oshawa, Ont. L1G 2B9

Irene Petrycia
Manitoba Medical Assoc.
125 Sherbrook Street
Winnipeg, Man. R3C 2E5

Tina Pichler
University of Toronto
Director
Institute of Health Management
McMurrich Building, 2nd Floor
Toronto, Ont. M5S 1A8

Lavada Pinder
Health and Welfare Canada
Jeanne Mance Building, Room 422
Tunney's Pasture
Ottawa, Ont. K1A 1B4

George Pink
University of Toronto
Department of Health Administration
McMurrich Building, 2nd Floor
Toronto, Ont. M5S 1A8

Richard Plain
University of Alberta
Dept. of Economics and Dept. HSA and CM
H.M. Tory Building, 8-14
Edmonton, Alberta T6G 2H4

G.H. Platt
Alberta Health
11010 - 101 Street, Box 2222
Hys Centre, 7th Floor
Edmonton, Alberta T5J 2P4

Sylvie Poirier
University of Maryland
20 N. Pine Avenue
Baltimore, Maryland 21201, U.S.A.

Graham L. Pollett
Halton Regional Health Department
465 Morden Road
Oakville, Ont. L6K 3W6

Anne Prémi
Ontario Ministry of Health
French Language Health Services
80 Grosvenor Street, Queen's Park
Hepburn Block, 7th Floor
Toronto, Ont. M7A 1R3

Marie Price
Algoma District Health Council
123 March Street, Suite 405
Sault Ste. Marie, Ont. P6A 2Z5

Michael M. Rachlis
Private Consultant
13 Langley Avenue
Toronto, Ont. M4K 1B4

Donald M. Raines
Vancouver General Hospital
855 West 12th Avenue
Vancouver, B.C. V5Z 1M9

Randy Rall
Alberta Hospital Association
10009 - 108 Street
Edmonton, Alberta T5J 3C5

Jack Reamy
Texas Woman's University
Dept. of Health Care Administration
1130 MD Anderson Blvd.
Houston, Texas 77030, U.S.A.

Gordon Redston
Livingston Pharmaceutical
Distribution Ltd.
405 The West Mall, Suite 200
Etobicoke, Ont. M9C 5K7

Norman Rees
Vice President, Financial Services
Centenary Hospital
2867 Ellesmere Road
Scarborough, Ont. M1E 4B9

R.H. Reid
Quorum Health Resources Ltd.
50 Burnhamthorpe Road West, Suite 606
Mississauga, Ont. L5B 3C2

Blair Richardson
Canadian Liquid Air Ltd.
1155 Sherbrooke Street West
Montreal, Quebec H3A 1H8

Kent Rondeau
Dalhousie University
School of Health Services Admin.
1234 Seymour Street
Halifax, N.S. B3H 3M3

Paul Rosenbaum
Evalusearch
P.O. Box 1231
Kingston, Ont. K7L 4Y8

Eleanor Ross
University of Toronto
Department of Health Administration
McMurrich Building, 2nd Floor
Toronto, Ont. M5S 1A8

Carl F. Roy
Asst. Exec. Director
Sudbury General Hospital
700 Paris Street
Sudbury, Ont. P3E 3B5

Dale A. Rublee
American Medical Association
535 N. Dearborn Street
Chicago, Illinois 60610, U.S.A.

A. Peter Ruderman
2 Charleston Road
Islington, Ont. M9B 4M7

Stephen E. Rudin
SER Associates
1231 Yonge Street
Toronto, Ont. M4T 2T8

Willis Rudy
Sr. Vice President, Member Services
Ontario Hospital Association
150 Ferrand Drive
Don Mills, Ont. M3C 1H6

Steve Russell
Ontario Ministry of Health
Provider Support Unit
15 Overlea Blvd., 2nd Floor
Toronto, Ont. M4H 1A9

Eva Ryten
Assoc. of Canadian Medical Colleges
151 Slater Street
Ottawa, Ont. K1P 5N1

Ahsan J. Sadiq
Ontario Ministry of Health
Claims Payment Division
Human Resources Planning
49 Place d'Armes, 3rd Floor
Kingston, Ont. K7L 5J3

John Saidak
Comp. Health System Planning Comm.
272 Dundas Street, 4th Floor
London, Ont. N6B 1T6

Norbert Salzberger
Ministry of Health
80 Grosvenor Street, Queen's Park
Hepburn Block, 8th Floor
Toronto, Ont. M7A 1R3

Claudia Sanmartin
University of Toronto
Department of Health Administration
McMurrich Building, 2nd Floor
Toronto, Ont. M5S 1A8

Ronald T. Sapsford
Ontario Ministry of Health
15 Overlea Blvd., 7th Floor
Toronto, Ont. M4H 1A9

Susan Schendel
Coord., Planning
Faculty of Medicine
University of Toronto
Toronto, Ont. M4S 1A8

Kathleen Scherer
Manitoba Department of Health
308 - 294 Portage Avenue
Winnipeg, Man. R3C 0B9

Cope Schwenger
University of Toronto
Centre for Studies of Aging
Toronto, Ont. M5S 2G8

Fernand Scopa
Senior Vice Pres.
Queensway General Hospital
150 Sherway Drive
Etobicoke, Ont. M9C 1A5

Richard Scotton
Monash University
Public Sector Management Institute
Clayton, Vic. 3168, Australia

Susan Seaby
Ontario Ministry of Health
CHC/HSO Program
15 Overlea Blvd., 6th Floor
Toronto, Ont. M4H 1A9

Ian E.W. Searle
Ontario Ministry of Health
Claims Payment Division
2195 Yonge Street, 6th Floor
Toronto, Ont. M4S 2B2

Denise Senk
Senior Finanancial Analyst
Maine Health Care Finance Commission
9 Green Street, State House Station 102
Augusta, Maine 04333, U.S.A.

Martin S. Serediak
Asst. Exec. Director
Alberta Medical Association
400, 12230 - 106 Avenue
Edmonton, Alberta T5N 3Z1

Evelyn Shapiro
University of Manitoba
Faculty of Medicine
Community Health Sciences
5113-750 Bannatyne Avenue
Winnipeg, Man. R3C 0W3

Roger Sharman
Orthopaedic and Arthritic Hospital
43 Wellesley Street East
Toronto, Ont. M4Y 1H1

Meg Sheehan
The Wellesley Hospital
160 Wellesley Street East
Toronto, Ont. M4Y 1J3

Heather Shilton
Haldimand War Memorial Hospital
206 John Street
Dunnville, Ont. N1A 2P7

Harold Shirley
Sudbury General Hospital
700 Paris Street
Sudbury, Ont. P3E 3B5

Hilary Short
Ontario Hospital Association
150 Ferrand Drive
Don Mills, Ont. M3C 1H6

Joseline Sikorski
V.P., Patient Services
Centenary Hospital
2867 Ellesmere Road
Scarborough, Ont. M1E 4B9

Brad Sinclair
Ontario Ministry of Health
Training and Research Branch
80 Grosvenor Street, Queen's Park
Hepburn Block, 8th Floor
Toronto, Ont. M7A 1R3

Jane E. Sisk
Office of Technology Assessment
U.S. Congress
Washington, D.C. 20510-8025, U.S.A.

Sharon E. Snell
Provincial Nursing Consultant
Alberta Health
P.O. Box 2222, 11010 - 101 Street
Hys Centre, 7th Floor
Edmonton, Alberta T5J 2P4

Lee Soderstrom
McGill University
Department of Economics
855 Sherbrooke Street West
Montréal, Québec H3A 2T7

Heather Stewart
The Ontario Council of Teaching Hospitals
56 Wellesley Street West, Suite 310
Toronto, Ont. M5S 2S3

Linda J. Stewart
Ontario Ministry of Health
Community Health Branch
15 Overlea Blvd., 7th Floor
Toronto, Ont. M4H 1A8

Greg Stoddart
McMaster University
Centre for Health Economics and
Policy Analysis
1200 Main Street West
Hamilton, Ont. L8N 3Z5

W. Vickery Stoughton
Duke University Medical Centre
P.O. Box 3708
Durham, NC 27710, U.S.A.

Fawne Stratford-Devai
McMaster University
Faculty of Health Sciences
Dept. of Clin. Epi. and Biostat.
1200 Main Street West, Room 2C5
Hamilton, Ont. L8N 3Z5

Wayne H. Sullivan
Dept. of Health and Fitness
P.O. Box 488
Halifax, N.S. B3J 2R8

Maurice Tabry
Merck Frosst Canada Inc.
P.O. Box 1005
Pointe Claire-Dorval, Quebec H9R 4P8

Richard W. Taylor
Livingston Pharmaceutical Distribution Ltd.
405 The West Mall, Suite 200
Etobicoke, Ont. M9C 5K7

Celso Teixeira
Thunder Bay District Health Council
516 E. Victoria Avenue, Suite 8
Thunder Bay, Ont. P7C 1A7

Kathleen Theocharis
V.P., Patient Services
Providence Centre
3276 St. Clair Avenue East
Scarborough, Ont. M1L 1W1

Helene Thibault
Children's Hospital of Eastern Ontario
401 Smyth Road
Ottawa, Ont. K1H 8L1

Bill Tholl
Canadian Medical Association
1867 Alta Vista Drive
Ottawa, Ont. K1G 3Y6

Tom Thomas
Christian Health Services
1701 E. Broadway
Columbia, MO 65201, U.S.A.

Gail Thompson
University of Toronto
Department of Health Administration
McMurrich Building, 2nd Floor
Toronto, Ont. M5S 1A8

Darrell Thomson
British Columbia Medical Association
115 - 1665 West Broadway
Vancouver, B.C. V6J 5A4

Mario Tino
Ontario Ministry of Health
15 Overlea Blvd., 7th Floor
Toronto, Ont. M4H 1A9

Gary Tompkins
University of Regina
Department of Economics
Regina, Sask. S4S 0A2

Paul Truscott
Chief of Staff
Centenary Hospital
2867 Ellesmere Road
Scarborough, Ont. M1E 4B9

Joann Trypuc
Ontario Hospital Association
150 Ferrand Drive
Don Mills, Ont. M3C 1H6

Jim Tsitanidis
Manitoba Health
308 - 294 Portage Avenue
Winnipeg, Man. R3C 0B9

A. Robert Turner
CRCS Blood Transfusion Services
University of Alberta
8249 - 114 Street
Edmonton, Alberta T6G 2R8

Anthony Ubaldi
Executive Director
Algoma District Health Council
123 March Street, Suite 405
Sault Ste. Marie, Ont. P6A 2Z5

Marica Varga
St. Joseph's Health Centre
30 The Queensway
Toronto, Ont. M6R 2X1

Judith A. Vestrup
Director, Trauma Services
Vancouver General Hospital
910 West 10th Avenue
Vancouver, B.C. V5Z 4E3

Jerry Vila
Economist
User Support Branch
Ontario Ministry of Health
15 Overlea Blvd., 2nd Floor
Toronto, Ont. M4H 1A9

Leslie Vincent
Mount Sinai Hospital
600 University Avenue, Room 342
Toronto, Ont. M5G 1X5

Barbara C. Voigt
Principal
RMC Resources Management
Consultants Ltd
2489 Bloor Street West, #100
Toronto, Ont. M6S 1R6

Hugh Walker
Alberta Occupational Health and Safety
10709 Jasper Avenue
Edmonton, Alberta T5J 3N3

Ray Walker
Chedoke-McMaster Hospitals
P.O. Box 2000, Station A
Hamilton, Ont. L8N 3Z5

Ronald Wall
Manitoba Centre for Health Policy
and Evaluation
Department of Community Health Sciences
University of Manitoba
Winnipeg, Manitoba R3E 0W3

William G. Weissert
University of Michigan
School of Public Health
1420 Washington Heights, Room M3174
Ann Arbor, Michigan 48109 -2029, U.S.A.

Pete Welch
Urban Institute
2100 M Street, N.W.
Washington, D.C. 20037, U.S.A.

Geoffrey R. Weller
V.P., Academic
Lakehead University
Oliver Road
Thunder Bay, Ont. P7B 5E1

Jim Whaley
Wellington-Dufferin D.H.C.
317 Speedvale Avenue East
Guelph, Ont. N1E 1N3

Mark Wheeler
Health and Welfare Canada
Brooke Claxton Building, Room 1405
Tunney's Pasture
Ottawa, Ont. K1A 0K9

Mary Wheeler
The Registered Nurses Association
of Ontario
33 Price Street
Toronto, Ont. M4W 1Z2

Sharon White
University Hospital
339 Windermere Road
London, Ont. N6A 5A5

Allan L. Whiting
President
Centenary Hospital
2867 Ellesmere Road
Scarborough, Ont. M1E 4B9

Mary Wiktorowicz
University of Toronto
Department of Health Administration
McMurrich Building, 2nd Floor
Toronto, Ont. M4Y 1R5

Machelle Wilchesky
Economist
Ontario Medical Association
250 Bloor Street East, Suite 600
Toronto, Ont. M4W 3P8

J. Ivan Williams
Sunnybrook Health Sciences Centre
Clinical Epidemiology Unit, A443
2075 Bayview Avenue
North York, Ont. M4N 3M5

Don Willison
McMaster University
Faculty of Health Sciences
Dept. of Family Medicine
1200 Main Street West
Hamilton, Ont. L8N 3Z5

Gordon Winsor
Department of Health, Newfoundland
P.O. Box 8700
West Block
St. John's, Nfld. A1B 4J6

Larry Wiser
Manitoba Ministry of Health
330 Graham Avenue, Suite 602
Winnipeg, Man. R3C 4A5

Harold Wodinsky
The Ont. Cancer Treatment and
Research Foundation
7 Overlea Blvd.
Toronto, Ont. M4H 1A8

Nancy Wolff
University of Wisconsin - Madison
Department of Preventive Medicine
504 North Walnut Street
Madison, Wisconsin 53705, U.S.A.

Anne Wood
371 MacKay Street, Apt. 2
Ottawa, Ont. K1M 2C3

Cathy Worthington
University of Toronto
Department of Health Administration
McMurrich Building, 2nd Floor
Toronto, Ont. M5S 1A8

Charles J. Wright
Vancouver General Hospital
855 West 12th Avenue
Vancouver, B.C. V5Z 1M9

Dorothy M. Wylie
University of Toronto
Faculty of Nursing
65 Scadding Avenue, #304
Toronto, Ont. M5A 4L1

Bob Youtz
Office for Senior Citizens' Affairs
76 College Street, 6th Floor
Toronto, Ont. M7A 1N3

Michael Zanin
Golden Rule Ins.
1339 Chestnut Blvd.
Cuyahoga Falls, Ohio 44223, U.S.A.

Jack Zwanziger
University of Rochester
Dept. of Community and
Preventive Medicine
P.O. Box 644, 601 Elmwood Avenue
Rochester, N.Y. 14642, U.S.A.

NOTE
Affiliations and addresses have been updated where revised information was available.